THE MENTAL IMPACT OF SPORTS INJURY

Much is known about the physical strain that athletes' bodies are subjected to and the dangerous aspects of competition immediately spring to mind. But why do athletes train the way they do, and why do they push the limits? Why do some recover well from injury while others struggle? Despite decades of medical and sport science research, a piece has been missing from this picture.

Until recently, the role of psychological factors in risk and rehabilitation has been poorly understood. Thankfully, there is increasing awareness of just how crucial these factors can be for predicting injury, improving recovery, developing prevention strategies, and supporting athletes' long-term health. Yet, research in this area is still in its infancy and it can be difficult to synthesize an ever-growing body of knowledge into practical injury management approaches.

Using analogies from everyday life, *The Mental Impact of Sports Injury* bridges the gap between academic research and practical settings in an informative, yet easy to follow guide to the psychology of sports injury. Addressing risk, rehabilitation, and prevention, it outlines key considerations for researchers and practitioners across all levels of sport. Alongside the fundamentals of injury psychology, emerging areas of importance are also discussed, including training load monitoring and the technological advances that are shaping modern sport medicine. Targeted examples highlight the challenges of preventing and managing injury in grassroots, elite, and professional contexts, with chapters dedicated to the under-served communities of youth and Para sport athletes. Stepping away from traditional texts, this unique book presents the landmark literature, major concepts, and athlete insights into sports injury psychology from a totally new perspective.

Carly D. McKay, PhD, is a Senior Lecturer in Injury Prevention at the University of Bath, United Kingdom.

THE MENTAL IMPACT OF SPORTS INJURY

Edited by Carly D. McKay

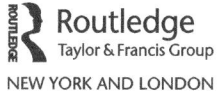

Routledge
Taylor & Francis Group

NEW YORK AND LONDON

Cover image: Laurence Griffiths/Staff/Getty Images

First published 2022
by Routledge
605 Third Avenue, New York, NY 10158

and by Routledge
2 Park Square, Milton Park, Abingdon, Oxon, OX14 4RN

Routledge is an imprint of the Taylor & Francis Group, an informa business

Library of Congress Cataloging-in-Publication Data
Names: McKay, Carly D., editor.
Title: The mental impact of sports injury / edited by Carly D. McKay.
Description: New York, NY: Routledge, 2022. | Includes bibliographical
references and index. |
Identifiers: LCCN 2021046753 (print) | LCCN 2021046754 (ebook) |
ISBN 9780367543600 (hardback) | ISBN 9780367370206 (paperback) |
ISBN 9781003088936 (ebook)
Subjects: LCSH: Sports injuries--Psychological aspects.
Classification: LCC RD97 .M46 2022 (print) | LCC RD97 (ebook) |
DDC 617.1/027--dc23/eng/20211021
LC record available at https://lccn.loc.gov/2021046753
LC ebook record available at https://lccn.loc.gov/2021046754

ISBN: 978-0-367-54360-0 (hbk)
ISBN: 978-0-367-37020-6 (pbk)
ISBN: 978-1-003-08893-6 (ebk)

DOI: 10.4324/9781003088936

Typeset in Bembo
by MPS Limited, Dehradun

This book is dedicated to Stephen West, who every day reminds me what all the hard work is for.

CONTENTS

FIGURES

TABLES

CONTRIBUTORS

Marelise Badenhorst, *Sports Performance Research Institute New Zealand (SPRINZ), Auckland University of Technology, New Zealand*

Caroline Bolling, *Amsterdam University Medical Centre, Netherlands*

Lisa Callaghan, *Ireland*

Wayne Derman, *Institute of Sport and Exercise Medicine, Stellenbosch University & IOC Research Center, South Africa*

Kirsten Dillon, *Western University, Canada*

Jordan D Herbison, *Queens University, Canada*

Luc J Martin, *Queens University, Canada*

Carly McKay, *University of Bath, England, United Kingdom*

Steve Mellalieu, *Cardiff Metropolitan University, Wales, United Kingdom*

Lee Moore, *University of Bath, England, United Kingdom*

Harry Prapavessis, *Western University, Canada*

Mason Raymond, *Canada*

Scott Rollo, *Children's Hospital of Eastern Ontario Research Institute, Canada*

Phoebe Runciman, *Stellenbosch University, South Africa*

Abby Tabor, *University of the West of England, England, United Kingdom*

Ulrika Tranaeus, *The Swedish School of Sport and Health Sciences, Sweden*

Nicol van Dyk, *Irish Rugby Football Union, Ireland*

Stephen West, *Sport Injury Prevention Research Centre, University of Calgary, Canada*

PREFACE

Vanity projects come in all shapes and sizes. When I originally set out to write this one, I had a very clear idea of the sort of book I wanted it to be. Not to give too much away, what you've got in front of you isn't what I had in mind. You might reasonably ask why, and all I can say is that I wrote it during a pandemic. Through 2020 and 2021, the world went completely sideways as I put these chapters together and that influenced the way I looked at the project entirely.

Being by turns locked down and quarantined in your home for months on end tends to make you miss a lot of things you've grown accustomed to in your everyday life. For me, as for many people, one of the most profound differences was the lack of face-to-face interaction. I have found very few activities as academically and personally inspiring as sitting down with a colleague over coffee for no other purpose than chatting. Having the time and space to toss ideas around and learn from each other, purely for the sake of interest, seems like such a luxury these days, but for me it's an irreplaceable part of my professional life. Some of my most exciting thoughts have come out of those informal discussions and nothing is quite so satisfying as dredging up a passing notion, months or years later, to form the key piece of an argument (or paper, lecture, grant, etc.). Not having the opportunity for these kinds of connections over a prolonged period left an indelible mark on the way I approached my work. (For anyone wondering why I couldn't have continued having virtual catchups, they are NOT the same thing.)

So, I decided that this book would become a kind of surrogate. I invited some of the most interesting people I know to sit down over a chapter with me to talk about what we're currently focusing on, the things we've been wondering about, and our musings about "what if?" In some sections, you'll hear mostly from my colleagues who are much better versed in certain areas that I am, and in others you'll be captive to my personal thoughts. Yes, it's indulgent and yes, it covers a lot of disparate topics, but hopefully the narrative is as amusing to you as it has been to us. It would be great if you learned a few new things, but mostly I hope that these pages spark an interest or insight that you hadn't had before. That's the value of a coffee conversation and, with any luck, the value of this book.

– Carly

ACKNOWLEDGEMENTS

Foremost, thank you to Lisa Callaghan, Mason Raymond, Cory Sarich, and Jason Wiemer for sharing their stories for this book. They've given voice to the athlete experience and, in doing so, have hopefully kickstarted a more inclusive conversation about sport injury psychology moving forward. Thanks also to Kathy and Glenn McKay for providing endless moral support, proofreading, and coffee when it was needed most. Finally, a debt of gratitude is owed to Marvel Studios for not only supplying much needed decompression during writing, but also the inspiration for exploring a complex and interconnected view of the world that speaks to the importance of sharing perspective, accounting for context, and looking out for the little guy.

1

INTRODUCTION: WHAT HAVE I GOTTEN MYSELF INTO?

Carly McKay

Setting the Scene

When you hear the term "sports injury," what comes to mind? Athletes hobbling on crutches, maybe a doctor rushing onto a field, or a stretcher being wheeled off? Injury is ubiquitous in sport settings and whether we've experienced one personally or have only borne witness as a spectator, it's an inherent part of sports for many people. Yet, for such a commonplace event, an injury can leave an indelible mark on an athlete and those around them. There are the obvious physical consequences, sure, but injuries can also trigger a cascade of cognitive, emotional, and social responses with the potential to affect both immediate and longer-term outcomes. As we're starting to better understand this and seek ways to minimize the risk of negative impacts on performance and health, sport injury psychology is emerging as a particularly hot topic in medical, coaching, and sport science circles. That's probably why you've picked up this book, right? Well, before we get into it, let's put this story into some firmer context as a starting point.

Historically, sport injury has been the domain of the medical professions, with a duty to assess the damage, repair it, and send athletes back out to compete again. To this end, Sport Medicine has developed as a distinct specialization and countless professional associations have evolved around the world to support its practitioners. This development rests upon the thousands of research studies devoted to identifying the best injury treatments, surgical techniques, and rehabilitation programmes, not to mention intense efforts toward injury prevention over the past several decades. Yet, despite all of this attention and resource, injury remains one of sport's biggest problems from grassroots levels right up through professional leagues. A narrow biomedical approach to injury management clearly doesn't seem to be solving this, so we're seeing increasing acknowledgement that injury isn't a purely physical phenomenon. This is where sport psychologists enter the story.[i]

DOI: 10.4324/9781003088936-1

There's a small but growing body of evidence, from both research and experiential sources, that shows us just how important the psychological elements of injury risk and rehabilitation can be. We'll take a journey through that information in the rest of the book, but first let's clear up one little issue that might be a barrier to anyone reading further. Without a doubt, "psychology" can be a little bit intimidating. For a lot of people, it comes across like a load of gibberish and made-up concepts that can't be directly measured. It can seem complex and confusing, and there are plenty of misconceptions out there about why people feel and act in certain ways. So, if the idea of injury psychology is a little off-putting, that's not surprising. But just because someone doesn't have a background in psychology, it doesn't mean they aren't intuitively aware of how athletes' thoughts, emotions, and behaviors can shape their injury experiences. We can hear it in the way they speak, see it in their body language and sport performance, and recognize the effects on their wellbeing. I can reassure you that this book isn't going to get into the esoteric debates that you might see in other branches of psychology, and you definitely don't need to be an expert in the area to follow along. Instead, the aim is to help make some of those abstract theoretical ideas a little more tangible and to define terms that get tossed around in conversation around sport injury. It's about making things accessible and easier to implement in practice – hopefully that's what you're here for.

Getting Your Bearings

One of the things you'll notice as you flip through the coming chapters is that this isn't meant to be a textbook. There are already plenty of really excellent ones out there, so if you want to look into the finer theoretical details or read a comprehensive review of the research literature, I'd point you toward one of those instead.[1-4] This book approaches the topic of sport injury psychology from a slightly more oblique direction. Why? Well, for starters, the worlds of sport medicine and sport psychology have merged relatively recently. It was only in the 1970s when a clear body of literature began to appear with a focus on the psychological effects of injury in sport. The field has expanded quickly since then but, on the grander scale of psychology, there still aren't all that many researchers or practitioners who are solely dedicated to this line of work. Of course, there are some very big names in the field (check out the authorship lists of the textbooks for a who's who), but many of us with a vested interest in the topic come at it from the medical end instead. In the sphere of injury prevention, for instance, the charge is mostly being led by epidemiologists, clinicians, and implementation scientists who are developing and delivering interventions in various sport contexts. This diversity brings to the conversation some interesting new perspectives and lessons learned that are valuable to understanding how research might be applied in practice, and that's where this book is coming from.

After personally spending more than a decade immersed in that world of sport injury prevention, a few things have become rather clear to me: foremost, psychological wellbeing is increasingly on the medical agenda as an important part of athlete health. Though it's still secondary to the physical aspects, the gap is narrowing and that's a good thing. But this also highlights that we have a long way to go before our understanding of injury psychology matches that of physiology, biomechanics, or medical science, and there are a few reasons why this presents an uphill challenge. Until now, researchers – and practitioners, to be fair – have largely operated in siloes, focusing on their particular area of expertise without fully integrating the disciplines in a way that mirrors the athlete's real-world context. After all, an athlete isn't just a limb segment or a cardiovascular system, they're a fully formed entity who lives within a particular social environment. We can't truly understand one element without accounting for how it functions in the presence of the others. Sport injury psychology has suffered from this limitation in the same measure as other disciplines, exploring cognitions, emotions, and be-haviors without a holistic consideration of the athlete and their surroundings. Though we've learned a lot about injuries from this single-minded approach, there's still much to be discovered by taking an interdisciplinary stance, and this can only improve our ability to support athletes through the injury process.[5]

The other consequence of this compartmentalized paradigm is that research to date has been undertaken in fits and starts. Unlike in more established fields of medicine, where there's been a systematic and strategic global effort to progress knowledge in a step-by-step fashion, sport injury psychology research hasn't yet been a coordinated effort. Much of the underlying theory is still untested and there hasn't been much consistency in the way studies have been designed.[5] This means that the literature is a little bit piecemeal, and we don't have the luxury of being able to compare between studies or pool their results together in the way we might have hoped. So, from a research perspective, there's a distance to go before we can be exceptionally confident that we have a good grasp of what's actually going on. This is a hurdle for evidence-informed practice, which is probably the bigger concern. Most of the theoretical models that we currently use in sport injury psychology are descriptive in nature, meaning that we have some hy-potheses about the mechanisms that lead to injury (or not) and positive recovery experiences (or not), but there isn't a set strategy for affecting those outcomes. Intervention is the ultimate goal if we hope to shape athletes' trajectories through the injury process and for now, we're relying on some fundamental psychological techniques that have been effective for enhancing sport performance but are largely untested for managing injury.[6] Given these challenges, this book cannot provide a how-to guide for reducing injury risk or speeding up rehabilitation. It can, however, take stock of where we're at and where we need to get to.

There's no doubt that meaningful progress will be made as research and practice develop further, but the first step in setting a direction of travel for the field is to speak openly about what we know and where the mysteries are. That's where this book comes in. It'll provide an overview of some key concepts and explore what they mean in practical terms, but through a nontraditional lens. A danger in any narrative lies in the balance of perspectives that help contribute to the story. When it's told from just one point of view, the key messages can be narrow and it's easy to miss important details. It's a bit like seeing an image with *forced perspective*. Take Hagrid from the Harry Potter films, or the Hobbits from the Lord of the Rings trilogy. Those characters were played by humans of average size, but camera angles (and a few other tricks) make them appear to be larger or smaller on screen. It's much the same with sport injury psychology. If we only hear from one group of stakeholders, our perception of the situation will be limited, and we might not fully grasp the nature of the situation. By including multiple perspectives (i.e., from different stakeholders), we have a much better chance of getting the whole picture.

With that in mind, this book isn't written from an entirely psychological standpoint. Instead, I've invited colleagues, friends, and subject-matter experts from a wide range of disciplines to weigh in on some of the big topics in injury psychology today. Some of them are leading academics in the field (to help keep the story grounded in evidence), but others are practitioners, clinicians, and policy makers who have unique views to share. Most importantly, we'll also hear from some athletes themselves, who can give us firsthand insight into their injury experiences. Together, we'll explore our current state of understanding with a critical eye, considering emerging issues in contemporary sport medicine that have the potential to shape injury risk and rehabilitation moving forward. We'll borrow from other fields of psychology here and there to explore some "what if?" scenarios, too. Oftentimes, having a fresh set of eyes on a problem will yield different solutions, so that's the approach I'm taking. With any luck, it'll be the starting point for some new research directions or practical approaches; if not, it'll be an interesting conversation to have anyway.

All in all, my hope is that this book will help to clarify some things if you're new to sport injury psychology, but mostly I want to share a few new ideas that might spark interest in the topic. There are so many potential avenues of research to be pursued and all kinds of opportunities to develop applied practice, but neither can happen without a wider community of invested stakeholders. Ideally, by the time you reach the last page, we can count you as part of the group. Wait, that sounds a little too serious, doesn't it? Reading in your spare time shouldn't feel like work or a commitment to something bigger, and it most certainly shouldn't be painful (though my sense of humour might be, in places). So, please, kick back, work your way through the story, and take from it what you can. With all of the growing attention on mental health in sport, psychology is filtering into a lot of what we do and we're not all experts in it. I hope this book is a friendly starting point and, at the very least, I hope you enjoy it.

Note

i That might be a little reductionist. Sport psychologists are certainly leading the charge, but sport sociologists, behavioural epidemiologists, implementation scientists, neuroscientists, and a whole host of mental skills coaches, counsellors, and other allied professionals are involved, too. This is a sport psychology book, though, so the psychologists get pride of place.

References

1 Wadey R. (ed.). *Sport injury psychology: cultural, relational, methodological, and applied considerations.* New York: Routledge 2020.

2 Arvinen-Barrow M, Walker N. (eds.). *The psychology of sport injury and rehabilitation.* New York: Routledge 2013.

3 Brewer BW, Redmond C. *Psychology of sport injury.* Champaign, IL: Human Kinetics 2016.

4 Gledhill A, Forsdyke D. *The psychology of sports injury: from risk to retirement.* London: Routledge 2021.

5 Almeida PL, Olmedilla A, Rubio VJ, et al. Psychology in the realm of sport injury: what it is all about. *Revista de Psicologia del Deporte* 2014;32:395–400.

6 Hall C, Duncan L, McKay C. *Psychological interventions in sport, exercise & injury rehabilitation.* Dubuque, IA: Kendall Hunt 2014.

2

THEORETICAL MODELS AND HOW TO READ THEIR INSTRUCTIONS: FLAT PACK PSYCHOLOGY

Carly McKay

We've all been there. We've come home with an innocent looking, brown cardboard box full of furniture parts and we're confident that they should be simple enough to assemble. After all, you only need a single screwdriver to do it! Then we open the box, find the incomprehensible pictures that pass as instructions, and spend the rest of the day cursing and looking for pieces that we swear are missing. Does that sound familiar? Well, for a lot of people, trying to understand a complex psychological theory results in much the same experience. There are all kinds of diagrams and, somehow, you're expected to figure out how everything fits together. Sometimes you're not even sure how to use it once you've figured it out!

Fear not. We're going to take a little tour through the prominent psychological theories of sport injury in a step-by-step way. For the nonpsychologists in the room, we'll start with the basics and go from there. If you do happen to have a background in the field, then you might be able to skip ahead a bit, but don't go too far! We'll end up referring back to this chapter throughout the rest of the book.

Who Follows the Directions Anyway?

People say things like "in theory, this should work" all the time. It usually means they're guessing about what might happen based on a rough idea or their own personal experience in a similar situation. That's perfectly fine for casual conversation but, in scientific circles, the term is used much more precisely. For researchers, a theory is developed based on evidence gathered over time. It provides a conceptual map of how variables are related to each other, and it's repeatedly confirmed through observation and/or experiment. So, it's not a collection of hunches and speculation, it's a substantiated explanation of some phenomenon in

DOI: 10.4324/9781003088936-2

the world. Theories are used to help us understand associations between specific concepts and they allow us to make predictions about events based on those associations. Take the legend of Newton sitting under an apple tree, for example. As he observed fruit falling to the ground, he wondered why objects would always descend perpendicularly to the earth and, based on a nearly infinite number of supporting observations (hold this book out and let go if you'd like to add another), the theory of gravitation was born. Of course, the actual theory and its development are a lot more complex than that, but a simple illustration serves our point: you don't need to drop this book in order to predict what would happen if you did. Even if you can't measure the speed at which it falls or calculate the angle at which it descends, you still know where it's going to end up. That's what theories provide. They help us make testable and falsifiable predictions about cause–effect relationships and, as we amass evidence to support them, they start to take away a lot of assumptions and guesswork about why things behave in the way they do.[1]

Some scientific theories, especially early on in their development, are incomplete or really specific to a particular situation. The more robust and generalizable they become, the more confident we can be in their predictions, and that makes them a whole lot more useful. To get to that point, most theories undergo a lot of testing where the goal is to verify their conceptual ideas about how variables affect one another by collecting data to support or refute them. Because some theories can be really complex and include a number of abstract concepts, this process can be quite challenging. It would be like if you called up a flat pack furniture store and had someone explain how to assemble your new item. Without a picture of the parts or how they're supposed to fit together, there would likely be a whole lot of trial and error (not to mention wasted effort and frustration). You could decide to wing it instead, relying on your own vague idea of the end goal and how to get there, but the results would probably be pretty hit-and-miss from person to person. And how would you know if there was a piece missing? It might become obvious straight away, or you might not realize it until you tried to use the furniture and had it collapse from under you. No, having instructions that can be referred back to is usually the way to go, and the same is true in research. We often need a more concrete idea of how a theory works, and for that we construct models.

A *model* is a visual representation of a theory. It distills all of the theory's complex ideas into their essential parts and presents a simplified diagram of how we think they relate to each other. Basically, a model helps us create a set of instructions, helping to make a theory testable. Let's take a look at this with a real example. The Health Action Process Approach (HAPA) is a theory of health behavior change that describes the process through which people start to engage in something healthy (e.g., exercising) or stop doing something that isn't good for them (e.g., smoking).[1] In brief, it proposes that there are two distinct phases to consider: forming an intention to change (a.k.a. the motivation phase) and then performing the action (a.k.a. the volitional phase).[2] The theory includes a number of precursors that influence whether or not someone will form an intention. Specifically, it predicts that if a person thinks they're at risk of a negative health outcome (risk perception), they're confident they can take on the new desired behavior or stop an unhealthy one (task self-efficacy), and that the change will lead to a preferred outcome (outcome expectancy), then they're more likely to form an intention.[2] The volitional phase also contains a number of component parts. A planning process is postulated to occur where a person turns their intention into concrete steps for behaving in a certain way (e.g., how, when, and the like), and additional forms of self-efficacy contribute to whether they're able to overcome barriers in maintaining the behavior (e.g., exercising even when it's raining) or getting back on the wagon after a relapse or time off.[2] There are likely a number of additional factors involved in the strength of the associations between all of these variables, too, such as a person's underlying health status, their age and experience with health behaviors, or any number of environmental or situational factors.

Right. After hearing that description, we can see just how complex the theory is and how many moving parts we'd need to account for. How would we go about testing it? We might not even know where to start. This is why a model can be helpful (Figure 2.1). It doesn't contain all of the detailed description of each concept that the theory actually contains, but it shows us the important elements and how current evidence suggests they fit together.

Now, you might be concerned that this looks suspiciously like those pictorial instructions in the furniture box, and, without words, there could be some ambiguity in how people go about piecing everything together. There are actually some universal symbols that are used in models to clarify how they're meant to be interpreted, which clears up a lot of that confusion. Lines and arrows, for example, are

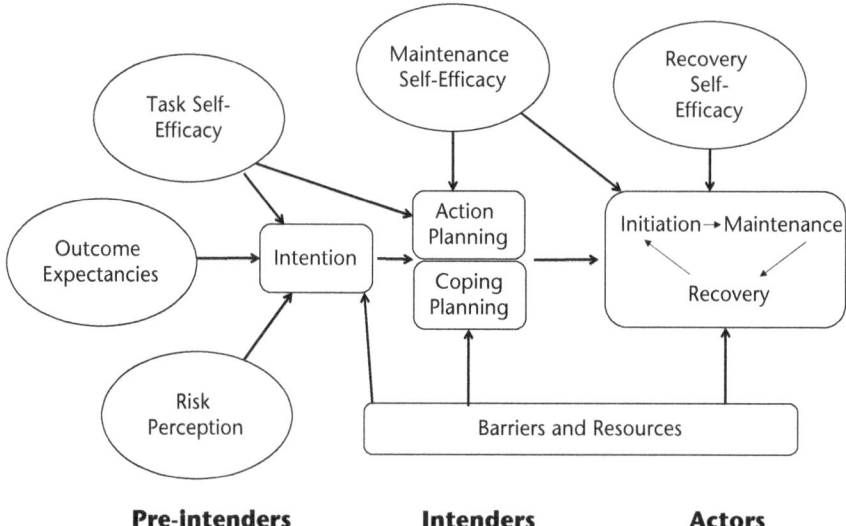

FIGURE 2.1 The Health Action Process Approach (HAPA) model.[2,3]

used to denote relationships between concepts. In the HAPA model, we can see unidirectional arrows indicating that one variable directly influences another, but it's a one-way effect. If the variables might influence each other, then the arrow would be bidirectional. In some fields, presenting concepts in circles means something different than presenting them in squares, too, but those rules aren't hard and fast (much like traffic signs are different shapes in different countries). The main point is that we end up with a clear schematic that can help us generate research questions and hypotheses (e.g., does higher task self-efficacy lead to stronger intentions?)

The final step in this evolution of making theories testable is using a model to design a research study. As you might imagine, it's often unrealistic to assess each and every part of a model in a single experiment. There are just too many elements to be able to account for them all in a rigorous and valid way, not to mention the number of observations you'd need to analyze. Instead, researchers often break models down into manageable chunks so they can be investigated in a well-controlled and systematic way. This is where *conceptual frameworks* come in. These provide structure and guidance about which specific variables need to be measured and what kinds of questions might be asked about their associations. They can also be useful when a single theory might not capture the whole picture.[1] For instance, if we're interested in the motivational phase of HAPA, our conceptual framework for a project could be trimmed to only include the variables that are salient to intention formation (Figure 2.2). We could also incorporate aspects of Self-

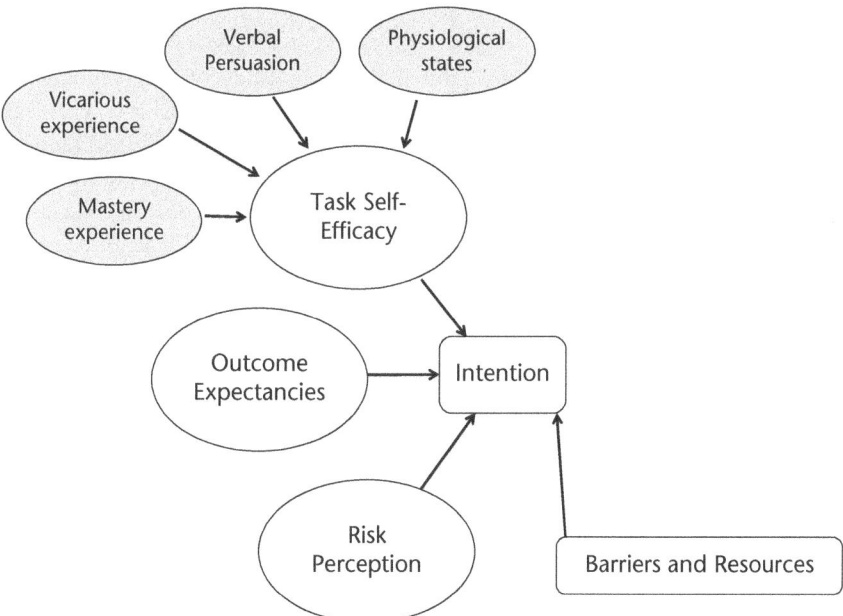

FIGURE 2.2 A hypothetical conceptual framework for a study investigating the motivational phase, combining HAPA and Self-Efficacy Theory.

Efficacy Theory by identifying four main sources of self-efficacy that could be manipulated (the gray circles in the figure).[4] Our study can then be set up to either observe associations between self-efficacy, outcome expectancy, risk perceptions, and intention, or we could provide additional verbal persuasion to boost self-efficacy and see if that results in stronger intentions. Either way, we'll be generating additional evidence to support or refute the main theory.

Creating a Blueprint

Now that we've got those fundamentals under control, we can consider the main theories and models that shape sport injury psychology research. For a relatively new field, there are a remarkable number of these in circulation, but that's not entirely surprising. Any time we encounter a new phenomenon, we try to make sense of it based on the information available to us, and then we fill in the gaps with logic. Since we all have slightly different perspectives, those initial explanations are likely to differ from person to person (or research group to research group). Theory development is a dynamic process and, as we accumulate more evidence, some of these theories will be discarded and others will be combined. This means that after an initial proliferation, the field will start to condense into a few well-established models to steer research and practice. For our purposes, there are four of these that we need to become familiar with.

The Stress-Injury Model

From an injury risk point of view, this is the granddaddy of all psychological models. Originally developed by Andersen and Williams in 1988,[5] it was revised ten years later[6] and is still directing the vast majority of research and intervention development in this area.[7] As you might anticipate from its name, the model is centered on athletes' stress responses. It suggests that when someone finds themself in a potentially stressful situation, the way they deal with it can increase or decrease their chances of being injured. Their responses will be affected by their personality, their history of stressors, and the coping resources available to them. For instance, take an athlete who has an anxious disposition. If they've recently had a major change in their life, or maybe a bunch of hassles have been adding up, they might be at the limit of their ability to cope. If they encounter a sport-related stressor at that moment, they may interpret it as particularly threatening, and that can trigger a number of responses. They may exhibit greater physiological activation and attentional disruption, typified by muscle tension, perceptual narrowing, and distractibility. It's hypothesized that these effects can lead to injury.[6]

Imagine a time when you were running late and needed to get out the door in a hurry. Maybe you're scrambling around getting ready, the phone is ringing, and someone in the house is trying to ask you for something. It's easy to see how you might get flustered under those circumstances, particularly if it's been a long day. If you're usually really organized or punctual, you might feel some added pressure as well. In that situation, it wouldn't be surprising if you missed what your house-mate was saying while you were concentrating on something else, or if you ab-sentmindedly put your keys on the table instead of in your pocket. You might even stub a toe on the coffee table while rushing around. The Stress-Injury Model operates on similar principles. When we feel stressed, we often miss things going on around us, we can be distracted easily, and we tend to clench up a bit. In everyday life, this might cause you to step off a curb when lost in your thoughts and end up in a near miss with a car. In sport, a lapse could mean a botched landing or collision. So, according to the model, injury risk comes down to how stressful we find a situation (based on our personality, what's been going on in our lives, and how tapped out we are), and how our body responds to that, at least from a psychological point of view.

We'll cover the research evidence around this some more in another chapter but suffice it to say there's been general support for the model. High life stress has been consistently associated with injury, and though there could be all kinds of mechanisms involved (e.g., impaired concentration and immune dysfunction), a variety of interventions based on stress reduction seem to be effective.[8,9] This backstop of sound evidence is why the theory had stood the test of time and is widely accepted within the injury psychology field.[7]

Integrated Model of Response to Sport Injury

Building on the Stress-Injury Model, Diane Weise-Bjornstal and colleagues developed the Integrated Model of Response to Sport Injury.[10] The model highlights that the factors affecting an athlete's susceptibility to injury (i.e., personality, history of stressors, and coping resources) can influence how they respond to one, as well. An injury is, after all, a major stressor in and of itself, so stress responses are equally salient after the fact. The Integrated Model then expands to consider how personal factors (e.g., demographics, physical health status, injury characteristics, motivations, and so on) and situational factors (e.g., level of competition, time in season, social interactions, the physical environment, and rehabilitation access) can affect the athlete's *cognitive appraisals* (i.e., how they interpret the meaning, impact, and consequences of the injury). They might make appraisals about what they think caused the injury, their rate of recovery, or their perceptions of themselves as an athlete, for example. These thoughts can then affect their emotions, triggering feelings like fear, tension, depression, or even optimism and a positive outlook, depending on the athlete. Thoughts and emotions can also influence behaviors, including adherence to rehabilitation or risk taking. The model explains that the primary direction of this cycle is for cognitive appraisal to affect emotions, which then determine behaviors, but it also indicates a secondary pathway where that order might be reversed.[10] (Anyone who's done something a little bit stupid in a social setting can probably relate to how a behavior might elicit certain emotional responses, causing you to reappraise yourself and the situation....)

This cycle is theorized to influence physical and psychosocial recovery after an injury, though the effects may be positive or negative. This is down to an athlete's stress response and their coping resources – those who can enact cognitive, emotional, or behavioral coping strategies to minimize stress will likely fare better than those who cannot, though there's no single, predictable response to sport injury. Personal and situational factors can change and adapt through rehabilitation, sometimes very quickly, so responses tend to fluctuate as a result.[11,12] To illustrate, let's think about a jockey who is thrown from a horse. If they aren't that experienced (personal factor) but are nearing an important race (situational factor) and have been under pressure to perform well (a history of stressors), then they may initially appraise the pain in their back as a serious and potentially career-altering injury (cognition). Fear and grief may result (emotional response), prompting withdrawal from those around them (behavioral response). However, if follow-up medical testing leads to a good prognosis, a reappraisal of the injury's consequences might lead to more positive feelings and renewed engagement with social support and rehabilitation activities. Things like setbacks in recovery, interaction with people in and outside of the sport environment, or even the athlete's sleeping patterns and symptoms can change the way they think, feel, and act. The Integrated Model, therefore, accounts for the fact that injury responses can be dynamic and highly individual.

There has been plenty of research in support of the overall structure and proposed relationships in the Integrated Model, suggesting it offers a flexible and testable theoretical framework. As such, it becomes one of the most influential models in the sport injury psychology field.[8,12] One of its limitations, though, is that it doesn't articulate any potential mechanisms by which factors might affect injury outcomes. This is where we might need to combine it with another theory if we want to fully understand what's going on.

Biopsychosocial Model

One candidate to address this gap is the Biopsychosocial Model.[13] Conceived to help explain how psychological and social factors might mechanistically determine rehabilitation outcomes, it proposes that injury characteristics (e.g., type and severity) and sociodemographic variables (e.g., age and sex/gender) can interactively affect *bio*logical factors (e.g., tissue repair and immune function), *psycho*logical factors (e.g., cognitions and behaviors), and *social*/contextual factors (e.g., life stress and social networks). These *biopsychosocial* factors have the potential to influence each other but, more importantly, they'll have an effect on intermediate injury outcomes like strength, pain, and endurance. These, in turn, will lead to overall rehabilitation outcomes including functional performance and return to sport. Furthermore, the model hypothesizes a pathway through which psychological factors might influence overall rehabilitation outcomes directly.[13] Some of this might seem a little farfetched – how can thoughts and feelings change the way we recover? – but we can walk through the process to see how it all fits together.

If we go back to our injured jockey, we can see how the kind of injury they sustained and their age or health status might determine their biological responses (e.g., how quickly they'll heal), as well as the way they appraise the situation and how much stress they experience. So, the first part of the model is remarkably similar to the Integrated Model of response to sport injury. From there, the association between their biological factors and intermediate rehabilitation outcomes is probably the most intuitive (tissue healing is clearly related to range of motion and rate of recovery). But what about the relationships between their psychological factors and injury outcomes? How might that work? Well, the model actually identifies four potential pathways through which these effects could occur.[14] In Path 1, psychological factors can directly affect rehabilitation outcomes that have a cognitive or affective component (e.g., pain, quality of life and symptom reports). It's not a stretch to think that psychological factors might also influence rehabilitation behaviors like adherence to treatment (as the Integrated Model would suggest), which would contribute to cognitive and affective outcomes (Path 2) or even physical outcomes (Path 3). Path 4 is perhaps the least straightforward, hypothesizing that psychological factors might actually change biological factors that determine physical outcomes. For instance, stress responses are known to cause differences in circulation and immune functioning, which could conceivably impact healing.[15,16] Evidence to support these theoretical relationships is limited, though causal links between psychological factors and rehabilitation outcomes have been found in a few small but well-controlled experimental studies.[14] So, this model has promise but it needs further validation before it can be confidently applied in practice.

Multilevel Model of Sport Injury

There are also a number of newer models that are poised to gain traction in the field, such as the Multilevel Model of Sport Injury (MMSI; props to the authors for finally giving us a model with a usable acronym!).[17] This addition to the toolkit was developed in response to the fact that injury-related research has predominantly been focused on athletes themselves, at a distinctly intrapersonal level. But, as other models have hinted at, injuries don't happen in isolation. They occur within a context characterized by interpersonal relationships, social structures, and organizational influence, and they can both be affected by/have effects at all these different levels. So, the MMSI presents a view of the broader sport environment where interdependencies between levels can affect the athlete and those around them.[17]

The model situates the athlete in the middle, surrounded by an interpersonal level of formal and informal social networks. This might include teammates, coaches, friends, and family. Up until now, research at this level has been mostly unidirectional – we ask about how social support can affect the athlete, but seldom think about how the athlete (or their injury) might affect those around them. Outcomes like vicarious trauma and vicarious growth are entirely possible, and the MMSI provides a structure through which to investigate them.[18] But we have to remember that athletes and their social circles exist within an institutional context, which is level three of the model. This covers things like sport culture, the physical environment, and various protocols (e.g., injury surveillance and rehabilitation services) that can impact injury experiences for everyone. Research at this level might have direct relevance to the development of professional practice, which represents a small, but growing, area of study. Beyond that, level four addresses larger cultural influences on injury, including the effects of the media, traditions, and value systems. This level is all about narratives and how they shape people's perspectives on what injuries mean and how they should be perceived. Finally, local and national policy sits at level five, encompassing societal structures that govern duty of care and legal or financial responsibilities when it comes to promoting or protecting athletes.[17]

The MMSI is a valuable addition to injury psychology canon, as it moves away from viewing injury as the sole responsibility of the athlete in recognizing it as a product of contextual factors. It doesn't minimize the necessity of research at the intraindividual level, but it does help to situate that evidence within a broader complex network of influences. This can help us better interpret how and why an individual athlete's personal and situational determinants interact in the way they do. Though the MMSI is the new kid on the injury psychology block, and consequently isn't as well supported as some of the other models just yet, it mirrors contemporary work in sport sociology and sport medicine where the contribution of cultural context to injury risk and rehabilitation is also being considered.[19] We'll talk more about that in Chapter 11.

Do-It-Yourself or Call a Professional?

So, if we bring all of these models together, the picture of sport injury psychology looks a little bit complex (Figure 2.3). From a research perspective, that's exciting

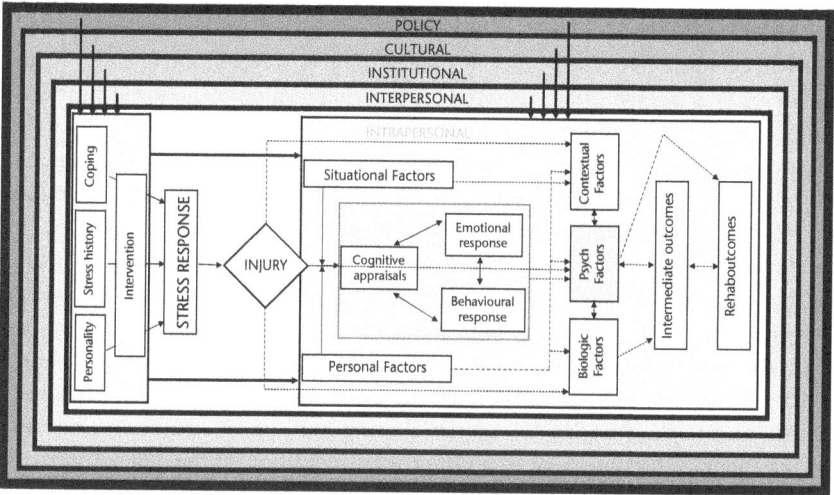

FIGURE 2.3   A superimposed schematic of the Stress-Injury Model, Integrated Model of Response to Sport Injury, Biopsychosocial Model, and MMSI. (Dotted lines represent proposed mechanistic pathways from the Biopsychosocial Model; blue boxes indicate where the psychological processes of the Integrated Model correspond with the same component of the Biopsychosocial Model.)

because there are so many questions to be asked and plenty of interesting directions to go in. From a practical point of view, though, it might be a little bit daunting. If the goal is to help athletes stay healthy and/or recover from their injuries, there seem to be some missing instructions.

As the inimitable Yogi Berra once said, *"in theory there is no difference between theory and practice. In practice there is."* Translating a theoretical model into the so-called "real world" comes with a set of challenges that we always need to bear in mind. For starters, the neat and tidy relationships that we depict on paper (or screens these days) are very rarely that clear cut in reality. For example, in the Integrated Model of response to sport injury, there appears to be a firm distinction between situational factors and cognitive appraisals. But it's actually really difficult to objectively measure situational factors like coach influences or social support provision. We often need to ask athletes to self-report that information. At that point, it becomes unclear whether we're truly assessing a situational factor or the athlete's cognitive appraisal of the situation, so the waters become increasingly muddy when we try to tease apart the effects of those variables.[8] It's also next to impossible to account for every single factor that might be important to injury risk or rehabilitation, and we don't yet understand which ones drive athlete outcomes the most. That means we're never getting a complete view of what's going on and there will be some inevitable noise in the signal, as it were. Consequently, there will always be a degree of imprecision and variability in how theorized relationships behave between athletes and/or settings.

If you happen to be a researcher, all this means is that there's work to be done in refining and developing these theories so we can figure out how best to use them when designing or delivering interventions. If you're not a researcher, though, it would be very sensible at this point to wonder why you'd bother with them at all. You'd be in good company if you did. There are plenty of sport psychologists and other practitioners who see theories and models as useful for knowledge creation but maybe less so for informing day-to-day practice. After all, they don't come with a user manual or provide step-by-step directions, and without a robust evidence base to draw on, there's a certain amount of interpretation necessary in applying them. What the theories do offer is an indication of the general sorts of things you want to keep an eye on when working with athletes (or as an athlete yourself). Their general premises have been empirically supported and, as we'll discover through the rest of the book, studies are finding that some of the finer details hold up as well. Therefore, they give some practical guidance on which red flags to look out for (e.g., pronounced stress responses, emotional distress, and unhelpful behaviors) and which factors might be modifiable in promoting positive injury outcomes.

As the necessity of psychological support for athletes is becoming more widely recognized, responsibility for providing it is quickly filtering into nonpsychologist roles. Coaches, medical practitioners, and others are increasingly in a position where they need to understand and apply basic psychological principles to minimize injury risk or, more often, help someone through their injury experience. Obviously, athletes with severe difficulties need to be referred to a specialist, but many turn to their immediate network for support. With that in mind, hopefully this chapter has provided a useful foundation. These key theories will shape the remainder of the book and are something you can always refer back to if the discussion becomes too abstract. Remember, though, that having a good grasp of theory doesn't always equate to being effective in practice and sometimes the way we think things should work isn't how it ends up at all. What do we mean by that? Well, check out the next chapter for an example.

Note

i This isn't the only health behavior change theory out there, but we're using it as an example because it'll come up again later in the book. Ooh, what a teaser! Yeah, it might not exactly fill you with suspense, but, in an academic book, there's only so much we can do....

References

1 Imenda S. Is there a conceptual difference between theoretical and conceptual frameworks? *J Soc Sci* 2014;38:185–195; doi: 10.1080/09718923.2014.11893249.

2 Schwarzer R. Self-efficacy in the adoption and maintenance of health behaviours: theoretical approaches and a new model. In: R Schwarzer (ed.). *Self-efficacy: thought control of action.* Washington: Taylor and Francis 1992.

3 Schwarzer R. The Health Action Process Approach (HAPA). Available at: http://www.hapa-model.de/ Accessed June 3, 2021.

4 Bandura A. Self-efficacy: toward a unifying theory of behavioral change. *Psychol Rev* 1977;84:191–215; doi: 10.1037/0033-295X.84.2.191.

5 Andersen MB, Williams JM. A model of stress and athletic injury: prediction and prevention. *J Sport Exerc Psychol* 1988;10:294–306; doi: 10.1123/jsep.10.3.294.

6 Williams JM, Andersen MB. Psychosocial antecedents of sport injury: review and critique of the stress and injury model. *J Appl Sport Psychol* 1998;10:5–25; doi: 10.1080/10413209808406375.

7 Johnson U. Psychosocial antecedents of sport injury, prevention, and intervention: an overview of theoretical approaches and empirical findings. *Int J Sport Exerc Psychol* 2007;5:352–369; doi: 10.1080/1612197X.2007.9671841.

8 Brewer BW. Psychology of sport injury rehabilitation. In: G Tenenbaum, RC Eklund (eds.). *Handbook of sport psychology.* New York: John Wiley & Sons, Inc 2007.

9 Gledhill A, Forsdyke D, Murray E. Psychological interventions used to reduce sports injuries: a systematic review of real-world effectiveness. *Br J Sports Med* 2018;52:967–971; doi: 10.1136/bjsports-2017-097694.

10 Wiese-Bjornstal DM, Smith AM, Shaffer SM, et al. An integrated model of response to sport injury: psychological and sociological dynamics. *J Appl Sport Psychol* 1998;10(1):46–69; doi: 10.1080/10413209808406377.

11 Wiese-Bjornstal DM. Personal and situational factors affecting psychological response to sport injuries. In: A Gledhill, D Forsdyke (eds.). *The psychology of sports injury: from risk to retirement.* London: Routledge 2021.

12 Wiese-Bjornstal DM, Wood KN, Kronzer JR. Sport injuries and psychological sequelae. In: G Tenenbaum, RC Eklund (eds.). *Handbook of sport psychology* (4th ed.). New York: John Wiley & Sons, Inc 2020.

13 Brewer BW, Andersen MB, Van Raalte JL. Psychological aspects of sport injury rehabilitation: toward a biopsychosocial approach. In: DL Mostofsky, LD Zaichkowsky (eds.). *Medical and psychological aspects of sport and exercise.* Morgantown, WV: Fitness Information Technology 2002.

14 Brewer BW. The role of psychological factors in sport injury rehabilitation outcomes. *Int Rev Sport Exerc Psychol* 2010;3:40–61; doi: 10.1080/17509840903301207.

15 Robinson H, Norton S, Jarrett P, et al. The effects of psychological interventions on wound healing: a systematic review of randomized trials. *Br J Health Psychol* 2017;22:805–835; doi:10.1111/bjhp.12257.

16 Walsh NP. Recommendations to maintain immune health in athletes. *Eur J Sport Sci* 2018;18:820–831; doi:10.1080/17461391.2018.1449895.

17 Wadey R, Day M, Cavallerio F, et al. Multilevel model of sport injury (MMSI): can coaches impact and be impacted by injury? In: R Thelwell, M Dicks (eds.). *Professional advances in sports coaching: research and practice.* London: Routledge 2018.

18 Martinelli LA, Day MC, Lowry RG. Sport coaches' experience of athlete injury: the development and regulation of guilt. *Sports Coaching Rev* 2016;6(2):162–720 178; doi: 10.1080/21640629.2016.1195550.
19 Bolling C, van Mechelen W, Pasman HR et al. Context matters: revisiting the first step of the 'sequence of prevention' of sports injuries. *Sports Med* 2018;48:2227–2234; doi: 10.1007/s40279-018-0953-x.

3

THE MYTH OF THE INJURY-PRONE ATHLETE: IT'S NOT JUST ABOUT PERSONALITY AFTER ALL

Carly McKay, Scott Rollo, Kirsten Dillon, and Harry Prapavessis

Anyone who participates in fantasy sports knows that, when the time comes to draft your team, there are certain athletes you avoid picking because they always seem to be injured. Unflattering terms get thrown around for these players and, after a while, we come to think of injury as a personal characteristic, as though being "injury prone" is simply part of who they are. But can that really be true? Are specific athletes genuinely more likely to be injured due to some inherent trait? Well, we need to think about how and why injuries happen before we can answer that question.

Injuries are multifactorial (see Figure 3.1). Athletes have various internal risk factors, like their age or physical parameters, that might predispose them to injury. Some of these are modifiable (e.g., strength) while others are not (e.g., bone structure). These *predisposed* athletes are then exposed to various external risk factors, such as the rules of the sport or the playing environment, and the inter- action between internal and external risk factors may make the athlete *susceptible* to injury. The final piece of the puzzle is an *inciting event* (e.g., a tackle or slip on a wet surface) that ultimately triggers the injury occurrence. In practice, this means that two athletes, who have different combinations of internal risk factors, may be more or less likely to experience an injury when exposed to the same external factors or inciting event.[1,2] So, yes, some athletes may in fact be at greater risk than others, and we can start to see the appeal of risk profiling in sport. But let's not get too carried away, because predicting injury isn't all that simple.

If quantifying individual athlete predisposition and susceptibility is the Holy Grail, then identifying specific risk factors for injury is a crucial first step.[i] Hence, enormous amounts of research have gone into finding key biomechanical and physiological variables associated with injury incidence, and our collective under- standing of these factors is improving all the time. Insight into psychological risk factors like personality are, however, lagging behind. Some of this can be attributed

DOI: 10.4324/9781003088936-3

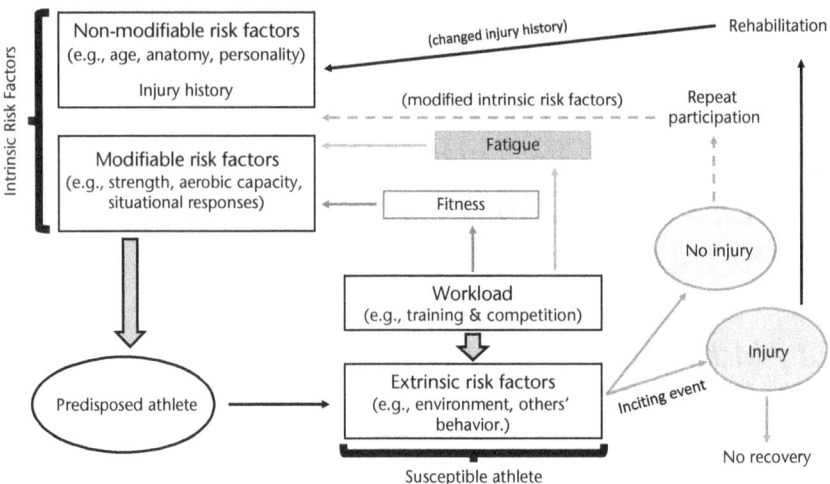

FIGURE 3.1 Schematic of the multifactorial etiology of sport injuries.[2]

to the context – when dealing with a physical problem, it makes sense to prioritize physical causes and physical solutions – but there also hasn't been a coordinated, systematic effort across the research community to progress this line of enquiry. Much of what we know comes from single studies or the collected works of a few research groups who are pushing the agenda forward. So, let's take a look at what we know at this point.

Personality-related Risk Factors

Consistent with the view of the "injury prone" athlete, researchers have been looking for psychological injury risk factors among individual differences in personality and temperament.[3] Now, personality can be conceptualized in several different ways but, for our purposes, we'll take it to mean a set of stable, enduring traits and tendencies to show consistent thoughts, feelings, and behaviors.[4] Perhaps not surprisingly then, one of the first hypotheses to be tested was that athletes with aggressive traits might be more frequently injured than their milder counterparts. The precise definition of "aggression" in the sport context has been hotly contested[5] but it has generally been characterized as *"purposeful physical, verbal or gestural acts, driven both by competitiveness and an intent to cause physiological or psychological harm."*[6] This has traditionally been broken down as either *instrumental* (premeditated and motivated by pursuit of a goal) or *hostile* (impulsive, angry, and motivated by a desire to hurt) aggression.[7] These forms can manifest through allowable actions like trying to knock an opponent out in boxing (pursuing a victory) or retaliatory violence like a fistfight in baseball (with the intent to harm). Either way, the relationship between aggression and injury is intuitive and studies have generally reported higher levels of aggression to be associated with greater injury risk.[8-10] Other researchers who have taken a broader view by investigating Type A personality traits, which include dominance, assertiveness, and anger, have found that athletes who score highly in Type A traits may also be at a higher injury risk or end up with injuries of greater severity.[11,12] It's speculated that such athletes tend to take greater risks or assume more central roles in sport situations, leading to negative health outcomes.

Yet, despite all of these positive associations, aggression and its immediate correlates tend to explain only small amounts of variance in injury risk. In other words, these intrinsic factors might increase predisposition, but on their own don't seem to be the primary drivers of injury incidence. This might be due to the highly variable way in which aggression is measured (using a mix of general and sport-specific tools), or because of the nature of the competitive setting itself – after all, some level of aggression is needed to prevail in physical contests and the line between aggression (with intent to harm) and assertiveness (no intent to harm) can be blurry.[5] Moreover, aggression is often defined using the *instrumental-hostile* dichotomy, which excludes behaviors with multiple motives.[7] This is problematic in sport. For example, an ice hockey player might bodycheck an opponent to gain a tactical advantage while simultaneously getting revenge for an earlier collision. Teasing apart these motives isn't straightforward and might partially account for the challenges in linking specific types of aggression to injury incidence. Plus, as you might have noticed, most of the early research focused on injuries to the aggressor. There's some logic to this, but the more obvious consequences of harmful behavior affect the person on the receiving end. Contemporary work has begun to address this gap, with greater emphasis on overtly violent acts.[13] Clearly, these have causal effects on injury and are a recognized problem in sport at all levels, but more nuanced forms of aggression can be difficult to operationalize and as such, their role as either an external risk factor or an inciting event may be difficult to measure. So, aggression is probably a personality factor we should consider when evaluating injury risk, but for now its contribution isn't well quantified.

Although aggression on its own might not be the best injury predictor, it's related to risk taking and that brings us to another personality trait: sensation-seeking. This is defined as *"the seeking of varied, novel, complex, and intense sensations and experiences, and the willingness to take physical, social, legal and financial risk for the sake of such experience."*[14] Basically, sensation-seekers love an adrenaline rush and go looking for ways to get it. Aggression and sensation-seeking have been correlated with one another in the literature;[15] however, unlike aggression, research findings for sensation-seeking have been inconsistent. Whereas several studies have observed that athletes low in sensation-seeking might be at a greater risk of injury,[15-17] others have found the opposite.[3,18] On the face of it, this could suggest that sensation-seeking isn't linked with injury risk after all (and Occam's Razor favors this conclusion). But a major confounder that hasn't been well considered is athlete skill level. Studies that have found low sensation-seekers to be at high risk included development and school-level athletes,[15,16] while those that found high sensation-seekers to be at high risk focused on expert/professional groups.[3,18] So, what might be going on here?

Sensation-seeking is a biologically based characteristic that reflects an individual's optimal levels of arousal. We wouldn't expect this to vary situationally, but people who have a lower tolerance for arousal tend to avoid unfamiliar or risky activities instead of trying to find them. This will cause an imbalance between personality types in different kinds of environments. We might, therefore, hypothesize that because success in sport requires a certain amount of risk-taking, athletes who make it to elite status may represent a "survivor cohort" of those who are most comfortable pushing boundaries. When someone with high skill/speed/size regularly puts themselves in dangerous situations, we would expect injury risk to go up. It's a logical preposition, but research has only partially borne this out. Some studies have found that athletes who report greater sensation-seeking also report more injuries.[18,19] Others have found a positive association between higher skill level and self-reported risky behavior, but not necessarily more injuries.[3,20–22] Skill level may be protective against injury to some extent, allowing more competent athletes to escape harm up to a point, or the greater physical fitness that often accompanies skill may offset some hazards. At the other end of the spectrum, less-skilled athletes with lower sensation-seeking scores may be at a higher risk of injury because fear or hesitancy could place them in vulnerable positions. For instance, a ten-year observational study reported that although beginner snowboarders displayed lower risk-taking behavior, they fell more frequently compared with advanced snowboarders.[21] Low skill combined with situational avoidance (e.g., "bailing out" partway through a maneuvre) could very easily increase injury risk. Of course, this is all a conjecture – future studies need to address the personality trait of sensation-seeking in relation to the years of experience and skill level if we hope to fully understand its effect on acute injury risk.

After reading that last paragraph you might be picturing some kind of catastrophic injury happening on a mountainside, and you wouldn't be too far off. Much of the research in this area has been focused on participation in extreme sports (e.g., skydiving and rock climbing). In fact, a meta-analysis of 39 studies revealed that athletes with high levels of sensation-seeking, extraversion, and impulsivity were significantly more likely to take part in high-risk sport.[23] The complex relationship between personality and risk-taking isn't confined to these dramatic environments, though. When we think about risk behaviors, they also include playing sport through pain or functional limitations that could result in chronic injury.[24–26] So, it isn't just about pushing major limits in pursuit of a thrill. Risk-taking occurs on a continuum relative to the individual's definition of risk (e.g., F1 drivers might have very different tolerance limits than recreational joggers), and this has yet to be fully accounted for when considering sensation-seeking and risk-taking as injury risk factors.

When we start to expand our tour of the personality-injury research from there, things become hit-and-miss simply because there aren't that many studies. A few researchers have examined the Big Five personality traits (conscientiousness, agreeableness, neuroticism, openness to experience, and extraversion)[27] and related variables like passion, locus of control, and hardiness, so we'll summarize the evidence here in brief. Neuroticism has been the subject of a few investigations, providing some fairly consistent evidence that it's a salient variable in the injury context. One study of 302 sportsmen determined that high neuroticism and extraversion scores were related to greater risk-taking in high-risk outdoor sport,[28] and athletes with chronic pain have been found to score higher in neuroticism than healthy matched controls.[29] In a sample of 170 adult competitive runners, both neuroticism and obsessive passion were significant, positive predictors of perceived injury susceptibility.[30] This is supported by another study that found obsessive passion was a risk factor for chronic injury in a sample of dance students.[31] Together, this small body of evidence suggests that athletes who have a tendency to quick emotional arousal and stress reactivity (neurotic characteristics), exhibit outgoing and energetic behavior (extraversion), and experience internal pressure to engage in an enjoyable activity (obsessive passion) may be at increased risk of injury. This makes intuitive sense; yet, with such small samples and a lack of corroboration across sport settings, these relationships are tenuous at best.

The other Big Five traits – conscientiousness, agreeableness, and openness to experience – haven't really been considered in the sport injury literature. There is some evidence that high-risk sport participants are more conscientious and open to experience than their low-risk sport counterparts,[32] but the importance of these variables to injury risk is poorly understood. It would make sense that athletes who are willing to try new things might be more apt to take risks, and those who are more conscientious might be more likely to wear protective equipment or behave in ways to minimize risk, but again these hypotheses have not been properly tested. A related concept is *locus of control*, which describes the degree to which people believe that they're in control of outcomes in their lives (internal LoC) rather than being at the mercy of external forces beyond their influence (external LoC). For athletes, this comes down to their belief about whether or not injuries can be prevented through their own actions. Research into locus of control has produced mixed findings. Having an external LoC was correlated with a higher injury rate among freshman college football players,[33] whereas Kolt and Kirkby[34] found that locus of control had no relationship with injury in a sample of non-elite gymnasts and an internal LoC was a significant injury predictor for elite gymnasts. Once again, some of this contradiction might be due to the moderating effect of athlete experience and skill, or inconsistencies in the way variables have been measured. Studies that have used general measurement tools have not found any relationship between locus of control and injury, but those using sport-specific measures have generally shown that external LoC is associated with more frequent or more severe injuries.[35,36] Therefore, understanding how this personality factor interacts with the sport environment is another important area for further investigation.

Okay, before we wrap up this discussion, we need to acknowledge the great big anxiety-shaped elephant in the room. Personality factors like trait anxiety and hardiness are by far the most well-researched in the sport injury literature,[37] so we would be remiss not to address them in a personality-focused chapter, right? Well, it turns out that although anxiety does have a small injury predictive effect[38] and hardiness has been shown to have a direct, negative relationship with injury incidence,[39] their true contribution to injury risk really becomes evident through interactions with situational (state) variables like stress appraisals and coping responses. So, fear not, we haven't ignored these important topics, we're just leaving them for the next chapter where we can talk about them in more detail.[ii]

And that sums it up. Genuinely, that's it, that's the body of literature we have to work with. Is there enough evidence to support the existence of an "injury-prone" personality profile? In a word, no. It's clear that in this domain, what we do know is far outweighed by what we don't know and we're miles away from injury prediction based on personality traits. In fact, a recent meta-analysis of 48 published studies examining the relationships between psychosocial variables and sport injury found poor evidence that personality or behavioral factors independently influenced injury rates.[40] This isn't a struggle limited to psychosocial research, though. Turns out, researchers from other disciplines aren't that much further ahead.

Why Has Personality Risk Profiling Been Unsuccessful?

The quest to reliably predict sport injury has been a long and difficult one. Incredible effort has been dedicated to finding key biomechanical and physiological risk factors from which to produce algorithms that identify "at-risk" athletes. But, despite a wealth of injury prediction studies in these areas, the summary result has been a collection of equations that are alright at categorizing risk factors but are largely incapable of flagging which specific athletes will be injured, or when an injury will happen.[41–43] This seems counterintuitive given how much research has gone into it, but there are some very good reasons why that's the case and we've actually touched on some of them already.

We've established that risk factors don't exist in a vacuum. Intrinsic and extrinsic variables interact dynamically to make athletes susceptible to injury. For example, a runner with poor ankle stability (intrinsic) might be predisposed to injury, but their susceptibility could be low on a treadmill and high on uneven terrain (extrinsic). This implies that any injury prediction attempt based on a single risk factor, rather than using a multivariable approach, will fail. There's also plenty of indication that the relationships between risk factors and injuries may be context-specific and are likely affected by inter-individual differences. For instance, our runner might manage uneven terrain well during self-paced training but less so when racing at a high speed, or a risk-taking runner may be more willing to sprint on a bumpy path than their risk-averse teammate. The inciting event that results in injury can also be situation-dependent (e.g., our runner might successfully traverse the same obstacle five times during a race, but on the sixth lap, it triggers a sprain). In other words, injury prediction isn't simply a matter of figuring out which risk factors are related to injury in a linear, unidirectional way.

Instead, injury causality is a complex web characterized by patterns of interactions between many variables.[44] This is why injury prediction is so difficult, and it forms the essence of *complexity theory*.

Well, this sounds complicated, right? Actually, a number of very readable applications of complexity theory have started emerging in the sport injury literature and they're worth a read if you're interested in big conceptual ideas.[44–46] Fundamentally, they describe the necessity of integrating biomechanical, physiological, and psychosocial factors, rather than looking at them separately, to improve our understanding of injury causation (Figure 3.2). We need to search for stable patterns in the way the variables interact with one another, not how they operate on their own, if we ever hope to quantify their contribution to risk. To illustrate, many of the personality traits that have been investigated appear to influence injury both directly and by driving risk behaviors, consequently accounting for little variance in injury incidence when considered by themselves. Instead, these factors may be better understood through a *complex systems* lens that accounts for their effects in combination with the effects of other risk factors. One of the key tenets of complexity theory is that small changes in a few factors can lead to dramatic and sometimes unexpected consequences elsewhere.[44] Therefore, it's possible that the small effects of personality traits seen in previous studies could magnify when considered as part of a larger system.[47,48]

Another reason that injury profiling hasn't been all that successful lies in the interpretation of existing research evidence. Most studies collect data from groups of athletes. Researchers pool all the data together and conduct statistical analyses

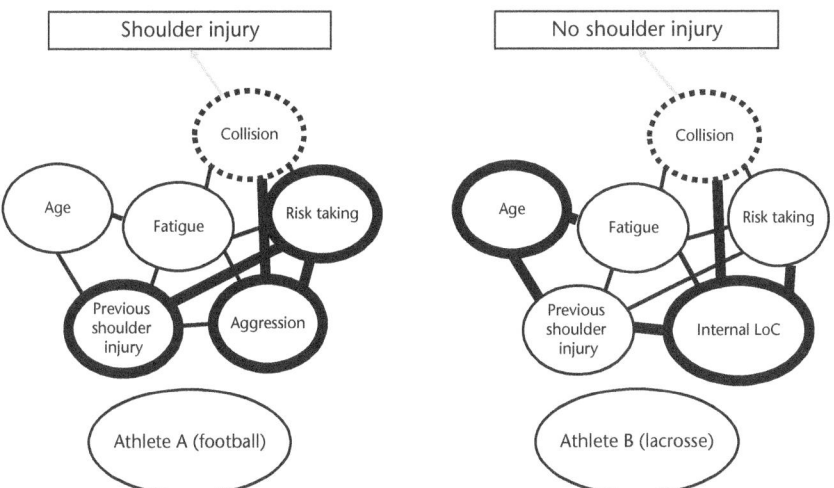

FIGURE 3.2   An illustration of complexity theory applied to sport injury (inspired by Bittencourt et al. 2016).[44] In different sport contexts, and with unique combinations of risk factors, some interaction effects may become more prominent than others (indicated by darker lines) and can lead to different outcomes.

based on the group's average values. This provides reliable information about how variables are related to each other at the group level, but we know that not all members of a group are the same and there's likely to be some variability in those relationships from person to person. For example, we might be interested in the association between some personality variable (let's call it *Personality Factor A,* or *PFA* for short) and injury risk. Some participants in the study have high levels of *PFA* and some have low levels of *PFA*, so the average value comes out somewhere in the middle. That's the value we use in the analysis, which shows that average *PFA* has a moderate association with injury; however, the relationship could actually be strongest for those with high *PFA* and weaker for those with low *PFA*. So, even though we're concluding that there's a moderate association between these variables, that may not represent the reality for participants at the upper or lower end of the distribution. Therefore, when we use this evidence to estimate someone's risk of injury, we're essentially making inferences about that person based on aggregate (group-level) data. This is known as an *ecological fallacy* and it's a key reason why risk factor models often don't work for individual-level prediction. Recalibrating expectations with the understanding that risk factors are not one-size-fits-all, and their contribution to injury might differ between athletes who have different sets of intrinsic and extrinsic risk factors, is important when interpreting and applying evidence in practice.

Improving on the Foundations

Needless to say, when it comes to identifying personality-related injury risk factors, there are currently far more questions than answers. This chapter has pointed out a few ways to progress this science, but first and foremost there needs to be more science to progress. Research volume is key to compiling robust, replicable evidence from which to draw firm conclusions, so more studies are needed to investigate how personality predictors interact with other psychosocial and system variables in injury risk. Future studies will also need to adopt different designs. An inherent limitation in the existing literature is that data have often been collected cross-sectionally (i.e., at a single time point), so it's difficult to determine whether the personality variables influenced the injury, or vice versa (e.g., did low sensation-seeking lead to injury, or did an injury make the athlete more risk-averse?). To avoid these chicken-and-egg problems, prospective studies that measure psychological factors (e.g., personality) at the beginning of the season and follow athletes forward for injury reports will enable the temporal association between variables to be established. As soon as we know which comes first, it becomes much easier to determine which personality factors might lead to injury and which behaviors are consequences thereof.

Another limitation with previous work is that data are usually collected at set time points, and we know that some personality-related variables (e.g., risk taking) can fluctuate rapidly and change from context to context. So, to identify athletes who are susceptible to injury, modern methods of assessing malleable psychosocial variables need to be explored and adopted. Recent technological advancements in mobile and sensor technologies, which can collect information in real-time, facilitate approaches such as Ecological Momentary Assessment (EMA). This involves using smartphones and web-based applications to gather real-world monitoring/self-report data on behaviors, emotional states, beliefs, attitudes, and perceptions as people go about their everyday lives. This method is more conducive to capturing phenomena that vary over time or space than the traditional cross-sectional and retrospective methods. For example, an EMA study might utilize periodic text messages to ask athletes about what they're experiencing at a given moment to get an idea of how their personality interacts with the particular environment they happen to be in at the time. This may allow for a more in-depth examination into not only inter-individual (i.e., between-person) differences in injury risk factors, but also whether there are intra-individual (i.e., within-person) effects that play an important part. This could yield new insights into the etiology of sport injury and inform the development of psychological interventions for injury prevention.

It's also clear that for the most accurate and informative risk profiles to be developed, the complex and dynamic nature of the sport environment needs to be accounted for. Injuries are multifactorial, and though things like the characteristics of the sport (e.g., rules and risk level) and its participants (e.g., skill level and experience) are usually considered, the interactions between these elements and other potential risk factors are not. Adopting a complex systems approach that embraces the integration of intrinsic/extrinsic and modifiable/non-modifiable risk factors, rather than using reductionist linear methods, would better characterize the context in which sport injuries occur.[46] This will require researchers and practitioners from a variety of disciplines to work in collaboration, with the goal of better understanding how psychological, biomechanical, physiological, and social factors combine to influence injury risk.

Risk Profiling in Practice

If personality-based injury prediction is an unrealistic goal (at least for the time being), it's easy to wonder if this whole enterprise is a dead end; however, there's plenty of additional value that can be gained by screening athletes for potential risk factors. Much like pre-participation movement assessment is lousy at predicting injury[42,43] but good for directing intervention toward athletes who are predisposed,[49] personality assessment might be best used in conjunction or together with other potential injury prediction variables to figure out which athletes would benefit most from injury prevention efforts. If we go back to the example of the risk-taking runner with the unstable ankle, understanding their intrinsic personality risk factors might not predict if or when they'll have a sprain, but it could determine what support they need to minimize its likelihood (e.g., stopping them from training through pain). Establishing an individual athlete's tendencies and needs is an important part of care, and something that can be done practically by using formal personality inventories and/or observing athlete behavior.

There is, of course, a danger with individually assessing people. Although we've pointed out that just because someone is predisposed to injury, it doesn't mean they'll go on to be injured, it's easy to fall into the trap of labeling individuals as "high-risk." On the surface, this sounds beneficial for targeting prevention efforts, but it can also land us right back where we started – not picking athletes in our fantasy pools because they're "injury prone." It's essential that those who work in sport recognize the potential stigma associated with personality risk factors. Awareness of mental health issues in sport has improved massively in recent years but as soon as someone is categorized as being at risk due to an inherent psychological trait, explicit and implicit biases can significantly affect them.[50] For instance, openly derogatory comments about "risky" athletes (explicit) or subtle differences in the way coaches speak to them (reflecting implicit biases) may serve to undermine their wellbeing and detrimentally affect their performance, reputation, and career prospects. Making sure that a risk profile doesn't unfairly impact athlete selection or treatment remains a concern and is something that practitioners must be vigilant against.

At the end of the day, the purpose of identifying predisposing factors is to figure out which athletes may be at greater risk of injury so that steps can be taken to manage that risk appropriately. To do that, researchers and practitioners need to work together to define, measure, and interpret the influence of psychological factors, including personality, on risk behaviors and injury outcomes in sport-specific contexts. Ultimately, this has the potential to inform effective screening and intervention strategies, though (if you'll forgive the quest metaphor) there's a long road ahead before we get to that point. And, as we'll see over the next couple of chapters, the psychology of injury risk involves more than just personality.

Notes

i For any Monty Python fans reading this, it seems like there should be a Black Knight joke in here somewhere. If you can do better than a "just a flesh wound" reference, feel free to have yourself a chuckle.
ii Hopefully the suspense isn't killing you….

References

1 Meeuwisse WH, Tyreman H, Hagel B, et al. A dynamic model of etiology in sport injury: the recursive nature of risk and causation. *Clin J Sport Med* 2007;17:215–219; doi: 10.1097/JSM.0b013e3180592a48.
2 Windt J, Gabbett TJ. How do training and competition workloads relate to injury? The workload—injury aetiology model. *Br J Sports Med* 2017;51(5):428–435; doi: 10.1136/bjsports-2016-096040.
3 Osborn ZH, Blanton PD, Schwebel DC. Personality and injury risk among professional hockey players. *J Inj Violence Res* 2009;1(1):15–19; doi: 10.5249/jivr.v1i1.8.
4 McCrae RR, Costa PT. Trait explanations in personality psychology. *Eur J Pers* 1995;9(4):231–252; doi: 10.1002/per.2410090402.

5 Sacks DN, Petscher Y, Stanley CT, et al. Aggression and violence in sport: moving beyond the debate. *Int J Sport Exerc Psychol* 2003;1(2):167–179; doi:10.1080/16121 97X.2003.9671710.

6 Sheldon JP, Aimar CM. The role aggression plays in successful and unsuccessful ice hockey behaviors. *Res Q Exerc Sport* 2001;72(3):304–309; doi: 10.1080/02701367.2001.10608965.

7 Bushman BJ, Anderson CA. Is it time to pull the plug on the hostile versus instrumental aggression dichotomy? *Psychol Rev* 2001;108(1):273–279; doi:10.1037/0033-295X.108.1 .273.

8 Cusimano MD, Nastis S, Zuccaro L. Effectiveness of interventions to reduce aggression and injuries among ice hockey players: a systematic review. *CMAJ* 2013;185(1):E57–E69; doi: 10.1503/cmaj.112017.

9 Cusimano MD, Ilie G, Mullen SJ, et al. Aggression, violence and injury in Minor League Ice Hockey: avenues for prevention of injury. *PloS One* 2016;11(6):e0156683; doi: 10.1371/journal.pone.0156683.

10 Thompson NJ, Morris RD. Predicting injury risk in adolescent football players: the importance of psychological variables. *J Pediatr Psychol* 1994;19(4):415–429; doi: 10.1 093/jpepsy/19.4.415.

11 Fields KB, Delaney M, Hinkle S. A prospective study of type A behavior and running injuries. *J Fam Pract* 1990;30:425–429; PMID: 2324695

12 Williams JM, Andersen MB. Psychosocial antecedents of sport injury and interventions for risk reduction. In: G Tenenbaum, RC Eklund (eds.). *Handbook of Sport Psychology*. New York: John Wiley & Sons, Inc 2007.

13 Parent S, Fortier K. Comprehensive overview of the problem of violence against athletes in sport. *J Sport Soc Issues* 2018;42(4):227–246; doi: 10.1177/0193723518759448.

14 Zuckerman M. Sensation seeking and sports. *Pers Individ Dif* 1983;4:285–292; doi: 10.1 002/9780470479216.corpsy0843.

15 Wilson LC, Scarpa A. The link between sensation seeking and aggression: a meta-analytic review. *Aggress Behav* 2011;37(1):81–90; doi: 10.1002/ab.20369.

16 Smith RE, Smoll FL, Ptacek JT. Conjunctive moderator variables in vulnerability and resiliency research: life stress, social support and coping skills, and adolescent sport injuries. *J Pers Soc Psychol* 1990;58(2):360–370; doi: 10.1037//0022-3514.58.2.360.

17 van Wijk CH. Mental health measures in predicting outcomes for the selection and training of navy divers. *Diving Hyperb Med* 2011;41(1):22–26; PMID: 21560981.

18 Niedermeier M, Ruedl G, Burtscher M, et al. Injury-related behavioral variables in alpine skiers, snowboarders, and ski tourers-a matched and enlarged re-analysis. *Int J Environ Res Public Health* 2019;16(20):3807; doi: 10.3390/ijerph16203807.

19 Ruedl G, Posch M, Niedermeier M, et al. Are risk-taking and ski helmet use associated with an ACL injury in recreational alpine skiing? *Int J Environ Res Public Health* 2019;16(17):3107; doi: 10.3390/ijerph16173107.

20 Goulet C, Régnier G, Valois P, et al. (2000). Injuries and risk taking in alpine skiing. In: R Johnson, P Zucco, J Shealy (eds.). *Skiing trauma and safety: thirteenth volume*. West Conshohocken, PA: ASTM International 2000.

21 Made C, Elmqvist LG. A 10-year study of snowboard injuries in Lapland Sweden. *Scand J Med Sci Sports* 2004;14(2):128–133; doi: 10.1111/j.1600-0838.2003.00342.x.

22 Ruedl G, Burtscher M, Wolf M, et al. Are self-reported risk-taking behavior and helmet use associated with injury causes among skiers and snowboarders? *Scand J Med Sci Sports* 2015;25(1):125–130; doi: 10.1111/sms.12139.

23 McEwan D, Boudreau P, Curran T, et al. Personality traits of high-risk sport participants: a meta-analysis. *J Res Pers* 2019;79:83–93; doi: 10.1016/j.jrp.2019.02.006.

24 Bahr R. No injuries, but plenty of pain? On the methodology for recording overuse symptoms in sports. *Br J Sports Med* 2009;43(13):966–972; doi: 10.1136/bjsm.2 009.066936.

25 Pluim BM, Loeffen FG, Clarsen B, et al. A one-season prospective study of injuries and illness in elite junior tennis. *Scand J Med Sci Sports* 2016;26(5):564–571; doi: 10.1111/ sms.12471.

26 Van der Sluis A, Brink MS, Pluim B, et al. Is risk-taking in talented junior tennis players related to overuse injuries? *Scand J Med Sci Sports* 2017;27(11):1347–1355; doi: 10.1111/sms.12729.

27 Costa PT, McCrae RR. *The NEO Personality Inventory manual.* Odessa, Florida: Psychological Assessment Resources 1985.

28 Castanier C, Le Scanff C, Woodman T. Who takes risks in high-risk sports? A typological personality approach. *Res Q Exerc Sport* 2010;81(4):478–484; doi: 10.1080/02 701367.2010.10599709.

29 San Antolín M, Rodríguez-Sanz D, Becerro de Bengoa Vallejo R, et al. Neuroticism traits and anxiety symptoms are exhibited in athletes with chronic gastrocnemius myofascial pain syndrome. *J Strength Cond Res* 2020;34(12):3377–3385; doi: 10.1519/ JSC.0000000000003838.

30 Stephan Y, Deroche T, Brewer BW, et al. Predictors of perceived susceptibility to sport-related injury among competitive runners: the role of previous experience, neuroticism, and passion for running. *Appl Psychol* 2009;58:672–687; doi: 10.1111/j.14 64-0597.2008.00373.x.

31 Rip B, Fortin S, Vallerand RJ. The relationship between passion and injury in dance students. *J Dance Med Sci* 2006;10:14–20.

32 Kajtna T, Tusak M, Baric R, et al. Personality in high-risk sports athletes. *Kinesiology* 2004;36:24–34.

33 Pargman D, Lunt SD. The relationship of self-concept and locus of control to the severity of injury in freshman collegiate football players. *Sports Med Train Rehab* 1989; 1(3):201–208; doi: 10.1080/15438628909511877.

34 Kolt G, Kirkby R. Injury in Australian female competitive gymnasts: a psychological perspective. *Aust J Physiother* 1996;42(2):121–126; doi: 10.1016/s0004-9514(14)60444-x.

35 Dalhauser M, Thomas MB. Visual disembedding and locus of control as variables associated with high school football injuries. *Percept Mot Skills* 1979;49(1):254; doi: 10.24 66/pms.1979.49.1.254.

36 Williams JM, Andersen MB. Psychosocial antecedents of sport injury: review and critique of the stress and injury model. *J Appl Sport Psychol* 1998;10(1):5–25; doi: 10.1 080/10413209808406375.

37 Ford JL, Ildefonso K, Jones ML, et al. Sport-related anxiety: current insights. *Open Access J Sports Med* 2017;8:205–212; doi: 10.2147/OAJSM.S125845.

38 Cagle A, Overcash K, Rowe D, et al. Trait anxiety as a risk factor for musculoskeletal injury in athletes: a critically appraised topic. *Int J Athl Train Ther* 2017;22(3):26–31; doi: 10.1123/ijatt.2016-0065.

39 Wadey R, Evans L, Hanton S, et al. An examination of hardiness throughout the sport injury process. *Br J Health Psych* 2012;17(1):103–128; doi: 10.1111/j.2044-8287.2011.02025.x.

40 Ivarsson A, Johnson U, Andersen MB, et al. Psychosocial factors and sport injuries: meta-analyses for prediction and prevention. *Sports Med* 2017;47:353–365; doi: 10.1 007/s40279-016-0578-x.

41 Drew MK, Cook J, Finch CF. Sports-related workload and injury risk: simply knowing the risks will not prevent injuries: narrative review. *Br J Sports Med* 2016;50:1306–1308; doi: 10.1136/bjsports-2015-095871.

42 Whittaker JL, Booysen N, de la Motte S, et al. Predicting sport and occupational lower extremity injury risk through movement quality screening: a systematic review. *Br J Sports Med* 2017;51(7):580–585; doi: 10.1136/bjsports-2016-096760.

43 Bahr R. Why screening tests to predict injury do not work – and probably never will: a critical review. *Br J Sports Med* 2016;50:776–780; doi: 10.1136/bjsports-2016-096256.

44 Bittencourt NFN, Meeuwisse WH, Mendonca LD, et al. Complex systems approach for sports injuries: moving from risk factor identification to injury pattern recognition – narrative review and new concept. *Br J Sports Med* 2016;50:1309–1314; doi:10.1136/bjsports-2016-095850.

45 Hulme A, Thompson J, Nielsen RO, et al. Towards a complex systems approach in sports injury research: simulating running-related injury development with agent-based modelling. *Br J Sports Med* 2019;53:560–569; doi: 10.1136/bjsports-2017-098871.

46 Bekker S, Clark AM. Bringing complexity to sports injury prevention research: from simplification to explanation. *Br J Sports Med* 2016;50:1489–1490; doi: 10.1136/bjsports-2016-096457.

47 Johnson U, Ekengren J, Andersen MB. Injury prevention in Sweden: helping soccer players at risk. *J Sport Exerc Psychol* 2005;27:32–38; doi: 10.1123/jsep.27.1.32.

48 Maddison R, Prapavessis H. A psychological approach to the prediction and prevention of athletic injury. *J Sport Exerc Psychol* 2005;27:289–310; doi: 10.1123/jsep.27.3.289.

49 Verhagen E, van Dyk N, Clark N, et al. Do not throw the baby out with the bathwater; screening can identify meaningful risk factors for sports injuries. *Br J Sports Med* 2018;52:1223–1224; doi: 10.1136/bjsports-2017-098547.

50 FitzGerald C, Hurst S. Implicit bias in healthcare professionals: a systematic review. *BMC Med Ethics* 2017;18:19; doi: 10.1186/s12910-017-0179-8.

4

THE LINK BETWEEN STRESS AND SPORTS INJURY: "I DIDN'T SEE IT COMING"

Carly McKay and Lee Moore

Sport is inherently stressful. Regardless of setting or competitive level, athletes frequently experience stressors associated with the competitive environment (e.g., expectations, rivalry), as well as their sporting organization (e.g., selection issues, coach conflict) and personal lives (e.g., relationship problems, family bereavement).[1] Now, the word "stress" is often treated as an umbrella term, and even scientists use it interchangeably to refer to both specific events or situations (e.g., giving a speech, losing your job) and the psychophysiological reactions to such situations (e.g., heightened anxiety, elevated heart rate). However, stress is best considered an emergent process that involves interactions between the athlete and environmental factors (e.g., team culture), historical and current events (e.g., daily hassles), and protective factors (e.g., coping strategies), which results in specific patterns of psychophysiological reactivity (e.g., increased stress hormones like cortisol).[2] While the experience of stress is highly individualistic, research has consistently linked it to negative outcomes including deteriorations in sports performance and poor athlete mental health.[3,4] Moreover, stress has been linked to sports injury.[5] Indeed, stress is at the centre of the most cited theoretical framework for explaining how psychosocial factors influence injury occurrence: the Stress–Injury Model.[6,7]

Revisiting the Model

If you remember our discussion of the Stress–Injury Model in chapter 2,[6] it suggests that the risk of an athlete becoming injured is influenced by the magnitude of their stress response to a potentially stressful situation (e.g., important sporting competition or key training session), and the scale of this stress response is determined by how the athlete cognitively appraises the situation (Figure 4.1). Specifically, when faced with a possibly stressful situation, the model suggests that

DOI: 10.4324/9781003088936-4

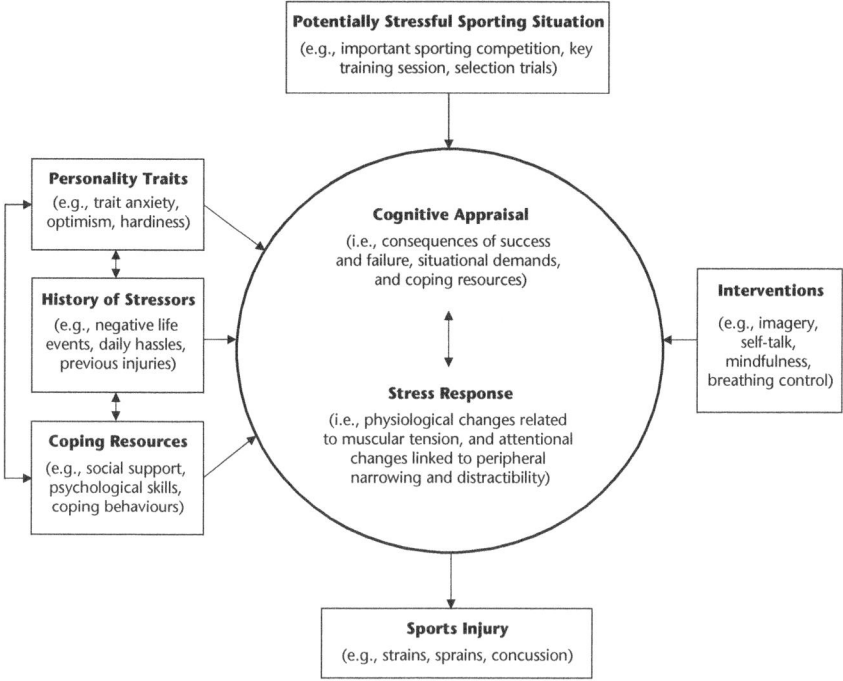

Potentially Stressful Sporting Situation
(e.g., important sporting competition, key training session, selection trials)

Personality Traits
(e.g., trait anxiety, optimism, hardiness)

History of Stressors
(e.g., negative life events, daily hassles, previous injuries)

Coping Resources
(e.g., social support, psychological skills, coping behaviours)

Cognitive Appraisal
(i.e., consequences of success and failure, situational demands, and coping resources)

Stress Response
(i.e., physiological changes related to muscular tension, and attentional changes linked to peripheral narrowing and distractibility)

Interventions
(e.g., imagery, self-talk, mindfulness, breathing control)

Sports Injury
(e.g., strains, sprains, concussion)

FIGURE 4.1   Model of stress and athletic injury (adapted).[6]

an athlete will assess the demands of the circumstances, whether they have the resources to cope with those demands, and the consequences of failure or success (e.g., deselection, trophies).[7] The net result of these cognitive appraisals will either evoke an exaggerated or attenuated stress response. For example, an elite skier who's in the starting gates and believes that the next run will have big implications for their career (e.g., Olympic qualification), and fears that they don't have the resources (e.g., skill, ability) to cope with the demands of the situation, is likely to experience an exaggerated stress response (e.g., greater muscular tension). In contrast, a skier who appraises the competition as less important and believes that they have the resources to cope with the situational demands, is likely to have a lower stress response.

An athletes' cognitive appraisal is therefore key in determining their injury risk in potentially stressful situations.[8] This isn't anything new in sport, though. Drawing on classic stress work,[9] other theories prominent in the sport perfor-mance literature have highlighted the importance of cognitive appraisals, too. For instance, the Biopsychosocial Model of Challenge and Threat[10,11] and theory of Challenge and Threat States in Athletes[12] link two different types of cognitive appraisals with distinct physiological, emotional, attentional, and behavioural outcomes. Challenge appraisals, in which athletes perceive that they have sufficient resources to cope with the demands of a potentially stressful situation, have been associated with more adaptive cardiovascular reactivity (e.g., higher cardiac activity and lower vascular resistance),[13] less negative emotion (e.g., cognitive anxiety),[14] more optimal attention (e.g., longer eye gaze durations),[15] and better performance (e.g., anaerobic power).[16] In contrast, threat appraisals, in which athletes perceive that the situational demands exceed their coping resources, have been related to less favourable outcomes.[3,17] We also know that consequences of success and failure are likely to feed into appraisals of situational demands,[12,18] with more severe consequences liable to prompt a higher perception of demands and evoke a threat appraisal. It seems, then, that similar processes are involved in performance and injury risk, which suggests that minimizing threat perceptions will have a double benefit for keeping athletes healthy and on the top of their game. So, given their importance, it's essential to understand what factors impact cognitive appraisals.

Key Contributors

Athletes' cognitive appraisals and stress responses are influenced by several psychosocial factors grouped into three broad categories; namely, personality characteristics, history of stressors, and coping resources (Figure 4.1).[7] The basic premise is that athletes with more maladaptive personality traits, a more extensive history of stressors, and fewer coping resources are more likely to appraise potentially stressful situations as a threat and have an exaggerated response.[19] We covered some important personality traits in the last chapter but research has shown that others are directly implicated in the way people handle stress. Those higher in *trait anxiety* (a stable tendency to experience fears and worries across many situations)[20], *external locus of control* (a belief that events are caused by factors outside of one's control),[21] and *perfectionism* (constant striving for flawlessness)[22] may be more susceptible to injury. The same is true for people lower in *hardiness* (tendency to respond to stress with commitment, control, and challenge),[23] *optimism* (positive outlook),[24] and *mental toughness* (resilience and strength).[25] As just one example, Johnson and Ivarsson[26] found that youth soccer players who reported greater trait anxiety were more likely to experience an injury during the competitive season. There are some additional personality characteristics that have been empirically related to challenge and threat appraisals but haven't yet been investigated in a sport injury context, including emotional intelligence, neuroticism, extraversion, agreeableness, and beliefs in a just world.[27] These bear some additional investigation as potentially important factors in the Stress-Injury Model.

Regarding history of stressors, research has demonstrated that athletes who have experienced more negative life events,[28] greater daily hassles,[29] and more injuries in the past[30] are more likely to sustain an injury. In a classic study, Bramwell et al.[31] found that 73% of American football players who reported experiencing high life stress incurred an injury during the competitive season, compared to 50% and 30% who reported moderate and low life stress, respectively. This pattern has been repeated in numerous studies since, to the point that life stress is the most robust psychological predictor of injury across sport settings. It makes intuitive sense, too. Imagine a cyclist who, in the lead-up to the Tour de France, goes through a significant adversity such as a family death, daily hassles related to childcare, and niggling injuries (e.g., knee pain). They're more likely to appraise the competition as a threat, experience an exaggerated stress response, and thus sustain an injury. However, it is worth noting that positive life events (e.g., marriage[i]) have also been linked to injury occurrence.[32] So, it may not only be negative things that cause stress, but disruptions in general. There's also some evidence that experiencing a moderate amount of life stress can lead to more positive responses following injury,[33] though more research is needed to understand why that might be the case.

In terms of coping resources, athletes who receive lower social support from significant others,[34] possess fewer psychological skills or techniques,[35] and have poorer general coping behaviours,[36] are more likely to get injured. Again, this relationship was demonstrated in a classic study where Smith et al.[37] found that basketball players, wrestlers, and gymnasts who reported lower levels of social support and fewer coping skills were at greatest risk of injury during a competitive season. Therefore, in line with the Stress-Injury Model,[6] we might hypothesize that an athlete who goes into draft testing or selection trials with limited support from their friends and family, very few mental skills such as goal-setting or self-talk, and having slept and eaten poorly for a few days is more likely to appraise the situation as a threat and have an amplified stress response, increasing their chance of getting injured. Interestingly, research has linked greater perceived social support with challenge appraisals,[38] showing that it's not just the actual receipt of support that's important, but the perception that support will be available.[39] So, even if our athlete at selection trials hasn't had much tangible support from their loved ones recently, just knowing it's there if they need it might make all the difference.

Despite the fact that we've talked about each of these psychosocial factors that influence cognitive appraisals, stress responses, and injury risk as distinct processes, in reality they interact with each other in complex ways.[6] Thus, while having particular personality traits might protect athletes from the negative effects of high life stress on injury, it's equally possible that greater exposure to life stress has helped athletes develop protective personality characteristics.[40] Similarly, although using specific coping strategies (e.g., slow breathing) might weaken the impact of high life stress on injury, experiencing more life stress might have led to the development and deployment of these coping strategies in the first place.[5] Finally, athletes with certain personality traits might have preferences for specific coping strategies (e.g., athletes higher in neuroticism tend to use more avoidance coping),[41] but equally, greater use of specific coping strategies might help shape an athletes' personality characteristics (e.g., mental toughness).[42] So, at the end of the day, we can't consider one without the other and teasing out which factors are most important is incredibly difficult.

How Does It All Work?

Ample research has linked stress with increased injury risk,[43] but we're still not sure precisely how it does so. According to the Stress-Injury Model,[6] appraising a potentially stressful situation as a threat heightens an athlete's risk of injury by increasing muscular tension, narrowing their visual attention, or increasing their distractibility. For instance, when viewing an important event as a threat, a cross-country runner may experience greater muscular tension (i.e., bracing), which limits their flexibility and disrupts their coordination, thus increasing their chances of strains or sprains. As well as feeling tense, a rugby player who appraises a crucial match as a threat might experience narrowing of their peripheral vision (i.e., tunnel vision) or become distracted by irrelevant stimuli (e.g., the crowd), leading to critical cues like a tackler being missed. Although research has struggled to make the connection between stress, muscular tension, and sports injury, some studies have supported the proposed attentional changes. For instance, Rogers and Landers[44] found that peripheral narrowing mediated the relationship between negative life events and injury.

These attentional mechanisms share similarities with the explanations offered by theories linking challenge and threat appraisals with sports performance. To illustrate, the Integrative Framework of Stress, Attention, and Visuomotor Performance,[45] states that challenge and threat appraisals impact performance via their effects on attentional control. Specifically, a threat appraisal causes athletes to become more distractible by task-irrelevant stimuli (e.g., the crowd or worrisome thoughts during a basketball free-throw), resulting in the suboptimal pick-up of visual information and poorer performance due to the stimulus-driven attentional system dominating the goal-directed system.[46] Research has supported this mechanism in various high-stress domains including sport,[13] aviation,[47] and surgery.[48] For example, Brimmell and colleagues[15] found that during a soccer penalty task, a threat appraisal was associated with worse performance and inferior attentional control, including less time visually fixating on the goal and shorter fixations on the ball prior to the run-up.[49] A threat appraisal has also been linked with more conscious processing or monitoring of movements,[12,16] which could have similar implications for injury because dangerous environmental cues may be missed while the athlete is focusing on their technique. How many times have we seen someone get hit while admiring the pass they just made or be blindsided whilst scrambling to recover a defensive position? Under stress, focusing on too many things or too few can be equally risky.

As well as cognitive appraisals impacting stress responses, there's a potential feedback loop in which stress responses such as physiological reactions (e.g., muscular tension) and attentional disruptions can influence cognitive appraisals (Figure 4.1).[6,7] For example, a pro golfer leading a major tournament going into the final hole might notice tightness in their muscles, butterflies in their stomach, and pay closer attention to negative thoughts (e.g., "you're going to mess up"), causing them to appraise the hole as a threat. It's widely thought that cognitive appraisals occur subconsciously and automatically (rather than consciously and deliberately) and are dynamic,[10] changing as new environmental information comes to light.[46] Recent research has offered some support for this notion, showing that while athletes have trait-like tendencies to appraise all potentially stressful situations as either a challenge or a threat, cognitive appraisals are primarily context-specific and change from situation to situation.[50] Given that cognitive appraisals, like stress responses, can fluctuate and are open to change, interventions can be used to alter them, thereby reducing athletes' injury risk.[51]

How Can We Combat Stress?

Despite considerable cross-sectional and prospective research supporting the link between stress and injury,[5,52] the most compelling empirical support comes from intervention studies. Here, we have two general approaches to consider. The first is focused on using techniques that help athletes appraise potentially stressful situations as a challenge and not a threat, using techniques like cognitive restructuring or confidence training. For instance, a swimmer could use thought stopping (i.e., telling themself to get a grip) to block negative thoughts prior to a crucial race, preventing them from making a threat appraisal. The second approach is aimed at equipping athletes with the skills to modify their responses to stress, enabling them to use these skills to reduce muscular tension or prevent disruptions in attention. For example, a soccer goalkeeper could use slow breathing before a penalty shootout to relax. These two approaches are not mutually exclusive and could be used together. Equally, intervention strategies could be targeted at the psychosocial factors proposed in the Stress-Injury Model, such as building positive personality traits (e.g., mental toughness), limiting exposure to pressurized training and competition during times of heightened life stress (e.g., during exams for youth athletes), bolstering the coping resources available to athletes (e.g., improving social support), or improving their general coping behaviours (e.g., stabilizing sleep patterns).[53–55]

Two reviews have summarized the findings from psychological interventions aimed at tackling stress and preventing injury.[5,56] In their meta-analysis, Ivarsson et al.[5] found that all seven studies showed fewer injuries in intervention groups relative to control groups, with a medium to large effect size ($d = -0.63$). Moderator analyses revealed that the interventions were even more effective with at-risk athletes (e.g., those who were less hardy, had experienced more life stress, possessed few coping strategies). Thus, when planning interventions, it's important for practitioners to use the psychosocial factors proposed by Stress-Injury Model to identify those athletes who could benefit most.[6] Similar findings were reported in a systematic review of 13 studies by Gledhill et al.[56], with 93% showing a decrease in injury rates following an intervention. The strategies shown to be effective included cognitive techniques such as confidence training and thought stopping,[57,58] somatic strategies including relaxation techniques and mindfulness,[59,60] and multimodal interventions like stress management training.[61,62] Of course, reviews are all well and good, but how might we apply these findings in practice? Well, in a prospective study of 470 rugby players, Maddison and Prapavessis[63] reported that low social support, coping style, and previous injury interacted conjunctively to maximize the relationship between life stress and injury. They followed up with 48 of the players who had an at-risk profile and randomized them to a cognitive behavioural stress management intervention or control group. The players who received the intervention missed less time due to injury during the subsequent season compared to controls and demonstrated an increase in coping resource and decreased worry. This goes to show that a system of identifying at-risk players and prioritizing them for intervention can be effective.

Inspiration for other untested psychological injury prevention interventions could come from the challenge and threat literature,[46] where strategies that boost an athletes' coping resources, like arousal reappraisal and self-talk, have been shown to promote a challenge state.[64,65] At the heart of many of these interventions is the prediction that high self-efficacy (situation-specific self-confidence), greater perceptions of control, and a focus on desirable outcomes helps athletes appraise potentially stressful situations as less threatening.[12] Indeed, research has shown that verbal instructions and imagery can be used to manipulate these antecedents and promote challenge appraisals.[66,67] Another intervention that's received empirical support is *pressure training*.[68] This involves manipulating the demands (e.g., equipment, space constraints, noise) and consequences (e.g., punishments, rewards, audience) of training to expose athletes to stress in a controlled and supportive manner, helping them develop coping strategies and view stressful competition as a challenge.[69] Van Rens et al.[70] provided proof of concept for this, in that cricket players' challenge appraisals improved following a pressure training intervention, though it hasn't yet been tested with a view to injury prevention. Finally, research has shown that athletes can be trained to resist the attentional disruptions typically seen in high-stress situations (e.g., via *quiet eye training* which works on visual gaze).[71] While such training holds promise for reducing injuries, further research is needed into their effectiveness.

Solving Some of the Mysteries

Despite the important applied implications of theory and research linking stress and sports injury, some limitations, gaps in the literature, and avenues for future research are worthy of discussion. First, the Stress-Injury Model[6] was developed as a framework to explain the psychosocial factors associated with acute injuries (e.g., sprained ankle). As a result, far less research has explored the psychosocial factors related to overuse injuries, despite these being common in some sports.[72] In fact, only a few studies have been conducted in this area to date,[73,74] finding that personality traits (e.g., perfectionism, risk-taking), history of stress, coping strategies, psychophysiological factors (e.g., mental fatigue, poor recovery), and sociocultural issues (e.g., team norms, coach-athlete relationship) influence the risk of overuse injuries.[75] Thus, to gain a more complete picture of the causes of sports injury, future research needs to expand with a more comprehensive injury definition in mind. Second, an under-researched area is the role of prior injury.[7] From an epidemiological perspective, having had an injury is the biggest predictor of sustaining another.[76] Though this may be for physiological or medical reasons, it also makes intuitive sense that athletes returning from injury who harbour fears of reinjury and concerns related to their performance (e.g., worries about their ability to execute skills, meeting others' expectations, reaching prior levels of performance)[77] should be more prone to threat appraisals and exaggerated stress responses. Little research has supported this proposition so far,[78] but it warrants a closer look so that better support can be offered to athletes returning from injury.[79]

Third, while the Stress-Injury Model[6] offers a relatively holistic view of stress, including the impact of life events, daily hassles, and responses to acutely stressful situations, it doesn't characterize the role of chronic stress particularly well. Though this might be wrapped up in an athlete's history of stressors, there's a conceptual difference between discrete stressors in the past that have been resolved and those that have been on-going for some time. Chronic stress is linked to conditions that present over a long period (e.g., caregiving, financial strain)[2] and is related to negative general health outcomes (e.g., depression).[80] Moreover, it's at the centre of athlete burnout,[81] which is defined by physical and emotional exhaustion, cynicism or devaluation toward sport, and a reduced sense of accomplishment,[82] which have all been linked to outcomes like sport dropout.[83] Thus, for a more comprehensive understanding of the stress-injury relationship, we need to know how chronic stress influences athletes' cognitive appraisals, stress responses, and injury risk. Fourth, in outlining the psychosocial factors that impact injury risk, the model focuses heavily on athlete-centred variables like personality traits and coping strategies,[7] largely ignoring environmental factors (e.g., cultural values, team pressures). Given recent research showing the importance of context,[84] we need to explore these factors further. Of particular interest could be the role of coaches and teammates in "passing on" stress to athletes,[85,86] a concept known as *stress contagion*,[87] or coaches and teammates assisting each other when stressed in a phenomenon called *communal coping*.[88]

Although central to the model of stress and athletic injury,[6] cognitive appraisals of potentially stressful situations have rarely been directly measured.[52] Thus, to offer further support for the predictions of this model, future research is encouraged to use both subjective and objective measures (e.g., cardiovascular reactivity [cardiac output, heart rate variability], changes in hormones [cortisol, testosterone], or fluctuations in brain activity [left and right prefrontal cortical areas]) of cognitive appraisals.[3,89] Including objective markers will overcome some of the limitations of self-report measures (e.g., social desirability bias) and could unearth more mechanisms that help explain the stress-injury relationship (e.g., elevated cortisol has been associated with riskier decision making).[90] Finally, while intervention studies have shown that psychological strategies related to stress management hold promise in preventing injury,[56] we still don't' really know how they work.[5] Therefore, future intervention studies are encouraged to assess their mechanisms of action to improve our understanding of how combatting stress reduces injury occurrence. Furthermore, future intervention studies should strive to improve the quality of their methodologies and reporting (e.g., clearer description of randomisation procedures, inclusion of comparative control groups, more details on adherence).[56] These improvements would give us more confidence in the evidence and provide guidance when scaling up promising interventions for use in practice.

Where Does That Leave Us?

Athletes frequently encounter stressors and are often required to perform to the best of their ability in potentially stressful situations. Evidence shows that the way they manage these kinds of demands is related to injury risk. An athlete who has unfavourable personality characteristics (e.g., high trait anxiety, low hardiness), has experienced or is currently experiencing high life stress (e.g., childhood adversity, daily hassles), and has insufficient coping resources (e.g., little social support, few mental skills), is more likely to appraise such situations as a threat (i.e., demands exceed resources) and react with maladaptive responses that increase their susceptibility to injury. This stress-injury relationship is at the heart of sport injury psychology, and we'll see that it fundamentally influences the way athletes respond to injuries after they happen, too. So, although research suggests that helping athletes combat stress via psychological interventions can be beneficial, we need to better understand how and why that's the case if we hope to confer lasting protection across an athlete's career. And, as we'll discuss in the next chapter, part of that is figuring out how psychological stress interacts with the other situational factors that define the sport context to either build athletes up or break them.

Note

i Though, as anyone who's planned a wedding can attest to, this treads a line between positive and negative stress depending on how smoothly the arrangements are going.

References

1 Sarkar M, Fletcher D. Psychological resilience in sport performers: a review of stressors and protective factors. *J Sports Sci* 2014;32:1419–1434; doi: 10.1080/02640414.2014.901551.

2 Epel ES, Crosswell AD, Mayer SE, et al. More than a feeling: a unified view of stress measurement for population science. *Front Neuroendocrinol* 2018;49:146–169; doi:10.1 016/j.yfrne.2018.03.001.

3 Hase A, O'Brien J, Moore LJ, et al. The relationship between challenge and threat states and performance: a systematic review. *Sport Exerc Perf Psychol* 2019;8:123–144; doi:10.1 037/spy0000132.

4 Rice SM, Purcell R, De Silva S, et al. The mental health of elite athletes: a narrative systematic review. *Sports Med* 2016;46:1333–1353; doi:10.1007/s40279-016-0492-2.

5 Ivarsson A, Johnson U, Andersen M, et al. Psychosocial factors and sport injuries: meta-analyses for prediction and prevention. *Sports Med* 2017;47:353–365; doi:10.1007/s402 79-016-0578-x.

6 Andersen MB, Williams JM. A model of stress and athletic injury: prediction and prevention. *J Sport Exerc Psychol* 1988;10:294–306; doi:10.1123/jsep.10.3.294.

7 Williams JM, Andersen MB. Psychosocial antecedents of sport injury: review and critique of the stress and injury model. *J Appl Sport Psychol* 1998;10:5–25; doi:10.1080/1 0413209808406375.

8 Johnson U, Ivarsson A. Psychosocial factors and sport injuries: prediction, prevention and future research directions. *Curr Opin Psychol* 2017;16:89–92; doi:10.1016/j.copsyc.201 7.04.023.

9 Lazarus RS, Folkman S. *Stress, appraisal, and coping.* New York, NY: Springer 1984.

10 Blascovich J. Challenge and threat. In: AJ Elliot (ed.). *Handbook of approach and avoidance motivation.* New York, NY: Psychology Press 2008.

11 Seery MD. Challenge or threat? Cardiovascular indexes of resilience and vulnerability to potential stress in humans. *Neurosci Biobehav Rev* 2011;35:1603–1610; doi:10.1016/ j.neubiorev.2011.03.003.

12 Jones M, Meijen C, McCarthy PJ, et al. A theory of challenge and threat states in athletes. *Int Rev Sport Exerc Psychol* 2009;2:161–180; doi:10.1080/17509840902829331.

13 Moore LJ, Vine SJ, Wilson MR, et al. The effect of challenge and threat states on performance: an examination of potential mechanisms. *Psychophysiol* 2012;49:1417–1425; doi:10.1111/j.1469-8986.2012.01449.x.

14 Moore LJ, Wilson MR, Vine SJ, et al. Champ or chump? Challenge and threat states during pressurized competition. *J Sport Exerc Psychol* 2013;35:551–562; doi:10.1123/ jsep.35.6.551.

15 Brimmell J, Parker J, Wilson MR, et al. Challenge and threat states, performance, and attentional control during a pressurized soccer penalty task. *Sport Exerc Perf Psychol* 2019;8:63–79; doi:10.1037/spy0000147.

16 Wood N, Parker J, Freeman P, et al. The relationship between challenge and threat states, anaerobic power, core affect, perceived exertion, and self-focused attention during a competitive sprint cycling task. *Prog Brain Res* 2018;240:1–17; doi:10.1016/ bs.pbr.2018.08.006.

17 Jamieson JP. Challenge and threat appraisals. In: AJ Elliot, CS Dweck, DS Yeager (eds.). *Handbook of competence and motivation: theory and application.* New York, NY: Guildford Press 2017.

18 Seery MD. The biopsychosocial model of challenge and threat: using the heart to measure the mind. *Soc Personal Psychol Compass* 2013;7:637–653; doi:10.1111/spc3.12 052.

19 Johnson U. Psychosocial antecedents of sport injury, prevention, and intervention: an overview of theoretical approaches and empirical findings. *Int J Sport Exerc Psychol* 2007;5:352–369; doi:10.1080/1612197X.2007.9671841.

20 Lavallee L, Flint F. The relationship of stress, competitive anxiety, mood state, and social support to athletic injury. *J Athl Train* 1996;31:296-296.

21 Pargman D, Lunt SD. The relationship of self-concept and locus of control to the severity of injury in freshman collegiate football players. *Sports Med Train Rehabil* 1989;1:201–208; doi:10.1080/15438628909511877.

22 Madigan DJ, Stoeber J, Forsdyke D, et al. Perfectionism predicts injury in junior athletes: preliminary evidence from a prospective study. *J Sports Sci* 2018;36:545–550; doi:1 0.1080/02640414.2017.1322709.

23 Wadey R, Evans L, Hanton S, et al. An examination of hardiness throughout the sport injury process. *Br J Health Psychol* 2012;17:103–128; doi:10.1111/j.2044-8287.2011.02 025.x.

24 Wadey R, Evans L, Hanton S, et al. Effect of dispositional optimism before and after injury. *Med Sci Sports Exerc* 2013;45:387–394; doi:10.1249/MSS.0b013e31826ea8e3.

25 Petrie TA, Deiters J, Harmison RJ. Mental toughness, social support, and athletic identity: moderators of the life stress–injury relationship in collegiate football players. *Sport Exerc Perf Psychol* 2014;3:13–27; doi:10.1037/a0032698.

26 Johnson U, Ivarsson A. Psychological predictors of sport injuries among junior soccer players. *Scand J Med Sci Sports* 2011;21:129–136; doi:10.1111/j.1600-0838.2009.01 057.x.

27 Kilby CJ, Sherman KA, Wuthrich V. Towards understanding interindividual differences in stressor appraisals: a systematic review. *Pers Individ Dif* 2018;135:92–100; doi:10.101 6/j.paid.2018.07.001.

28 Ivarsson A, Johnson U, Podlog L. Psychological predictors of injury occurrence: a prospective investigation of professional Swedish soccer players. *J Sport Rehabil* 2013;22:19–26.

29 Ivarsson A, Johnson U, Lindwall M, et al. Psychosocial stress as a predictor of injury in elite junior soccer: a latent growth curve analysis. *J Sci Med Sport* 2014;17:366–370; doi:10.1016/j.jsams.2013.10.242.

30 Devantier C. Psychological predictors of injury among professional soccer players. *Sport Sci Rev* 2011;20:5–36.

31 Bramwell ST, Masuda M, Wagner NH, et al. Psychological factors in athletic injuries: development and application of the Social and Athletic Readjustment Rating Scale (SARRS). *J Human Stress* 1975;1:6–20; doi:10.1080/0097840X.1975.9940404.

32 Petrie TA. Coping skills, competitive trait anxiety, and playing status: Moderating effects of the life stress-injury relationship. *J Sport Exerc Psychol* 1993;15:261–274; doi:1 0.1123/jsep.15.3.261.

33 Wadey R, Evans L, Hanton S, et al. Can pre-injury adversity affect post-injury responses? A 5-year prospective, multi-Study analysis. *Front Psychol* 2019;10:1411; doi:1 0.3389/fpsyg.2019.01411.

34 Hardy, CJ, Richman JM, Rosenfeld LB. The role of social support in the life stress/injury relationship. *Sport Psychol* 1991;5:128–139; doi:10.1123/tsp.5.2.128.

35 Hanson SJ, McCullagh P, Tonymon P. The relationship of personality characteristics, life stress, and coping resources to athletic injury. *J Sport Exercise Psychol* 1992;14:262–272; doi:10.1123/jsep.14.3.262.

36 Williams JM, Tonymon P, Wadsworth WA. Relationship of stress to injury in intercollegiate volleyball. *J Human Stress* 1986;12:38–43; doi:10.1080/0097840X.1986.993 6763.

37 Smith RE, Smoll EL, Ptacek JT. Conjunctive moderator variables in vulnerability and resiliency research: life stress, social support, and coping skills, and adolescent sport injuries. *J Pers Soc Psychol* 1990;58:360–369; doi:10.1037/0022-3514.58.2.360.

38 Freeman P, Rees T. How does perceived support lead to better performance? An examination of potential mechanisms. *J Appl Sport Psychol* 2009;21:429–441; doi:10.1 080/10413200903222913.

39 Freeman, P. Social support. In R. Arnold, D. Fletcher (eds.). *Stress, well-being, and performance in sport*. Abingdon, UK: Routledge 2021.

40 Tranaeus U, Ivarsson A, Johnson U. Stress and injuries in elite sport. In: R Fuchs, M Gerber. *Handbuch stressregulation und sport*. London, UK: Springer 2018.

41 Kaiseler M, Polman RCJ, Nicholls AR. Effects of the Big Five personality dimensions on appraisal coping, and coping effectiveness in sport. *Eur J Sport Sci* 2012;12:62–72; doi:10.1080/17461391.2010.551410.

42 Ponnusamy V, Lines RLJ, Zhang C, et al. Latent profiles of elite Malaysian athletes' use of psychological skills and techniques and relations with mental toughness. *PeerJ* 2018;6:4778; doi:10.7717/peerj.4778.

43 Clement D, Ivarsson A, Tranaeus U, et al. Investigating the influence of intraindividual changes in perceived stress symptoms on injury risk in soccer. *Scand J Med Sci Sports* 2018;28:1461–1466; doi:10.1111/sms.13048.

44 Rogers TJ, Landers DM. Mediating effects of peripheral vision in the life event stress/athletic injury relationship. *J Sport Exerc Psychol* 2005;27:271–288; doi:10.1123/jsep.2 7.3.271.

45 Vine SJ, Moore LJ, Wilson MR. An integrative framework of stress, attention, and visuomotor performance. *Front Psychol* 2016;7:1–10; doi:10.3389/fpsyg.2016.01671.

46 Moore LJ, Vine SJ, Wilson MR. Stress, attention, and visuomotor performance. In: R Arnold, D Fletcher (eds.). *Stress, well-being, and performance in sport.* Abingdon, UK: Routledge 2021.

47 Vine SJ, Uiga L, Lavric A, et al. Individual reactions to stress predict performance during a critical aviation incident. *Anxiety, Stress, & Coping* 2015;28:467–477; doi:10.1080/1 0615806.2014.986722.

48 Vine SJ, Freeman P, Moore LJ, et al. Evaluating stress as a challenge is associated with superior attentional control and motor skill performance: testing the predictions of the biopsychosocial model of challenge and threat. *J Exp Psychol* 2013;19:185–194; doi:10.1 037/a0034106.

49 Vickers JN. Origins and current issues in quiet eye research. *Curr Iss Sports Sci* 2016;1:101; doi:10.15203/CISS_2016.101.

50 Moore LJ, Freeman P, Hase A, et al. How consistent are challenge and threat evaluations? A generalizability analysis. *Front Psychol* 2019; doi:10.3389/fpsyg.2019.01778.

51 Williams SE, Cumming J, Balanos GM. The use of imagery to manipulate challenge and threat appraisals in athletes. *J Sport Exerc Psychol* 2010;32:339–358.

52 Singh H, Conroy DE. Systematic review of stress-related injury vulnerability in athletic and occupational contexts. *Psychol Sport Exerc* 2012;33:37–44; doi:10.1016/j.psychsport.2 017.08.001.

53 Bergeron MF, Mountjoy M, Armstrong N, et al. International Olympic Committee consensus statement on youth athletic development. *Br J Sports Med* 2015;49:843–851; doi: 10.1136/bjsports-2015-094962.

54 Forsdyke D. Are you a buffer or an amplifier? The role of social support in the effective return to sport following injury. In: A Gledhill, D Forsdyke D. (eds.). *The psychology of sports injury: from risk to retirement.* Abingdon, UK: Routledge 2021.

55 Bonnar D, Bartel K, Kakoschke N, et al. Sleep interventions designed to improve athletic performance and recovery: a systematic review of current approaches. *Sports Med* 2018;48:683–703; doi:10.1007/s40279-017-0832-x.

56 Gledhill A, Forsdyke D, Murray E. Psychological interventions used to reduce sports injuries: a systematic review of real-world effectiveness. *Br J Sports Med* 2018;52:967–971; doi: 10.1136/bjsports-2017-097694.

57 Johnson U, Ekengren J, Andersen MB. Injury prevention in Sweden: helping soccer players at risk. *J Sport Exerc Psychol* 2005;27:32–38; doi:10.1123/jsep.27.1.32.

58 Kerr G, Goss J. The effects of a stress management program on injuries and stress levels. *J Appl Sport Psychol* 1996;8:109–117; doi:10.1080/10413209608406312.

59 Ivarsson A, Johnson U, Andersen MB, et al. It pays to pay attention: a mindfulness-based program for injury prevention with soccer players. *J Appl Sport Psychol* 2015;27:319–334; doi:10.1080/10413200.2015.1008072.

60 Kolt GS, Hume PA, Smith P, et al. Effects of a stress-management program on injury and stress of competitive gymnasts. *Percept Mot Skills* 2004;99:195–207; doi:10.2466/pms.99.1.195-207.

61 Edvardsson A, Ivarsson A, Johnson U. Is a cognitive-behavioural biofeedback intervention useful to reduce injury risk in junior football players? *J Sports Sci Med* 2012;11:331–338.

62 Tranaeus U, Johnson U, Engström B, et al. A psychological injury prevention group intervention in Swedish floorball. *Knee Surg Sports Traumatol Arthrosc* 2015;23:3414–3420; doi:10.1007/s00167-014-3133-z.

63 Maddison R, Prapavessis H. A psychological approach to the prediction and prevention of athletic injury. *J Sport Exerc Psychol* 2005;27:289–310; doi:10.1123/jsep.27.3.289.

64 Hase A, Hood J, Moore LJ, et al. The influence of self-talk on challenge and threat states and performance. *Psychol Sport Exerc* 2019;45:101550; doi:10.1016/j.psychsport.2019.101550.

65 Sammy N, Anstiss PA, Moore LJ, et al. The effects of arousal reappraisal on stress responses, performance, and attention. *Anx Stress Coping Int J* 2017;30:619–662; doi:10.1080/10615806.2017.1330952.

66 Turner MJ, Jones MV, Sheffield D, et al. Manipulating cardiovascular indices of challenge and threat using resource appraisals. *Int J Psychophysiol* 2014;94:9–18; doi:10.1016/j.ijpsycho.2014.07.004.

67 Williams SE, Van Zanten JJCS, Trotman GP, et al. Challenge and threat imagery manipulates heart rate and anxiety responses to stress. *Int J Psychophysiol* 2017;117:111–118; doi:10.1016/j.ijpsycho.2017.04.011.

68 Kent S, Devonport TJ, Lane AM, et al. Implementing a pressure training program to improve decision-making and execution of skill among premier league academy soccer players. *J Appl Sport Psychol* 2021; doi:10.1080/10413200.2020.1868618.

69 Stoker M, Lindsay P, Butt J, et al. Elite coaches' experiences of creating pressure training environments for performance enhancement. *Int J Sport Psychol* 2016;47:262–281.

70 Van Rens FECA, Burgin M, Morris-Binelli K. Implementing a pressure inurement training program to optimize cognitive appraisal, emotion regulation, and sport self-confidence in a women's state cricket team. *J Appl Sport Psychol* 2020; doi:10.1080/10413200.2019.1706664.

71 Vine SJ, Moore LJ, Wilson MR. Quiet eye training: the acquisition, refinement and resilient performance of targeting skills. *Eur J Sport Sci* 2014;14:S235–S242; doi:10.1080/17461391.2012.683815.

72 Spiker AM, Dixit S, Cosgarea AJ. Triathlon: running injuries. *Sports Med Arthrosc Rev* 2012;20:206–213; doi: 10.1097/JSA.0b013e31825ca79f.

73 Tranaeus U, Johnson U, Engstrom B, et al. Psychological antecedents of overuse injuries in Swedish elite floorball players. *Athletic Insight* 2014;6:155–172.

74 Van Der Sluis A, Brink MS, Pluim B, et al. Is risk-taking in talented junior tennis players related to overuse injuries? *Scand J Med Sci Sports* 2017;27:1347–1355; doi:10.1111/sms.12729.

75 Martin S, Johnson U, McCall A, et al. Psychological risk profile for overuse injuries in sport: an exploratory study. *J Sports Sci* 2021; doi:10.1080/02640414.2021.1907904.

76 Toohey LA, Drew MK, Cook JL, et al. Is subsequent lower limb injury associated with previous injury? A systematic review and meta-analysis. *Br J Sports Med* 2017;51:1670–1678; doi: 10.1136/bjsports-2017-097500.

77 Podlog L, Dimmock J, Miller J. A review of return to sport concerns following injury rehabilitation: practitioner strategies for enhancing recovery outcomes. *Phys Ther Sport* 2011;12:36–42; doi:10.1016/j.ptsp.2010.07.005.

78 Christakou A, Stavrou NA, Psychountaki M, et al. Re-injury worry, confidence and attention as predictors of a sport re-injury during a competitive season. *Research in Sports Medicine* 2020;1–11; doi:10.1080/15438627.2020.1853542.

79 Hsu CJ, Meierbachtol A, George SZ, et al. Fear of reinjury in athletes: implications for rehabilitation. *Sports Health* 2017;9:162–167; doi:10.1177/1941738116666813.

80 Juster RP, McEwen BS, Lupien SJ. Allostatic load biomarkers of chronic stress and impact on health and cognition. *Neurosci Biobehav Rev* 2010;35:2–16; doi:10.1016/j.neubiorev.2009.10.002.

81 Raedeke TD, Smith AL. Development and preliminary validation of an athlete burnout measure. *J Sport Exerc Psychol* 2001;23:281–306; doi:10.1123/jsep.23.4.281.

82 Madigan DJ, Gustafsson H, Smith A, et al. The BASES expert statement on burnout in sport. *The Sport and Exercise Scientist* 2019;61:6–7.

83 Isoard-Gautheur S, Guillet-Descas E, Gustafsson H. Athlete burnout and the risk of dropout among young elite handball players. *Sport Psychol* 2016;30:123–130; doi:10.1123/tsp.2014-0140.

84 Li C, Ivarsson A, Lam LT, et al. Basic psychological needs satisfaction and frustration, stress, and sports injury among university athletes: a four-wave prospective survey. *Front Psychol* 2019;10:665; doi: 10.3389/fpsyg.2019.00665.

85 Pensgaard AM, Ivarsson A, Nilstad A, et al. Psychosocial stress factors, including the relationship with the coach, and their influence on acute and overuse injury risk in elite female football players. *BMJ Open Sport Exerc Med* 2018;4; doi:10.1136/bmjsem-2017-000317.

86 Thelwell RC, Wagstaff CRD, Rayner A, et al. Exploring athletes' perceptions of coach stress in elite sport environments. *J Sports Sci* 2017;35:44–55; doi:10.1080/02640414.2016.1154979.

87 Engert V, Linz R, Grant JA. Embodied stress: the physiological resonance of psycho-social stress. *Psychoneuroendocrinology* 2019;105:138–146; doi:10.1016/j.psyneuen.2018.12.221.

88 Leprince C, D'Arripe-Longueville F, Doron J. Coping in teams: exploring athletes' communal coping strategies to deal with shared stressors. *Front Psychol* 2018;9:1908; doi:10.3389/fpsyg.2018.01908.

89 Mendes WB, Park J. Neurobiological concomitants of motivational states. *Advances in Motivational Science* 2014;1:233–270; doi:10.1016/bs.adms.2014.09.001.

90 Van den Bos R, Harteveld M, Stoop H. Stress and decision-making in humans: performance is related to cortisol reactivity, albeit differently in men and women. *Psychoneuroendocrinology* 2009;34:1449–1458; doi.10.1016/j.psyneuen.2009.04.016.

5

STRESS, COPING, AND THE MISSING LINK IN TRAINING LOAD: CAMEL, MEET STRAW

Carly McKay and Stephen West

Let's do a little experiment. Think back to a time in your life when there was *a lot* going on. Pick the busiest time you can remember and try to list all of the pressures that were sitting on your shoulders (e.g., competing deadlines, family/social responsibilities, work tasks, major events, a never-ending to do list …) Odds are, your list will include a combination of things from different parts of your life that all seemed to be happening at the same time. Now, what word would you use to describe your experience at that moment? Does "overloaded" capture it?

Interestingly, the term "load" and its derivatives (workload, training load, etc.) have become increasingly common in sports science and medicine. In the modern world of data-driven athlete monitoring, they've become synonymous with some kind of aggregate measure of what athletes are exposed to in training and competition (e.g., training frequency, intensity and duration, and competition minutes). But, unlike the way we use these terms in everyday conversation, in sport, they have both positive and negative connotations. For instance, training load has specifically been described as *"the input variable in a training system that coaches and scientists most commonly manipulate to elicit the desired training response."*[1] So, in the context of physical loads, this amounts to *"the cumulative amount of stress placed on an individual from multiple training sessions and games over a period of time."*[2] Importantly, though, training load incorporates aspects of both the physical work undertaken by the athlete (*external load*) as well as their physiological and psychological responses to that work (*internal load*).[3] So, in simple terms, "load" really refers to all of the stressors and demands applied to athletes,[4] plus how they react to them.

External loads are the easiest to conceptualize because they're specific to the sporting discipline and include resistance, power output, distance, and speed. Internal loads, on the other hand, are specific to the athlete themselves (e.g., heart rate, lactate) and can be highly variable in different situations. To use an analogy, the system is like a car: while the brakes, suspension, wheels and frame endure the

DOI: 10.4324/9781003088936-5

external load (accelerations, distance, decelerations), the car also demonstrates an internal response to that load (fuel consumption), which fluctuates depending on the road and weather conditions. If we want to understand how well the car is performing, we need to capture both aspects, and it's the same for athletes. Here, it's important to recognize that when applying the same external load across multiple athletes, their internal loads can be substantially different, kind of like driving a pickup truck versus a scooter up the same hill. Internal load is therefore often regarded as the more important metric as it better represents the functional outcome of training at an individual level.[5]

Of course, when an athlete (or a car, for that matter) can't withstand the demands of the situation, they break down. So, there's a logical link between physical load and injury risk: when you apply a load that exceeds the load-bearing capacity of a structure, that structure will fail.[6] We might therefore expect a direct causal link between training load and injury, but that's not what the evidence is telling us. Despite substantial resource allocated to investigating this relationship, results have been widely contrasting and inconsistent.[7] Exposure to matches has shown clear associations with injury incidence, with match congestion,[8,9] turnaround time between matches,[10] and overall exposure to match play[11] all implicated as risk factors. Conversely, research into the relative contributions of acute and chronic training loads to injury risk has yielded highly variable results depending on which calculations are used, suggesting that the strength of the relationship reflects a statistical artefact rather than a causal association.[12,13] We know that injury is multifactorial in nature (see Chapter 3), and training load is likely just one of many variables in the causal web. Figuring out how it interacts with other intrinsic and extrinsic factors is the next step in sorting out exactly how it fits into the puzzle; however, as research on the topic is booming, there's a danger of putting the cart before the horse. Before we can hope to understand why some athletes respond well to certain training loads whilst others end up at greater risk of injury, we need to be very clear about exactly what we're measuring when we try to capture load variables.

Measuring What We Can't See

Quantifying external load can be a fairly straightforward exercise – we can measure distance traveled, speed, or weight lifted without too much difficulty. Internal loads are a little trickier. Some methods involve objective measurements taken at the time of loading exposure using tools that are relatively easy to come by (e.g., heart rate or lactate monitors). These have the advantage of being accessible and interpretable by amateur and elite athletes alike, but they only provide part of the story. Sure, they'll tell you how the athlete is responding physiologically to their training, but they can't tell you why they're having that response. For example, a runner might see decreased heart rate variability (HRV) as an indicator of fatigue,[14–16] but studies have also shown decreased HRV in response to heightened excitement or anxiety (e.g., pre-race jitters).[16,17] Understanding the relative contribution of physiological adaptations and cognitive or emotional states is complex and relying on a single objective metric to capture internal load can oversimplify things.

With that in mind, many researchers and practitioners favor the session Rating of Perceived Exertion (sRPE) method,[4,5,18] which represents a proxy measure for internal load that's collected after a training session. It determines how difficult the athlete *perceived* the external load to be (hence the name). This means that it accounts for the athlete's cognitive appraisal of the situational demands, their emotional/coping response to those demands, and their interpretation of physiological indicators of stress (e.g., heart rate as a product of fitness/fatigue + sympathetic nervous system input). Altogether, this yields a more comprehensive picture of internal load, particularly when used alongside other objective measures. The method is easy to apply, too. After the session, the athlete is asked to rate its intensity on a 10-point scale ranging from 0 ("rest") to 10 ("maximal"). This number is multiplied by how many minutes were in the session to produce a single load score.[19] The use of differential RPE has also been suggested to distinguish between the perceptual demands of different activities within a single session.[20,21] These scores are collected in the same manner and represent sRPE-B (breathlessness), sRPE-L (leg muscle exertion), sRPE-U (upper body exertion), sRPE-T (cognitive technical demands). This approach gives athletes and practitioners a more nuanced appreciation for the loads associated with specific components of their sport.

The sRPE measure is widely used for several reasons, including its applicability to multiple session types. It's been found reliable in steady-state aerobic training,[22] intermittent aerobic training,[22] and strength training.[23,24] Furthermore, it's comparable with other commonly used internal load metrics including heart rate (r=0.89),[25] and lactate (r=0.86).[25] A recent review of sRPE even demonstrated its validity and reliability in a wide range of team and individual sports.[26] All in all, not bad. But, as with any measure, sRPE has its limitations. Age, fitness, environmental factors, and even personality traits have been shown to affect scores.[26] As it turns out, extroverts tend to overestimate work intensity and people high in neuroticism or with anxiety or depression tend to underestimate intensity.[27] Listening to music or watching videos can also decrease perceived exertion, and the presence of coaches or other athletes can prompt socially desirable responses (i.e., under-rating intensity to make oneself appear fitter).[26,28] Therefore, whilst sRPE can be a valuable tool for determining how much internal load an athlete is experiencing, it can be challenging to disentangle the load construct from the factors that affect it.

The Other Side of the Equation

So far, we've talked mostly about training load in terms of the physical work athletes need to do to prepare for competition, and that's how it's been viewed in most of the research literature. But it's also evident that perceptions of load can be shaped by the context in which they're being measured, and this has significant implications for understanding injury risk. This is especially true when we consider that the features of that context may themselves be a load upon the athlete. As outlined in a review of player management in professional rugby union, Quarrie and colleagues noted that load cannot be viewed as a single stressor; it's a composite of a number of constituent factors in and outside of sport that add up on a daily basis (Figure 5.1).[4]

This was echoed in a 2016 International Olympic Committee consensus statement on load management in sport, where load was defined as *"the sport and non-sport burden (single or multiple physiological, psychological or mechanical stressors)."*[29] In other words, psychological stressors outside of sport are part of the "life load" that impacts an athlete's responses to training and consequent injury risk. Wait a second, we've heard some of this before.

It's easy to think about athletes as existing within the confines of their sport, and we sometimes forget that they're faced with the same major life events and daily hassles as everyone else. In the last chapter we established that life event stress is the most well evidenced and consistently reported psychosocial risk factor for injury, particularly for those with low coping resources.[29,30] Well, a sure-fire way to deplete someone's coping resources is to keep piling on the demands. When stressors begin to accumulate or a number of life events occur in close proximity to one another, chronic or acute life loads can affect an athlete's physical health (fatigue and feelings of insufficient rest, muscle tension and vulnerability are common).[29] They may also perceive their ordinary training demands as more challenging (i.e., providing higher sRPE scores). When an athlete who is already managing a number of personal stressors is exposed to additional loads in their professional sphere, this can quickly exceed their physical and psychological capacity, leading to performance impairments and/or injuries.

The possible mechanisms by which psychological stressors may lead to injury risk have been well outlined in the Stress-Injury Model proposed by Andersen and Williams[30] and in subsequent work. These include increased muscle tension, narrowing of the visual field, increased distractibility, fatigue and reduced timing/co-ordination.[29] Our trusty car analogy is getting pretty strained at this point, but we can imagine that the vehicle drives along just fine on a smooth road. When potholes appear, it has to swerve. If the potholes are spaced apart, the car can steer around them but when a big one appears, or a lot of small ones in quick succession, the car must slow down or risk a crash. If the driver is tired or distracted – or simply doesn't see them coming – the chances of hitting one increases. Similarly, when athletes hit bumps in their road, they sometimes experience short-term speed wobbles (e.g., lapses in concentration or performance). When these stretch out over time or a major stressor pops up, an adverse outcome is more likely to occur.

Injury is often the primary worry when athletes find themselves overwhelmed by a combination of life and sport loads, but another significant concern is *burnout*. This is a multidimensional cognitive-affective syndrome characterized by a

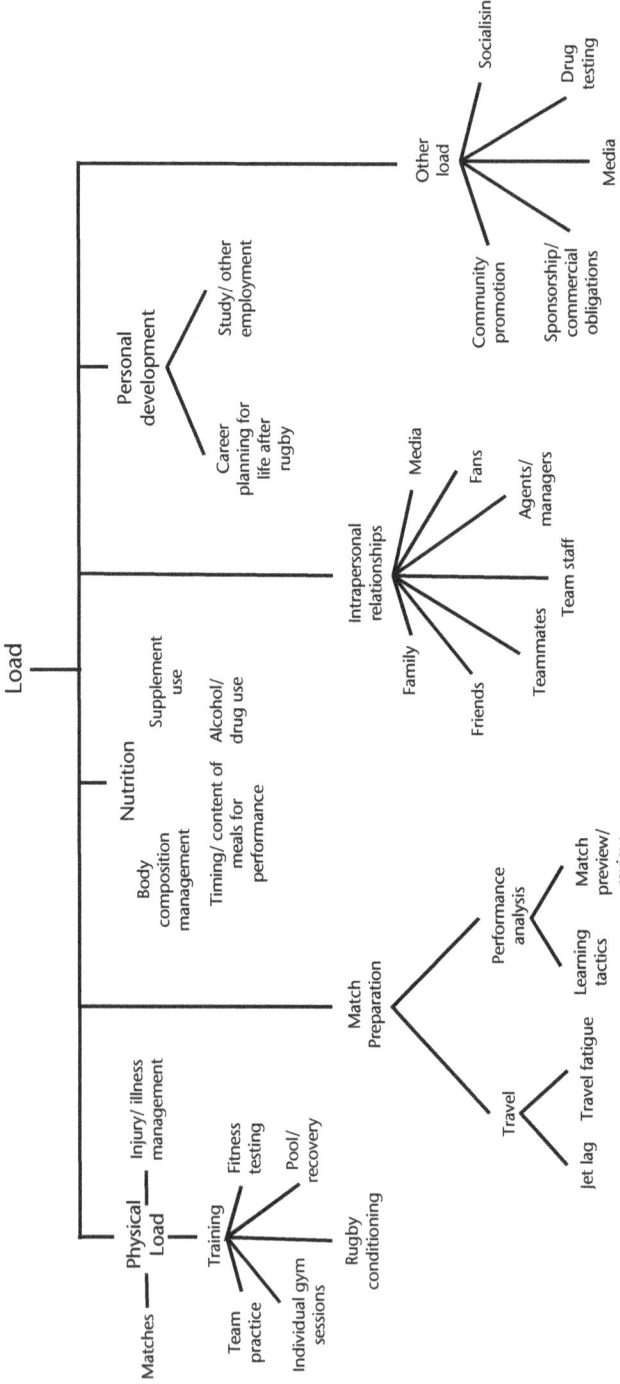

FIGURE 5.1 Loads to which professional rugby players are subjected. [4]

reduced sense of accomplishment, sport devaluation and, crucially, emotional and physical exhaustion. Athletes experiencing burnout often perceive a depletion of their personal (emotional and physical) resources, brought on by training and competing under conditions of chronic stress.[31,32] Studies have shown that this can lead to performance decrements, depression, and decreased self-regulation,[32] and the risk of burnout seems to be higher for those with strong athletic identity, performance-based self-esteem, and perfectionistic concerns (e.g., self-criticism, high personal standards).[32] If we think about this with respect to the load-injury relationship, there's a pathway by which high training and life loads can directly contribute to injury risk while also pushing the athlete toward a burnt-out state. This in turn may exacerbate feelings of fatigue and limited coping resource, causing a vicious spiral toward elevated sRPE, injury, and impaired quality of life. Curiously, research into the association between burnout and injury is sparse, despite obvious implications for athlete health and wellbeing. While we wait for evidence in this area to build, athletes and practitioners need to consider how best to monitor life loads to prevent such negative consequences.

Contemporary Approaches to Athlete Monitoring

From a practical point of view, it makes sense to collect life load data alongside physical load metrics when working with athletes, and to monitor how things change day-to-day and over the longer term. This can identify sudden changes or trends indicative of injury and/or burnout risk. Of course, assessing life stress isn't new from a sport psychology point of view, but in the modern era of professional sport where athletes are under greater scrutiny than ever, this approach is being heralded as the new kid on the block for maximizing performance. Simultaneously, the technological boom in athlete monitoring has driven the desire to capture more elements of the dose-response effects of training and matches. Consequently, in-creasing demand for the measurement of psychological/life load has triggered an increase in the use of a wide variety of tools for this purpose.

Although measures of psychological stressors have been developed mostly in the context of the general population, several existing instruments have been adapted for use in sport (Table 5.1).[33] Subjective measures have been found to be more responsive to changes in training load than objective measures, meaning that self-reported mood, stress and recovery are deemed useful by many sport practi-tioners for tailoring load management strategies for individual athletes.[34] One of the most commonly used tools in this context is the Profile of Mood States (POMS) which was developed to assess the constructs of global mood as well as tension, depression, anger, fatigue, and confusion.[35] Since the original POMS was introduced, numerous iterations have emerged to be shorter in length or directed at a target population (e.g., youth) and these have been applied in a variety of sports. Indeed, a meta-analysis of 25 articles (n=1497) found that POMS and its versions have been used in sport performance research since 1975, providing valid and reliable performance predictions across a number of competitive

TABLE 5.1 Psychological load monitoring tools that have been used in sport[33]

Measure	Primary Dimension	General or Sport Specific
Profile of Mood States (POMS)	Mood	G
POMS-Short Form (POMS-SF)	Mood	G
POMS-Abbreviated (POMS-A)	Mood	G
POMS – Adolescents/ Brunel Mood Scale (BRUMS)	Mood	G
Brief Assessment of Mood (BAM)	Mood	G
POMS energy index	Mood	G
POMS training distress scale	Mood	G
Multicomponent Training Distress Scale (MTDS)	Mood, stress, symptoms	G,S
Daily Analysis of Life Demands for Athletes (DALDA)	Stress, symptoms	G,S
Training Distress Scale (TDS)	Symptoms	G,S
Perceived Stress Scale (PSS)	Stress	G
Recovery-Stress Questionnaire for Athletes (RESTQ-Sport)	Stress, recovery	G,S
Acute Recovery and Stress Scale (ARSS)	Stress, recovery	S
Short Recovery Stress Scale (SRSS)	Stress, recovery	S
Recovery-Cue	Stress, recovery	G,S
Perceived Recovery Status Scale (PRS)	Recovery	S
Emotional Recovery Questionnaire (EmRecQ)	Emotions	G

G: general well-being; S: sport-specific well-being.

settings.[36]There's also evidence that the questionnaire provides robust estimates in both training and competition, making it well suited to use for athlete monitoring purposes.[37] It's important to remember that mood state can be highly variable, though, influenced by factors both central and peripheral to the sport context. This makes POMS a good omnibus indicator of what the athlete is experiencing at a given moment, but it cannot distinguish the contributions of different types of load – it measures the symptoms but not their cause.[34] In that sense, it's a great way to tell when something's wrong, but it doesn't tell you what the problem is.

Other prominent athlete monitoring tools, designed to capture stress and re-covery, are the Daily Analyses of Life Demands for Athletes (DALDA) ques-tionnaire,[38] the Recovery-Stress Questionnaire for Athletes (REST-Q Sport),[39] the Acute Recovery Stress Scale (ARSS),[40] and the Short Recovery Stress Scale (SRSS).[40,41] These instruments differentiate perceived stressors from the athlete's reaction to them, and/or gauge recovery in both nonspecific and sport-specific areas, yielding more easily interpretable scores.[42,43] Research has shown that they consistently identify impaired wellbeing with acute increases in training load (and improved wellbeing with training load reductions), though again it can be difficult to figure out whether the tool is capturing the effects of physical stress or the combined effects of training and life loads. Nonetheless, when combined with mood data, which are also responsive to changes in training load,[42] these measures can help to inform training periodization and individual prescription.

So, how does all of this come together into a practical athlete monitoring plan? Well, we've seen that not only can an athlete's psychological state influence their training load, but it's also possible for the opposite to happen. So, there's clearly a need to capture training load and life load, as well as the athlete's responses to them, in a way that facilitates both performance and injury risk management. At least from a subjective measurement point of view, the typical approach is for practitioners to ask for sRPE following training sessions to get an idea of the athlete's perceptions of that specific physical stimulus. This is kind of like doing a quick check of your car's brakes and lights during a roadtrip to see if anything needs adjusting on the fly. Collecting daily wellbeing data using POMS, DALDA, or other questionnaires is often undertaken as well, akin to keeping a car maintenance record. These are typically administered through smartphone apps or online forms that athletes complete at a set time during the day. Daily score fluctuations and trends over time can be indicators of underlying problems that need to be addressed through strategic periods of rest to maintain a manageable stress balance.

That's all well and good, but before becoming entirely reliant on tools and technology to assess how athletes are dealing with the various loads placed upon them, it's important for practitioners (and athletes themselves) to take a step back. You can actually get a pretty good sense of someone's psychological state by simply having a conversation with them. In many cases, practitioners rely on personal communication and building relationships with athletes to identify when things are "not normal." Vital to this approach is having an open dialogue that empowers athletes to discuss what's going on in their lives in and outside of sport. That requires significant trust from everyone involved but, in the modern world of sport where everything needs to be quantified, often a chat over a coffee will tell you more about an athlete's wellbeing than any number of questionnaires. Remember, athletes are people, not robots (or cars, for that matter).

The Irony of Load Monitoring

Naturally, having just made a plea for human interaction, we expect that everyone's going to keep collecting load metrics anyway. Such is life. Since the advent of the first heart rate monitors, the quantification of "load" has grown exponentially. Though this is generally regarded as a positive change in how athletes are managed, it's also led to a huge amount of money and resource being poured into capturing, analysing, interpreting, and communicating data. For example, in professional sport it's common to record load data several times every day, including both objective and subjective measures (e.g., GPS, performance metrics, questionnaires, etc). While this not only places a burden on athletes, staff have to deal with a constant stream of information that needs to be processed nearly in real-time.[i] While data collection is almost always undertaken with the best interests of the athlete in mind, it's also got some downsides. The load of load monitoring itself is one of them.

Moreover, the number of available monitoring tools has grown significantly in recent years, resulting in a kind of technological arms race where everyone's trying to use the newest metric or most precise equipment. Not only does this generate more data than is reasonable to sift through, let alone synthesize and understand, it raises the question of validity. A tool's performance (psychometrics) needs to be evaluated for the specific environment in which it's being applied, and this step is often missed out when teams are trying to keep up with the Joneses. Add in the challenges of "monitoring fatigue", where athletes may rush or falsify their responses due to frustration, ambivalence, or concerns about how the data will be used, and suddenly "evidence-informed" decisions about load management are anything but. Given all this, some tools may need to be used more infrequently. For example, Coutts and Cormack[42] recommend psychological inventories be used only on a weekly or monthly basis, with more frequent assessment during times when psychological load may be particularly high (e.g., during a playoff run). This obviously limits the ability to detect some acute responses to changes in load, but the trade-off may be worth it.

In fast moving practical environments, there's a serious risk of collecting data for the sake of collecting data. It's imperative that practitioners have a means of analysing and interpreting it in a timely and meaningful way to inform player welfare strategies; otherwise, we can capture as many metrics as we want, it still won't help us prevent injuries or burnout. In the past decade, extensive research has been undertaken to develop and validate complex statistical methodologies for informing decision making using load data.[44,45] These often require specialist understanding and a fair bit of technical know-how, meaning that they're impractical in all but the most well-resourced settings. Simpler systems can be used on a daily basis by the rest of us, for instance by flagging athletes for follow-up if their responses are out of character or demonstrate a downward trend. Over time, being able to recognize patterns in an athlete's responses to particular stressors will enable more proactive strategies to support them through challenging situations. That's the next big step, though. How do we help athletes manage their various loads in a healthy and adaptive way?

Training for Stress

It's well established that to achieve adaptation in a system, an element of overload is required, followed by adequate recovery time before a successive stimulus is applied.[46] In terms of physical loads, we know that we need to push people toward their limits if they want to get stronger or faster. But, to allow adaptation to occur and to avoid overtraining/injury, they need some downtime as well. In the past decade, the training load-injury relationship has become one of the hottest topics in sport because load is seen as a modifiable risk factor − we can optimize the balance between training and recovery to promote efficient progression whilst protecting the athlete. This gets a little more challenging when we consider life loads, though. Some things just aren't in anyone's control (e.g., daily hassles are unavoidable). Athletes typically don't get the luxury of recovery time between major life events and, as these pile up, adding a physical training stimulus might just be the straw that breaks the camel's back.

Sport psychologists have had this issue on their radar for some time, but the emergence and increasing interest in life load in the athlete monitoring sphere represents an exciting new opportunity to consider how the stress-injury relationship plays out in an applied context. First off, it's worth remembering that the life loads that impact an athlete are mostly unique to that individual, though there are some common features of the sport environment that will affect everyone. As outlined in Figure 5.1, professional athletes have a particular set of loads that are a product of participating at that level. Interestingly, in the context of amateur sport, some of these stressors exist in the same way. For example, interpersonal relationships and traveling to matches are still salient factors, regardless of one's competitive level. In a similar way, sports participation for youth athletes comes with certain psychological stressors. In instances where a young athlete is particularly talented, they may be part of school, club, provincial and national teams, sometimes in multiple sports. Performance expectations, not wanting to let people down, and being pulled in different directions by their coaches creates a highly demanding atmosphere.[46] Well, these issues can plague professionals and adult amateurs, too. No matter the sport setting or level, some stressors just come with the territory. There are some common non-sport stressors to look out for too, such as competing demands (e.g., work or school), poor sleep quality (for any number of reasons), and family/social pressures. Although it's difficult to plan for major life events that occur less regularly, such as bereavements or pandemics[ii], we can bank on some of these other things cropping up from time to time.

The main issue for athletes and practitioners is figuring out how to stop these accumulated life loads from exceeding personal coping resources. The obvious approach would be to adjust training load and other modifiable features of the sport environment to compensate (e.g., losing some cargo to keep the car traveling at speed), though this isn't the only solution. It isn't always possible for athletes to take time off or to ease up on their physical preparation, so helping them to build capacity for load can provide some buffer. Alongside classic stress-management interventions for this purpose (imagery, goal setting, attribution training, self-talk, etc.), more exotic approaches like *stress inoculation training (SIT)* have also been trialled. SIT is often used in clinical psychology to expose people to milder forms of stress in order to arouse their defensive mechanisms (e.g., coping processes) without overwhelming them. Much like a vaccine, this is thought to improve coping responses and raise the person's confidence in using them, bolstering their preparedness for when serious stressors appear.[47] As a tailored form of cognitive-behavioral therapy, this rests on the idea that not all stressors are the same. Some are *acute time-limited stressors* (e.g., preparing for a particular event), some are *chronic intermittent stressors* (e.g., repeated evaluations or tasks), others are *chronic continual stressors* (e.g., ongoing physical or situational conditions), and sometimes they're a *sequence of stressful events* (e.g., changes that happen after a significant life event).[47] SIT focuses on enabling individuals to identify and apply appropriate coping strategies for the specific combination of stressor types present in their own lives.

Does it work? Maybe. Evidence from medical and psychiatric populations shows that SIT is moderately successful in improving stress responses and behavioral adjustment,[47] so this led to a lot of interest from the sport community in the 1980s and 1990s. When applied to performance, it appeared to improve athletes' anxiety management[48] and a handful of studies indicated that it could help injured athletes manage post-surgical pain.[49] A single study explored a SIT-inspired stress management program with 24 elite gymnasts and over an eight-month intervention period they reported clinically meaningful reductions in stress and injury compared to a control group.[50] Despite this initial promise, however, research dropped off. Yet, with the rise of load monitoring practices, we might be primed for a resurgence. We're now able to assess how athletes are responding to stress on a regular basis and can identify thresholds in their capacity based on performance and wellbeing data. Manipulating acute and chronic loads to introduce some progressive overload, with periods of respite built in, may be a means of capitalizing on the 'inoculation' concept. In other words, it might be possible to use monitoring data to tailor a SIT intervention based on the athlete's unique stress profile and demonstrated coping reserve. Naturally, this would need to be done by a qualified psychologist – we can't go micro-dosing athletes with stress (or anything else) without relevant expertise – but it's an interesting application that could be explored in future research.

That's a big blue-sky idea, though, and it doesn't help anyone working in the field right now. Immediately useful techniques for stress/load management include problem-focused coping (addressing the stressors and not just the symptoms) and promoting social support. Research has found a low-moderate inverse relationship between social support and burnout, and we know that social support can modify the stress-injury relationship, so fostering positive peer interactions, supportive coaching climates, and diffuse social networking outside of sport can all be beneficial.[51] Proceed cautiously, though – the relationship between athletes and their friends, families and teammates can have both positive and negative consequences. When they're functioning well, these relationships blunt the deleterious effects of stress, but they can also be a source of conflict or distraction. Therefore, relying on social support as an athlete's primary resource is tenuous and developing other psychological stress-management skills is strongly advised.

It's also important to consider the reasons why people engage in sport in the first place. For amateurs, it may be a means of reducing life stress, a cathartic opportunity to burn off emotional tension, gain relief from work commitments, and have a social outlet. Conversely, at the professional level, sport may in fact be a source of considerable stress. At the end of the day, the goal of load monitoring (and subsequent intervention) should be to keep athletes operating in a state of demand-resource balance, a 'sweet spot' where they're able to perform well and enjoy participating. It's easy to lose sight of this as quantification becomes all-consuming and there's a risk of trying to reduce absolute load without considering that it's actually a relative construct. It wouldn't do any good to reduce training load if sport itself is someone's coping strategy, would it?

Answering Loaded Questions[iii]

The concept of life event stress is not a new one, but under the shiny banner of "life load" there's now more widespread acknowledgement of its importance for both performance and injury. And, in an age where data-based metrics are held in such high regard, advancing technology means we now have more ability than ever to assess its effects and truly explore the complex interactions between stressors, coping strategies, and the physical demands of sport. Understanding athletes' internal responses to combinations of physical and life loads may be the key to unlocking the potential of athlete monitoring as a whole and presents interesting avenues for psychological approaches to injury prevention. This is likely to be a vital area for research and practice in the years to come, with plenty of unanswered questions yet to be addressed.

Notes

i Staff burnout is a real danger, too. Just ask any sport performance intern or PhD student.
ii We wrote this chapter in 2020 at the height of the COVID-19 pandemic, so it seemed a topical example. Here's hoping it ages well.
iii Forgive us, we couldn't resist the pun.

References

1 Coutts AJ, Crowcroft S, Kempton T. Developing athlete monitoring systems: theoretical basis and practical applications. In: M Kellmann, J Beckmann. (eds.). *Sport, recovery and performance: interdisciplinary insights*. Abingdon: Routledge 2018.
2 Gabbett TJ, Whyte DG, Hartwig TB, et al. (2014). The relationship between workloads, physical performance, injury and illness in adolescent male football players. *Sports Med* 2014;44:989–1003; doi: 10.1007/s40279-014-0179-5.
3 Halson SL. (2014). Monitoring training load to understand fatigue in athletes. *Sports Med* 2014;44(2):139–147; doi: 10.1007/s40279-014-0253-z.
4 Quarrie KL, Raftery M, Blackie J, et al. Managing player load in professional rugby union: a review of current knowledge and practices. *Br J Sports Med* 2017;51:421–427; doi: 10.1136/bjsports-2016-096191.
5 Impellizzeri FM, Marcora SM, Coutts AJ. *Int J Sports Physiol Perform* 2019;14:270–273; doi: 10.1123/ijspp.2018-0935.
6 Kalkhoven JT, Watsford ML, Impellizzeri FM. A conceptual model and detailed framework for stress-related, strain related, and overuse athletic injury. *J Sci Med Sport* 2020;23:726–734; doi: 10.1016/j.jsams.2020.02.002.

7 Eckard TG, Padua DA, Hearn D, et al. The relationship between training load and injury in athletes: a systematic review. *Sports Med* 2018;48:1929–1961; doi: 10.1007/s4 0279-018-0951-z.

8 Dupont G, Nedelec M, McCall A, et al. Effect of 2 soccer matches in a week on physical performance and injury rate. *Am J Sports Med* 2010;38:1752–1758; doi: 10.11 77/0363546510361236.

9 Dellal A, Lago-Penas C, Rey E, et al. The effects of a congested fixture period on physical performance, technical activity and injury rate during matches in a professional soccer team. *Br J Sports Med* 2015;49:390–394; doi:

10 Murray NB, Gabbett TJ, Chamari K. Effect of different between-match recovery times on the activity profiles and injury rates of national rugby league players. *J Strength Cond Res* 2014;28:3476–3483; doi: 10.1519/JSC.0000000000000603.

11 Williams S, Trewartha G, Kemp SPT, et al. How much rugby is too much? A seven-season prospective cohort study of match exposure and injury risk in professional rugby union players. *Sports Med* 2017;47:2395–2402; doi: 10.1007/s40279-017-0721-3.

12 Dalen-Lorentsen T, Andersen TE, Bjorneboe J, et al. A cherry, ripe for picking: the relationship between the acute-chronic workload ratio and health problems. *J Orthop Sports Phys Ther* 2021;51:162–173; doi: 10.2519/jospt.2021.9893.

13 West SW, Williams S, Cazzola D, et al. Training load and injury risk in elite rugby union: the largest investigation to date. *Int J Sports Med* 2020; doi: 10.1055/a-1300-2 703.

14 Plews DJ, Laursen PB, Kilding AE, et al. Heart rate variability and training intensity distribution in elite rowers. *Int J Sports Physiol Perform* 2014;9:1026–1032; doi: 10.1123/ ijspp.2013-0497.

15 Chen JL, Yeh DP, Lee JP, et al. Parasympathetic nervous activity mirrors recovery status in weightlifting performance after training. *J Strength Cond Res* 2011;25(6):1546–1552; doi: 10.1519/JSC.0b013e3181da7858.

16 Edmonds RC, Sinclair WH, Leicht AS. The effect of weekly training and a game on heart rate variability in elite youth rugby league players. *Int J Sports Med* 2013;34:1087–1092; doi: 10.1055/s-0033-1333720.

17 Morales J, Garcia V, García-Massó X, et al. (2013). The use of heart rate variability in assessing precompetitive stress in high-standard judo athletes. *Int J Sports Med* 2013;34:144–151; doi: 10.1055/s-0032-1323719.

18 Drew MK, Finch CF. The relationship between training load and injury, illness and soreness: a systematic and literature review. *Sports Med* 2016;46:861–883; doi: 10.1007/ s40279-015-0459-8.

19 Foster C. Monitoring training in athletes with reference to overtraining syndrome. *Med Sci Sports Exerc* 1998;30:1164–1168; doi: 10.1097/00005768-199807000-00023.

20 Weston M. (2013). Difficulties in determining the dose-response nature of competitive soccer matches. *J Athl Enhanc* 2013;2:1–2.

21 McLaren SJ, Smith A, Spears IR, et al. A detailed quantification of differential ratings of perceived exertion during team-sport training. *J Sci Med Sport* 2017;20:290–295; doi: 10.1016/j.jsams.2016.06.011.

22 Foster C, Florhaug JA, Franklin J, et al. A new approach to monitoring exercise training. *J Strength Cond Res* 2001;15:109–115; PMID: 11708692.

23 Day ML, McGuigan MR, Brice G, et al. Monitoring exercise intensity during resistance training using the session RPE scale. *J Strength Cond Res* 2004;18:353–358; doi: 10.151 9/R-13113.1.

24 Comyns T, Flanagan EP. Applications of the session rating of perceived exertion system in professional rugby union. *Strength Cond J* 2013;35:78–85.

25 Gabbett TJ, Domrow N. Relationships between training load, injury, and fitness in sub-elite collision sport athletes. *J Sports Sci* 2007;25:1507–1519; doi: 10.1080/0264041 0701215066.

26 Haddad M, Stylianides G, Djaoui L, et al. Session-RPE method for training load monitoring: validity, ecological usefulness, and influencing factors. *Front Neurosci* 2017; doi: 10.3389/fnins.2017.00612.

27 Morgan WP. Psychological factors influencing perceived exertion. *Med Sci Sports* 1973;5:97–103; doi: 10.1249/00005768-197300520-00019.

28 Comyns T, Hannon A. Strength and conditioning coaches' application of the session rating of perceived exertion method of monitoring within professional rugby union. *J Hum Kinet* 2018;23:155–166; doi: 10.1515/hukin-2017-0118.

29 Soligard T, Schwellnus M, Alonso JM, et al. How much is too much? (Part 1) International Olympic Committee consensus statement on load in sport and risk of injury. *Br J Sports Med* 2016;50:1030–1041; doi: 10.1136/bjsports-2016-096581.

30 Andersen MB, Williams JM. A model of stress and athletic injury: prediction and prevention. *J Sport Exerc Psychol* 1988;10:294–306; doi: 10.1123/jsep.10.3.294.

31 Gustafsson H, DeFreese JD, Madigan DJ. Athlete burnout: review and recommendations. *Curr Opin Psychol* 2017;16:109–113; doi: 10.1016/j.copsyc.2017.05.002.

32 Crowell D, Madigan DJ. Perfectionistic concerns cognitions predict burnout in college athletes: a three-month longitudinal study. *Int J Sport Exerc Psychol* 2020; doi: 10.1080/1 612197X.2020.1869802.

33 Saw AE, Kellmann M, Main LC, Gastin PB. Athlete self-report measures in research and practice: considerations for the discerning reader and fastidious practitioner. *Int J Sports Physiol Perform.* 2017 Apr;12 (2); doi: 10.1123/ijspp.2016-0395.

34 Saw AE, Main LC, Gastin PB. Monitoring the athlete training response: subjective self-reported measures trump commonly used objective measures: a systematic review. *Br J Sports Med* 2016;50:281–291; doi: 10.1136/bjsports-2015-094758.

35 McNair DM, Lorr M, Droppleman LF. *Manual for the profile of mood states.* San Diego, CA: Educational and Industrial Testing Services 1971.

36 Lochbaum M, Zanatta T, Kirschling D, et al. The Profile of Moods States and athletic performance: a meta-analysis of published studies. *Eur J Investig Health Psychol Educ* 2021;11:50–70; doi: 10.3390/ejihpe11010005.

37 Andrade E, Rodríguez D. Factor structure of mood over time frames and circumstances of measurement: two studies on the Profile of Mood States questionnaire. *Plos One* 2018;13(10):e0205892; doi: 10.1371/journal.pone.0205892.

38 Rushall BS. *Daily analyses of life demands for athletes.* Spring Valley, CA: Sports Science Associates-Canada 1987.

39 Kellmann M, Kallus K. *Recovery-stress questionnaire for athletes: user manual.* Champaign, IL: Human Kinetics 2001.

40 Kellmann M, Kolling S, Hitzschke, B. *The acute measure and short scale of recovery and stress for sports: manual.* Koln, Germany: Sportverlag Strauß 2016.

41 Hitzschke B, Kolling S, Ferrauti A, et al. Development of the Short Recovery and Stress Scale for Sports (SSRS). *Zeitschrift fur Sportpsychologie* 2015;22:146–162; doi: 10.1026/1 612-5010/a000150.

42 Coutts AJ, Cormack S. Monitoring the training response. In: D Joyce, D Lewingdon (eds.). *High-performance training for sports.* Champaign, IL: Human Kinetics 2014.

43 Kellmann M, Bertollo M, Bosquet L, et al. Recovery and performance in sport: consensus statement. *Int J Sports Physiol Perform* 2018;13:240–245; doi: 10.1123/ijspp.2017-0759.

44 Ward P, Coutts AJ, Pruna R, et al. Putting the 'I' back in team. *Int J Sports Physiol Perform* 2018;13:1–14; doi: 10.1123/ijspp.2018-0154.

45 Windt J, Ardern CL, Gabbett TJ, et al. Getting the most out of intensive longitudinal data: a methodological review of workload-injury studies. *BMJ Open* 2018;8:e022626; doi: 10.1136/bmjopen-2018-022626.

46 Meeusen R, Duclos M, Foster C, et al. Prevention, diagnosis, and treatment of the overtraining syndrome: joint consensus statement of the European College of Sport Science and the American College of Sports Medicine. *Med Sci Sports Exerc* 2013;45:186–205; doi: 10.1249/MSS.0b013e318279a10a.

47 Meichenbaum D. Stress inoculation training. In: D Meichenbaum. *The evolution of cognitive behavior therapy: a personal and professional journey with Don Meichenbaum.* New York: Routledge 2017.

48 Saunders T, Driskell JE, Johnston JH, et al. The effect of stress inoculation training on anxiety and performance. *J Occup Health Psychol* 1996;1:170–186; doi: 10.1037/1076-8998.1.2.170.

49 Ross MJ, Berger RS. Effects of stress inoculation training on athletes' postsurgical pain and rehabilitation after orthopedic injury. *J Consult Clin Psychol* 1996;64:406–410; doi: 10.1037/0022-006X.64.2.406.

50 Kerr G, Goss J. The effects of a stress management program on injuries and stress levels. *J Appl Sport Psychol* 1996;8:109–117; doi: 10.1080/10413209608406312.

51 Freeman P. Social support. In: Arnold R, Fletcher D. *Stress, well-being, and performance in sport.* New York: Routledge 2021; doi: 10.4324/9780429295874.

6

EXPLORING THE COMPLEXITIES OF PAIN: WHY IT ISN'T "ALL IN YOUR HEAD"

Carly McKay and Abby Tabor

More Than a Feeling

"Walk it off!" "Battle through it!" "It's a long way from your heart!" If you've been involved in sport for any length of time, you've probably heard things like that, often said in an offhand way in response to someone's visible signs of agony or exhaustion. They're phrases that have gone beyond cliché and become maxims, rules to live by if you want to reach peak performance. But how often do we stop to think about what they actually mean? Athletes often recognize pain as a part of their everyday lives, with coaches, spectators, and companies glorifying it as the mark of physical superiority. But, as we learn more about what pain actually is, how it's interpreted, and what happens when it's normalized, suddenly those phrases start to lose some of their lustre. Intuition tells us that pain is a hallmark symptom of injury, part and parcel of physical pursuits, but it's so much more than just an indication that something's wrong. Instead of being a purely physical sensation that we can shrug off, it's a sophisticated and integral part of the way we experience the world, reflecting our dynamic biology, cognitive and emotional domains, even our social interactions.

Let's look at this in the context of sport. Often an inevitable consequence of pushing ourselves to the limit, pain is broadly accepted as an indicator of what condition our body is in. It's historically been synonymous with tissue damage, a sign that we've hurt ourselves and should probably stop what we're doing. Although this common sense interpretation seems logical, in what follows, we will explore why we need to look beyond injury to understand and effectively treat pain. From an evolutionary point of view, the function of pain is to change behavior.[1] It demands attention and aims to interrupt what we're doing or thinking, directing us to behave in a way that will reduce potential harm. In this sense, pain is really more about future action than the current state of our body, a mechanism that tells us to

DOI: 10.4324/9781003088936-6

protect our future selves.[2] Of course, it doesn't tell us what to do, only that we need to do something. That means we need to rely on our previous experiences, current multisensory information, and predictions about what might happen in order to make sense of the pain and act appropriately.[3–5] The main upshot of this is that our experience of pain is not a direct reflection of tissue health but is instead an amalgam of information influenced by the past, situated in the present, and directed toward the future.[2]

Integrating information from different sources makes us very efficient at interpreting what is going on in our bodies and in the world – we tend to react instinctively and make very quick judgments – but they aren't necessarily accurate. Think of visual illusions, like an image of a hollow mask rotating in the air. We see it as being convex in both directions, which clearly can't be true, and even when we're in on the secret it's tough to stop seeing it that way.[6,i] That's because what we see is influenced by our expectations, not simply the information at hand. As humans, we've evolved to deal with uncertainty, so we fill in gaps, selectively attend to certain information, and unconsciously prime relevant details.[3,8,9] It's no different for pain. In the lab, presenting people with alternating red and blue lights at the same time as prodding them with a very cold steel rod designed to induce pain through specialist nerve endings can bias the pain experience such that higher pain is reported with the red stimulus (we associate the color red with "hot" and "danger") compared to the blue one (associated with "cool" and "calm").[10] Patients also report enhanced pain when viewing visual stimuli that manipulate the size, color, shape, and tactile input to a painful body part.[11–13] More recently, the use of virtual reality has shown that our perceptual systems can be tricked. In patients with neck pain, viewing a scene through virtual reality that exaggerated how far their neck had turned caused the experience of pain to occur earlier[14,15] In other words, they felt pain when they thought they were nearing the point where their neck typically hurt, despite not having reached it yet. Work outside of pain has demonstrated how malleable our experiences are, too. For example, hearing a creaky door in association with consistent pressure applied through the lower back results in an enhanced experience of stiffness.[16] So, our experiences reflect a combination of the information we have access to, and that has implications for the way we interpret pain in sport.

What we're essentially saying is that all experience is determined by context. In this case, pain is influenced by the way biology interacts with factors in the environment, and the way we interpret it can depend on our cognitive and emotional responses as well as the social situation we find ourselves in. For example, athletes sometimes injure themselves quite seriously but don't even realize it until after the competition is over, or sometimes what seems to be an innocuous injury keeps someone from the lineup. The context in which these injuries happen (e.g., whether it's an Olympic final or a pick-up game with friends) will shape how an athlete experiences pain, the meaning they assign to it, and how they respond.

Knowing all this, "pain" becomes a little bit trickier to define: Is it a physical sensation? An interpretation of the environment? An emotion? A mental phenomenon? All of the above? In 2020, the International Association for the Study of Pain extended their existing definition,[17] which was "*an unpleasant sensory and emotional experience associated with, or resembling that associated with, actual or potential tissue damage,*" to incorporate six additional key elements:

1. Pain is always a personal experience that is influenced to varying degrees by biological, psychological, and social factors.
2. Pain and *nociception* (specialized part of the sensory system for responding to dangerous information from heat, chemicals, pressure) are different phenomena. Pain cannot be inferred solely from activity in sensory neurons.
3. Through their life experiences, individuals learn the concept of pain.
4. A person's report of an experience of pain should be respected.
5. Although pain usually serves an adaptive role, it may have adverse effects on the function and social and psychological well-being.
6. Verbal description is only one of several behaviors to express pain; inability to communicate does not negate the possibility that a human or a non-human animal experiences pain.

There's a lot to unpack there. The definition establishes that pain isn't just a bodily sensation, but an experience that is both *embodied* (defined by action, extending beyond the brain and nervous system) and *embedded* (situated in place and time). More specifically, three core domains of the experience have been identified: *inference, liminality* and *defense*.[18] *Inference* is all about trying to work out what's going on with the body given multiple sources of information. As we've seen, the experience of pain draws on all sorts of information and we infer the need to protect ourselves from our previous experiences (e.g., this is how I sprained my ankle last time), current sensory information (my ankle looks as swollen as it did when I sprained it badly), and predictions about the future (last time this happened I was out for three months). *Liminality* is about transition from one situation to another. Pain is ordinarily a short-lived, transitory state, aiming to return us to within our bodily limits as quickly as possible. But sometimes it persists, reflecting a system that continues to perceive threats to its integrity. Recognizing disruptions to pain transitions is paramount to recovery, but more on that later. *Defense* is action, a collection of conscious and non-conscious behaviors that attempt to resolve the potential threat to the body, ranging from limping all the way to the cellular action of inflammation at the site of the injury. Defense often focuses on constraint, helping to aid recovery; however, prolonged defense stops us from accessing new information. For example, not wiggling an injured ankle from time to time increases our uncertainty about the state of our body and how to act.

In many ways this approach to pain, which describes it as a call for protective action in order to maintain the integrity of the body, sits at odds with the experience of pain commonly encountered in sport. In that context, pain is expected, frequently tolerated through training and competition as a necessary part of the process

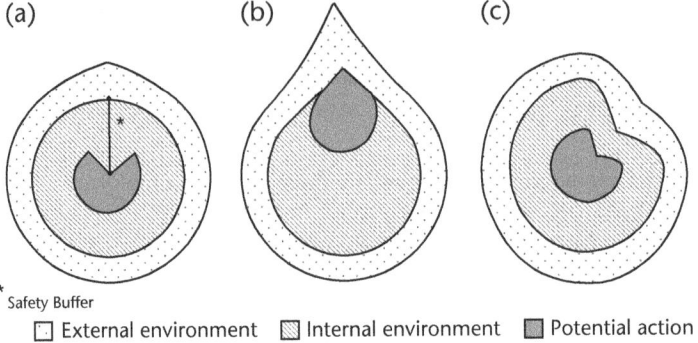

FIGURE 6.1 Schematic representation of altered "safety-buffer" and potential action in different individuals.[19]

in pushing one's bodily boundaries to reach the top. We can visualize this scenario using a simple graphic (Figure 6.1).

Here, individual (a) is an average person who has reasonably accurate interpretations related to their internal environment, but they're also fearful of what pain means. Placed in a novel external environment like a sprint exercise task (dotted area), they're required to infer the state of their body (checked area) in relation to their environment and predict the consequences of potential action. In this case, potential action is reduced (grey area) to minimise changes in bodily arousal (e.g., fear sets limits on how far the person is willing to push things). Individual (b) is an elite athlete, and the sprint exercise task is a familiar environment for them. Thanks to their training, they know what changes in bodily arousal will occur and have refined predictions about the consequences of their potential actions. In this case, the athlete is able to push bodily limits, reducing the 'safety-buffer' and enhancing the action output. Finally, let's say an individual with a sprained ankle (c) is placed into a known environment. As a consequence of their injury, their bodily state is altered, and even familiar environments become challenging. They must predict the consequences of their actions (e.g., weight bearing through the ankle) and infer the appropriate potential actions. In acute injury, these potential actions will be reduced as a protective mechanism, but their 'safety-buffer' may still be smaller than for a non-athlete. These schematics reflect a malleable interaction between the world and the individual, constantly reforming to reflect change (fear, training, injury)

So, we're saying that pain functions as a warning system and directs our actions in a self-protective way, but for athletes it's a little bit different. They commonly report pain in the course of training and competition, and it doesn't always trigger defensive action. To understand how that happens, let's take a look at what we know about the underlying biology, psychology, and sociology of pain, and how these might shape daily versus injury-related pain experiences in sport.

Protect and Survive

Most people think of pain as being driven by neural activity. Specifically, *nociceptors* (special sensory receptors that carry information about potentially dangerous stimuli) project into our skin and soft tissues to detect extremes in temperature, mechanical, and chemical signals, which alert us to potential dangers. However, there has been a crucial shift in understanding that reflects the inadequacy of this simple view of the pain experience. Pain can occur in the absence of nociception (e.g., phantom limb pain) and sometimes people don't feel pain in the presence of nociception (e.g., injury that isn't noticed until after a competition). So, while we can recognize that pain is associated with tissue damage, there is both clinical and laboratory evidence demonstrating there's not a straightforward relationship between special sensory activation and pain. This partly because we have particular pathways in the brain and nervous system which decrease activity of (or *modulate*) these receptors, for example when extreme emotion prevents people from feeling pain.[20] This is a survival function, preventing pain from dominating action in emergency situations. So, pain really emerges not as a simple sensation, but as part of an integrated experience shaped by what have been referred to as *sub-systems*.[21]

The biological aspect of pain, spanning peripheral and central components of our bodies, extend across neurological, immune, and endocrine sub-systems. These interact to ensure the on-going protection of the body by effectively responding to stressors and maintaining *homeostasis* (a stable equilibrium). Injury is an example of a perturbation that pushes our bodies beyond homeostatic limits. It disturbs local tissue, resulting in a cascade of multi-system activity that includes transmission of sensory information, immune response, and altered blood flow. This adaptive and integrated process, helping us to regain or maintain homeostasis, is known as *allostasis*.[22]

The Nervous System

The nervous system prioritizes the detection and defense of the body. Nociceptors not only signal tissue injury but release substances that initiate inflammatory processes, which in turn change the threshold of the nociceptors themselves. Working in conjunction with the immune system like this, a *sensitization* in the periphery occurs in response to injury, which means that the protection systems of the body are hyper alert, responding to both dangerous and non-dangerous stimuli. This is usually short-lasting, aiming to prioritize protection from future harm. As we go further up the nervous system pathway, we find a structure in the spinal cord known as the dorsal horn. This is particularly important in the integration of multisensory information from the periphery as well as signals from the brain. The dorsal horn can both facilitate and inhibit responses to potential danger, prioritizing these based on the context of the situation.[21,23] For example, when athletes are injured during a big game, activity in the dorsal horn can help to inhibit information relating to danger to allow them to keep playing. As we reach the brain, we find that the process of integration is both broadened and deepened. Here, connectivity across brain regions puts sensory information about the body and the world into context. The brain brings together memories of past experiences and current information to help make sense of our current state, helping us to selectively attend to information, assign it value, and learn from it.[24]

Although genetics determine much of the structure and function of the nervous system, it's continually refined through interactions with the world. For instance, significant exposures, particularly in early life, have the ability to influence how flexible the system is.[25] We don't really know the optimal balance of developing the ultimate nervous system; however, a variety of experiences including stressful ones (whether they be biological, psychological, or social) during development determine how well the system responds. Much the same way as dealing with stressors can build an athlete's coping resources or deplete them, there's the potential that challenges to the nervous system can either create capacity or lock in negative response patterns. This is currently an area of research interest.

The Immune System

The immune system is linked with the nervous system and the endocrine system, working together to actively maintain homeostasis. In the acute phase of injury, the immune response involves releasing substances that facilitate local inflammation and sensitization. These act to reduce movement and increase pain. Importantly, this process is bidirectional, so the nervous system can modulate the immune response (e.g., reduce inflammation and sensitization) if necessary. The central nervous system also interacts with specialist immune cells known collectively as *glial cells*. Under ordinary circumstances these cells provide support and protection for the nervous system, but when stressors such as injury threaten homeostasis, glial cells also trigger inflammatory responses.[26] These contribute to an increased sensitivity to non-dangerous stimuli (*allodynia*) as well as a heightened response to dangerous stimuli (*hyperalgesia*), which put the body on high alert until the threat can be assessed and acted upon.[27] Like the acute response in the nervous system, this process is usually short-lived; however in circumstances where pain persists, dysregulation of the immune system may be the culprit.[28]

The Endocrine System

The endocrine system orchestrates our body's response to stressors, which falls broadly into two categories.[21] The first is *defensive arousal*, the second is *recovery*. *Defensive arousal* involves the release of hormones that heighten our vigilance, attention, and fear, interacting with our autonomic nervous system to engage defensive behavior. The *recovery* phase aims to preserve the resources often depleted in the arousal phase, regulating initial defensive reactions to minimize the costs of allostasis. The concept of a cost to allostasis is an important one in athletes and in the context of sport. Often, sports performance requires operating in the presence of multiple stressors repetitively and over time (e.g., injury, pain, anxiety, depression, and illness). As a result, there's potential for persistent allostatic load placed on the system. This load may deplete vital resources that, without sufficient recovery, can lead to a dysregulation of future stress responses and a reduced ability to adapt to change. For athletes, this may manifest in persistent pain during their career, or an altered aging process beyond their career.[22]

Pain Modulation in Athletes

The pain system is modulated by neuroimmune and neuroendocrine mechanisms throughout the lifespan (i.e., they can upregulate or downregulate its responses, depending on the situation).[29] The reciprocal interactions between these systems over time is how we're able to accommodate exposure to a wide range of stressors, such as physical injury and infection. Such stressors activate the endocrine system as well as peripheral and central immune responses and reorganize the sensitivity of the nervous system to potential threats. There's evidence that athletes have consistently higher pain tolerance relative to other groups, possibly because exercise can reduce pain sensitivity[30] or because repeated pain exposures lead to greater modulation of the pain system.[31] This is really helpful while training and competing, but it comes with risks as well. Research has demonstrated that persistent neuroimmune activation contributes to long term pathological states. This is of particular relevance to athletes, as on-going exposure to stressors can affect the system in ways that will only manifest later in life (e.g., chronic pain).[32]

Although there's clearly a strong underlying biology associated with bodily protection, it's only when we view these components of pain within the context of the individual that we're able to appreciate the bigger picture. The psychosocial environment comprises multiple sources of stressors that perturb the individual and demand an allostatic response. Understanding how these factors operate reciprocally with the biological part of the system is essential if we want to help athletes manage pain, so let's take a look at how psychological processes and social interactions help to shape the experience.

Under Pressure

The interpretation of sensory information and the meaning attributed to the experience of pain typically fall under the remit of psychology. Considerations in this domain span a broad range of cognitions, as well as directed attentional processes which selectively seek information based on a person's short- and long-term goals. These processes are linked to the biology of pain, but they aren't entirely dependent upon it. That means the way we interpret pain isn't just based on the intensity of the danger or how suddenly it comes on. Instead, there's a continual process of gathering information about the condition of our body, what's happening in our immediate environment, and what has happened in the relevant past, which informs the way we experience pain. Okay, that's a little bit abstract so let's put it into more concrete terms.

In sport, the information gathering process is focused on pushing bodily limits in the pursuit of performance excellence. Through training, an athlete learns to predict the consequences of their actions in different situations, finding their current pain thresholds, and working to extend them as an indicator of improved endurance, strength, or flexibility. This fits into the "no pain, no gain" concept, like when athletes want to feel their muscles aching as a sign that they're creating positive change in their bodies. Yet, the same sensations can also be interpreted as threatening in a different context: if it's something they've never felt before, if they are carrying an injury, if it occurs suddenly, or if they're in in a risky environment (e.g., trying a new skill or competing), it might trigger a protective response. In a sporting context, then, pain is often conceptualized as a valuable source of performance feedback on the one hand ("good pain"), and an indication that the potential threat posed to the body is beyond control ("bad pain").

This interpretive duality presents some unique circumstances for athletes and the broader sporting community. In the general population, pain fundamentally demands attention, interfering with day-to-day cognitive processes (e.g., preventing multitasking and impairing executive function);[33–35] but for athletes, their focus has to be on performance even in the presence of pain.[36] This redirection of attention away from pain counteracts the evolutionary function of the system (to change one's actions in order to protect the body). So, when pain is telling an athlete to stop, they very often make the conscious choice to ignore it, or reframe its meaning (e.g., "good pain"), and keep going. This raises an interesting question: in disengaging from the evolved function of pain, do athletes expose themselves to long-term risk in the pursuit of short-term gains?

Well, we might hypothesize that constantly ignoring pain might make athletes more vulnerable to injury both during sport participation and later in life. Though there isn't any specific evidence around this, we do know that overuse injury is a significant burden in many sport settings so there may be some truth to it.[37] Conversely, athletes constantly scan their bodies and interpret painful sensations as either something that requires action or not. This behavior is actually a hallmark of persistent pain conditions, where we see *hypervigilance* to pain-related stimuli.[38] This means that individuals are always on the alert for the smallest sensation of discomfort and have difficulty disengaging from threatening stimuli. It could be that by developing a highly attuned awareness of their bodily sensations, athletes are priming their systems for hypervigilance once their careers are over. There's some indication that this might happen, as it's been shown that athletes with pain-related anxiety show patterns of attentional bias toward threatening stimuli and could be vulnerable to chronic pain problems.[39,40] Though techniques like attentional retraining and mindfulness meditation may be functionally helpful in minimizing the intrusiveness of hypervigilance,[41] allowing athletes to perform in spite of it, we don't know what the effects might be on post-sport pain responses.

Gauging the long-term impact of attending and disattending to pain in athlete populations is therefore an important future research direction.

The appraisal process that the athlete undertakes when their body is threatened directs attention, to be sure, but it also assigns value and meaning. This interpretation is influenced by a range of higher-level cognitions including learning and memory. Some cognitive-emotional responses like anxiety, fear, and catastrophizing, can bias attention toward pain.[39] Attending to pain and pain-related information is one thing, but the interpretation of this information has a crucial bearing on the transition from arousal to recovery. Adaptive cognitions promote a downregulation of the pain experience, whereas maladaptive cognitions can prevent the body from moving into a recovery state. For instance, pain is often accompanied with fear of particular movements. Although this is intuitive in the initial phases of potential bodily threat, as a protective mechanism, fear-avoidance can play a prominent role in the persistence of pain following injury.[42] The *fear-avoidance model* is a theoretical framework that describes how following a painful episode, some people end up in a vicious loop where hypervigilance leads to reduced activity in the longer term, which is associated with pain persistence and emotional distress.[43] In severe cases, this can cause lasting performance decrements or even prevent athletes from returning to sport.[42] A related psychological process that has been shown to predict distress in response to pain is *pain catastrophizing*. This is defined as "*an appraisal process where individuals focus excessively on pain sensations, exaggerate the threat value of painful sensations, and perceive themselves as unable to cope effectively with the pain situation.*"[44] Catastrophic thinking is associated with increased pain intensity and has been linked to negative responses including emotional difficulties and decreased rehabilitation engagement.[45,46] Addressing fear and catastrophizing is therefore an important consideration for effective rehabilitation.[46]

Whether they be adaptive or maladaptive, psychological elements of the pain experience are themselves a source of stress that demand resource (i.e., carry allostatic load). In this way, pain management is not simply an issue of "mind over matter" and when athletes are told to "suck it up," sometimes they can't. If the system has sufficient evidence, whether through current sensory information or previous experiences, that the integrity of the body is threatened, then protective mechanisms including pain will emerge. Indeed, even in the absence of injury, sufficient information about threat may exist to warrant an on-going protective response. This has been described as a "stickiness" where the system deploys a "better safe than sorry" principle[47] that can be accompanied by multisystem dysregulation. Here, a protective state is maintained because there is enough evidence of continued danger. This could result from a sufficiently large bodily perturbation or sustained low level perturbation, which may be biological, psychological or social in nature. So, if an athlete is under substantial psychosocial stress, ordinarily minor physical events may cause particularly large or lasting pain responses. To an outsider, this might seem like an over-reaction, but the athlete's experience is very real and definitely not "all in their head."

Our understanding of the role of psychological factors in pain has dramatically increased over the last 50 years, indeed so much so that a focus on pain cognitions in psychology often neglects the rest of the bodily systems.[18] Yet, accounting for the psychological aspects highlights the influence of brain-based mechanisms in the experience of pain. Processes like attention, fear, catastrophizing, goal setting, anxiety, coping, and depression are integrated within the neurobiological pain system and can exert influence over the nervous, immune, and endocrine subsystems, or vice versa. Therefore, psychological factors are inextricably linked with the biological processes of pain from the outset, and both parts should always be considered in tandem when treating sport injury.[20] How best to do this, however, is poorly understood. Almost all of the research in this area has been completed in non-sporting environments and given the unique dual meaning of pain in sport, more context-specific consideration is sorely needed.

Everybody Loves a Winner

About that context, then. So far, we've looked at the biology and the psychology of pain, and to complete the picture we have to embrace the social. As fundamentally social beings, our experiences of pain are informed by the interpersonal relationships we form. Considering the athlete in pain therefore requires a conceptualization that incorporates the network of people they interact with, the actions they take in this network, and the setting and ideologies of the network.[48] In sport, pain is often dismissed as "part of game," with the expectation that athletes will play and train through it.[49,50] In this environment, research has shown that normal social learning processes dictate pain experiences, shaped by the fact that expressing pain in an athlete's network (e.g., to coaches, family, peers) may result in decreased playing time and separation from the team.[51] It's unsurprising then, that learning within this social environment can result in altered and even hidden pain narratives.

Sports participation is synonymous with a culture of risk, whereby athletes are often willing to repeatedly place their bodies in harm's way by training in pain, competing whilst injured, or returning to play before being completely recovered.[52] This highlights an almost impossible balance that must be struck by the athlete: to push their bodily limits while maintaining bodily integrity. In the social domain, we see external pressures that induce risk-taking behaviors, denouncing pain as part and parcel of the sporting world. This repetitive demand placed across the athlete's biological, psychological, and social resources clearly has significant potential to affect their long-term wellbeing. We often think of this in terms of physical and mental health, but there can be consequences for their social health as well.

According to Karos et al.,[53] pain compromises three core aspects of the social self: *the need for autonomy, the need to belong, the need for justice/fairness*. In applying these considerations in the sporting context, we can reveal how sport may enhance threats across all three domains. To begin with, athletes strive for *autonomy*through maintaining control over their actions and the consequences of those actions in sport. Pain often puts this control in jeopardy and requires athletes to rely on others in order to meet their goals. For instance, a player may need to be substituted if they cannot continue, shifting their ability to affect the outcome of the match onto their teammates. Moreover, humans have evolved in social groups that communicate needs and elicit help. In sport, communication around pain is often silenced or reformulated in a way that discourages athletes from asking for help. In such circumstances, feelings of helplessness and uncontrollability can manifest, having negative influences on pain (and injury) experiences.

From a social perspective, people have a pervasive drive to form and maintain relationships. Given that often an athlete's world is tied up in the sport they play, pain has the potential to interfere dramatically with their sense of *belonging*. Social isolation is often reported as one of the most difficult aspects of sport injury[48] and it's known to impact biological and social domains, leading to problems ranging from immune dysregulation to depression.[54] The attributed cause of an athlete's pain can have a profound effect on the pain experience as well. Perceived injustice has been conceptualized as a set of cognitions comprising attributions of blame, and the magnitude or irreparability of a loss. If justice or fairness is comprised, for instance in an injury resulting from an illegal tackle, this could lead to the persistence of pain over the longer term. Together, these issues demonstrate that the social context of sport can shape the meaning of pain, its intensity and duration, and its overall effects on an athlete's health and wellbeing. We therefore need to be mindful that helping athletes to manage pain is not only a matter of addressing its source, but also the factors that amplify its internal meaning whilst silencing its external expression.

Good Times, Bad Times

Although frequently associated with injury, the experience of pain is multifaceted. That means supporting injured athletes requires us to consider the broader context in which they experience pain and what learned relationship they have with it. When assessing an athlete in pain, we therefore need to adopt a full biopsychosocial approach. This is recognized by a consensus statement from the International Olympic Committee,[20] which specifies that treatment should address all contributors to pain including underlying pathophysiology, biomechanical abnormalities, and psychosocial issues. This highlights that injury may occur without pain and pain may occur without evidence of injury, and both are valid experiences requiring treatment.

Alongside pharmacological therapies, it's the responsibility of frontline clinicians to identify and address inaccurate conceptualizations of pain and injury, including psychosocial and contextual influences. Interventions that seek to educate athletes about the causes of pain, as well as providing cognitive support to mitigate feelings of anxiety and catastrophic thought processes are paramount to successful rehabilitation.[20] Yet, more specific guidance for athletes is currently missing.[55] Guided imagery thought stopping/reframing, and other strategies to improve coping responses may help, though these address only part of the pain experience and evidence for their efficacy in pain management is largely anecdotal.[56] It's also important to remember that many athletes report pain that persists beyond injury rehabilitation, so interventions may need to stretch well into the return to sport phase. Finding approaches which athletes can self-manage outside of traditional therapeutic settings could therefore dramatically improve current provision, but for now this represents another gap in our understanding.[55]

Now, we've considered the acute response to injury and pain, as well as circumstances in which pain persists. The concept of allostatic load is particularly poignant in this regard, as we also need to think about the impact pain may have on the athlete beyond their playing career. Experiencing repetitive stressors is likely to have long-term consequences for wellbeing, particularly because balancing short-term risk against the long-term sustainability of any biological system is a continual trade-off. It's possible to run with a deficit in resource for a time, but the system will inevitably begin to shut down or malfunction without appropriate rest. We simply don't know when that point will be reached and there's a risk that athletes who suppress their pain experiences throughout their careers will end up paying for it later in life. Through that lens, the experience of pain becomes far removed from simple tissue damage. Instead, it emerges as an indicator of an allostatic process that looks to maintain the long-term integrity of the individual. How we reconcile this with the role pain plays in sport is something we'll need to think more carefully about in research and practice if we hope to treat athletes and not just injuries.

For What It's Worth[ii]

The more we learn about pain, the more we realize that it cannot be reduced to simply a physical sensation. Instead, it's a phenomenon that spans biological, psychological, and social realms. It's a continually evolving process, informed by the past, situated in the present and oriented toward the future. It reflects a highly efficient process of defensive action but it's not necessarily an accurate reflection of present danger. It's also an experience that carries a cost. Western sporting culture positions pain as part of attaining success, demanding that it be simultaneously silenced and used as a badge of honour. In both cases the function of pain is at odds with a system that adaptively aims to protect, and what remains unknown is the toll that this takes further down the line. Here, we run headlong into the uncomfortable relationship between the experience of pain and the pursuit of success in sport. Enhanced load across the life of the athlete is an important moral and ethical dilemma. How do we sufficiently manage pain and injury in a way that's conducive to health across their entire lifespan, not just up to the point of retirement? That's the big question that research now needs to address.

Note

i You can see this classic illusion with a simple web search for "hollow mask illusion", but the description by Professor Richard Gregory is a particularly good watch.

ii If you've been thinking that the section headings in this chapter sound kind of familiar, you've caught us – we've created a mini playlist for you: 1. "More than a feeling" (Boston, 1976) / 2. "Protect and survive" (Jethro Tull, 1980) / 3. "Under pressure" (David Bowie & Queen, 1981) / 4. "Everybody loves a winner" (U2 & Maria McKee, 2011) / 5. "Good times, bad times" (Led Zeppelin, 1969) / 6. "For what it's worth" (Buffalo Springfield, 1966). Consider it a little treat for getting 1/3 of the way through the book!

References

1 de C Williams AC. What can evolutionary theory tell us about chronic pain? *Pain* 2016;157:788–790; doi:10.1097/j.pain.0000000000000464.

2 Tabor A, Burr C. Bayesian learning models of pain: a call to action. *Curr Opin Behav Sci* 2019;26:54–61; doi:10.1016/j.cobeha.2018.10.006.

3 Körding KP, Beierholm U, Ma WJ, et al. Causal inference in multisensory perception. *PLoS One* 2007;2:e943; doi:10.1371/journal.pone.0000943.

4 Tabor A, Thacker MA, Moseley GL, et al. Pain: a statistical account. *PLoS Comput Biol* 2017;13:e1005142; doi:10.1371/journal.pcbi.1005142.

5 Seymour B. Pain: a precision signal for reinforcement learning and control. *Neuron* 2019;101:1029–1041; doi:10.1016/j.neuron.2019.01.055.

6 Grosjean M, Rinkenauer G, Jainta S. Where do the eyes really go in the hollow-face illusion? *PLoS One* 2012;7:e44706; doi:10.1371/journal.pone.0044706.

7 Gregory R. Hollow mask - brain illusion. Available at: https://youtu.be/6YIPtJlCbIA Accessed June 15, 2021.

8 Knill DC, Pouget A. The Bayesian brain: the role of uncertainty in neural coding and computation. *Trends Neurosci* 2004;27:712–719; doi:10.1016/j.tins.2004.10.007.

9 Vilares I, Kording K. Bayesian models: the structure of the world, uncertainty, behaviour, and then brain. *Ann N Y Acad Sci* 2011;1224(1):22–39; doi:10.1111/j.1749-6632.2011.05 965.x.

10 Moseley GL, Arntz A. The context of a noxious stimulus affects the pain it evokes. *Pain* 2007;133:64–71; doi:10.1016/j.pain.2007.03.002.

11 Bayer TL, Baer PE, Early C. Situational and psychophysiological factors in psychologically induced pain. *Pain* 1991;44:45–50; doi:10.1016/0304-3959(91)90145-N.

12 Acerra NE, Moseley GL. Dysynchiria: watching the mirror image of the unaffected limb elicits pain on the affected side. *Neurology* 2005;65:751–753; doi:10.1212/01 .wnl.0000178745.11996.8c.

13 Moseley GL, Parsons TJ, Spence C. Visual distortion of a limb modulates the pain and swelling evoked by movement. *Curr Biol* 2008;18:R1047–R1048; doi:10.1016/j.cub.2 008.09.031.

14 Harvie DS, Broecker M, Smith RT, et al. Bogus visual feedback alters onset of movement-evoked pain in people with neck pain. *Psychol Sci* 2015;26:385–392; doi:1 0.1177/0956797614563393.

15 Harvie DS, Smith RT, Hunter EV, et al. Using visuo-kinetic virtual reality to induce illusory spinal movement: the MoOVi Illusion. *PeerJ* 2017;5:e3023; doi:10.7717/ peerj.3023.

16 Stanton TR, Moseley GL, Wong AY, et al. Feeling stiffness in the back: a protective perceptual inference in chronic back pain. *Sci Rep* 2017;7(1):1–12; doi:10.1038/s415 98-017-09429-1.

17 Raja SN, Carr DB, Cohen M, et al. The revised International Association for the Study of Pain definition of pain: concepts, challenges, and compromises. *Pain* 2020;161:1976–1982; doi:10.1097/j.pain.0000000000001939.

18 Tabor A, Keogh E, Eccleston C. Embodied pain—negotiating the boundaries of possible action. *Pain* 2017;158:1007–1011; doi:10.1097/j.pain.0000000000000875.

19 Tabor A, Vollaard N, Keogh E, et al. Predicting the consequences of physical activity: an investigation into the relationship between anxiety sensitivity, interoceptive accuracy and action. *PLoS One* 2019;14:e0210853; doi:10.1371/journal.pone.0210853.

20 Hainline B, Derman W, Vernec A, et al. International Olympic Committee consensus statement on pain management in elite athletes. *Br J Sports Med* 2017;51:1245–1258; doi:10.1136/bjsports-2017-097884.

21 Chapman CR, Tuckett RP, Song CW. Pain and stress in a systems perspective: reciprocal neural, endocrine, and immune interactions. *J Pain* 2008;9:122–145; doi:10.1 016/j.jpain.2007.09.006.

22 McEwen BS. Allostasis and the epigenetics of brain and body health over the life course: the brain on stress. *JAMA Psychiatry* 2017;74:551–552; doi:10.1001/jamapsychiatry.201 7.0270.

23 Todd AJ. Neuronal circuitry for pain processing in the dorsal horn. *Nat Rev Neurosci* 2010;11:823–836; doi:10.1038/nrn2947.

24 Wiech K, Ploner M, Tracey I. Neurocognitive aspects of pain perception. *Trends Cogn Sci* 2008;12:306–313; doi:10.1016/j.tics.2008.05.005.

25 Korgaonkar MS, Antees C, Williams LM, et al. Early exposure to traumatic stressors impairs emotional brain circuitry. *PLoS One* 2013;8: e75524; doi:10.1371/journal.pone.0075524.

26 Watkins LR, Maier SF. Beyond neurons: evidence that immune and glial cells contribute to pathological pain states. *Physiol Rev* 2002;82:981–1011; doi:10.1152/physrev.00011.2002.

27 Marchand F, Perretti M, McMahon SB. Role of the immune system in chronic pain. *Nat Rev Neurosci* 2005;6:521–532; doi:10.1038/nrn1700.

28 Xu M, Bennett DL, Querol LA, et al. Pain and the immune system: emerging concepts of IgG-mediated autoimmune pain and immunotherapies. *J Neurol Neurosurg Psychiatry* 2020;91:177–188; doi:10.1136/jnnp-2018-318556.

29 Zouikr I, Karshikoff B. Lifetime modulation of the pain system via neuroimmune and neuroendocrine interactions. *Front Immunol* 2017;8:276; doi:10.3389/fimmu.2017.00276.

30 Vaegter HB, Fehrmann E, Gajsar H, et al. Endogenous modulation of pain: the role of exercise, stress, and cognitions in humans. *Clin J Pain* 2020;36:150–161; doi:10.1097/AJP.0000000000000788.

31 Tesarz J, Schuster AK, Hartmann M, et al. Pain perception in athletes compared to normally active controls: a systematic review with meta-analysis. *Pain* 2012;153:1253–1262; doi:10.1016/j.pain.2012.03.005.

32 Vineis P, Avendano-Pabon M, Barros H, et al. Special report: the biology of inequalities in health: the lifepath consortium. *Front Public Health* 2020;8:118; doi:10.3389/fpubh.2 020.00118.

33 Crombez G, Eccleston C, Baeyens F, et al. Habituation and the interference of pain with task performance. *Pain* 1997:70:149–154; doi:10.1016/s0304-3959(96)03304-0.

34 Eccleston C, Crombez G. Pain demands attention: a cognitive–affective model of the interruptive function of pain. *Psychol Bull* 1999;125:356; doi:10.1037/0033-2909.125.3.356.

35 Berryman C, Stanton TR, Bowering KJ, et al. Do people with chronic pain have impaired executive function? A meta-analytical review. *Clin Psychol Rev* 2014;34:563–579; doi:10.1016/j.cpr.2014.08.003.

36 Deroche T, Woodman T, Stephan Y, et al. Athletes' inclination to play through pain: a coping perspective. *Anxiety Stress Coping* 2011;24:579–587; doi:10.1080/10615806.2011.552717.

37 Rio E, Moseley L, Purdam C, et al. The pain of tendinopathy: physiological or pathophysiological? *Sports Med* 2014;44: 9–23; doi:10.1007/s40279-013-0096-z.

38 Crombez G, Van Damme S, Eccleston C. Hypervigilance to pain: an experimental and clinical analysis. *Pain* 2005;116:4–7; doi:10.1016/j.pain.2005.03.035.

39 Bardel MH, Woodman T, Perreaut-Pierre E, et al. The role of athletes' pain-related anxiety in pain-related attentional processes. *Anxiety Stress Coping* 2013;26:573–583; doi:10.1080/10615806.2012.757306.

40 Bar-Haim Y, Lamy D, Pergamin L, et al. Threat-related attentional bias in anxious and nonanxious individuals: a meta-analytic study. *Psychol Bull* 2007;133:1–24; doi:10.1037/0033-2909.133.1.1.

41 Garland EL, Howard MO. Mindfulness-oriented recovery enhancement reduces pain attentional bias in chronic pain patients. *Psychother Psychosom* 2013;82:311–318; doi:10.1159/000348868.

42 Fischerauer SF, Talaei-Khoei M, Vissers FL, et al. Pain anxiety differentially mediates the association of pain intensity with function depending on level of intolerance of uncertainty. *J Psychiatr Res* 2018;97:30–37; doi:10.1016/j.jpsychires.2017.11.006.

43 Vlaeyen JW, Linton SJ. Fear-avoidance model of chronic musculoskeletal pain: 12 years on. *Pain* 2012;153:1144–1147; doi:10.1016/j.pain.2011.12.009.

44 Sullivan MJ, Bishop SR, Pivik J. The pain catastrophizing scale: development and validation. *Psychol Assess* 1995;7:524; doi:10.1037/1040-3590.7.4.524.

45 Udry E, Gould D, Bridges D, et al. Down but not out: athlete responses to season-ending injuries. *J Sport Exerc Psychol* 1997;19:229–248; doi:10.1123/jsep.19.3.229.

46 Sullivan MJ, Tripp DA, Rodgers WM, et al. Catastrophizing and pain perception in sport participants. *J Appl Sport Psychol* 2000;12:151–167; doi:10.1080/10413200008404220.

47 Borsook D, Youssef AM, Simons L, et al. When pain gets stuck: the evolution of pain chronification and treatment resistance. *Pain* 2018;159:2421; doi:10.1097/j.pain/0000000000001401.

48 Killick L, Davenport TE. Pain worlds: towards the integration of a sociocultural perspective of pain in clinical physical therapy. *Physiother Res Int* 2014;19:193–204; doi:10.1002/pri.1583.

49 Nixon HL. A social network analysys of influences on athletes to play with pain and injuries. *J Sport Soc Issues* 1992;16:127–135; doi:10.1177/019372359201600208.

50 Hughes R, Coakley J. Positive deviance among athletes: the implications of overconformity to the sport ethic. *Sociol Sport J* 1991;8:307–325; doi:10.1123/ssj.8.4.307.

51 Killick L. *Walking the fine line? Young people, athletic risk, health and embodied identities* (dissertation). Loughborough University 2009.

52 Charlesworth H, Young K. Why English female university athletes play with pain. In: K Young (ed.). *Athletic bodies, damaged selves: sociological studies of sports related injury.* Oxford, UK: Elsevier Science Press 2004.

53 Karos K, Williams ACDC, Meulders A, et al. Pain as a threat to the social self: a motivational account. *Pain* 2018;159:1690–1695; doi:10.1097/j.pain.0000000000001257.

54 Jaremka LM, Fagundes CP, Glaser R, et al. Loneliness predicts pain, depression, and fatigue: understanding the role of immune dysregulation. *Psychoneuroendocrinology* 2013;38:1310–1317; doi:10.1016/j.psyneuen.2012.11.016.

55 Zideman DA, Derman W, Hainline B, et al. Management of pain in elite athletes: identified gaps in knowledge and future research directions. *Clin J Sport Med* 2018;28:485–489; doi: 10.1097/JSM.0000000000000618.

56 Hainline B, Turner JA, Caneiro JP. Pain in elite athletes—neurophysiological, biomechanical and psychosocial considerations: a narrative review. *Br J Sports Med* 2017;51:1259–1264; doi:10.1136/bjsports-2017-097890.

7

HOW INJURY CAN BE A POSITIVE THING: SOME PEOPLE ARE JUST GOOD AT EVERYTHING

Carly McKay and Mason Raymond

Mapping the Recovery Process

If we recall the Integrated Model of Response to Sport Injury proposed by Wiese-Bjornstal and colleagues[1] (quick, flip back to Chapter 2 if you need a reminder), there are a number of factors that influence an athlete's post-injury experiences. Personal factors like their injury history, personality, and motivations can affect the way they cognitively appraise the situation. So can the nature of their injury (e.g., what kind of injury it is, how severe it is, and how it happened). For instance, someone with a mild overuse injury who has had similar injuries in the past may have a very different view than an athlete with a severe traumatic injury who has never experienced anything like it before. Other environmental variables, such as their sport setting, the time in the season, the influence of coaches and teammates, or even their access to rehabilitation services can shape how stressful the injury is, as well. The appraisals that the athlete forms about the cause of their injury, how quickly they might recover, or how detrimental it is to their career go on to drive emotional responses and behaviors that ultimately determine how well they manage.

There are obviously a few different ways for this process to turn out. In some cases, it ends up being a difficult journey of negative cognitive appraisals, anxiety, and frustration, and diminishing motivation to stick with a rehabilitation program. Considerable attention has been focused on these kinds of stories, putting a spotlight on just how devastating a sport injury can be.[2] But what about cases that go in the complete opposite direction? We don't hear about those quite as often, but some athletes seem to sail through rehabilitation and come out the other side stronger, more driven, and in better shape than ever before. We might chalk this up to luck or good genetics but in reality, these outcomes are the product of adaptive responses and proactive approaches to recovery. Sure, these might come

DOI: 10.4324/9781003088936-7

more naturally to some folks than others, but a lot of factors in the post-injury period are modifiable and can be developed to improve any athlete's chance of success. We can say pretty confidently that an injury is never going to be an enjoyable event, but we can learn a lot from people who've had positive experiences. Why don't we take a look at some examples and think about how we can borrow their strategies to make the recovery process a little bit easier for everyone.

Just a Bump in the Road

Let's take an extreme example to begin with. We know that some athletes, following incredibly serious injuries, manage to fully recover and return to sport as though nothing ever happened. Compared to their peers who struggle to regain form after similar injuries, they seem to have special powers of recovery. Dutch professional road cyclist Annemiek van Vleuten is one of these people. Road cycling carries an obvious risk of severe injury, with the high speeds, treacherous weather conditions, and hard landing surfaces that define the competitive landscape. So, it's probably not surprising that her career has been marked by several significant injuries, with the most dramatic occurring in the 2016 Olympic road race. While in the lead and just 12km from the finish line, van Vleuten crashed on a sharp descending bend.[3] The video of the crash was genuinely horrifying to watch and there was immediate concern that everyone had just witnessed a catastrophic or potentially fatal event.[4] In the aftermath, it was confirmed that she had three spinal fractures and a severe concussion, not to mention extensive bruising and road rash.[5] Now, ordinary people would take a considerable amount of time to recover from such injuries. The physical healing process aside, there would likely be a host of cognitive and emotional wounds to work through as well (e.g., fear, anxiety, possibly depression). Apparently not for van Vleuten, though. She was riding her bike again within 10 days of the crash, and within a month she took the overall victory and two stage wins at the Lotto Belisol Belgium Tour. Her success didn't end there, either. She was the 2017 and 2018 World Road Cycling Champion, too.

How does that happen? Well, some of it will come down to physiology – personal characteristics like age and overall health, as well as injury treatment, can change healing times.[6,7] This doesn't account for all of the variability in recovery between athletes, though. There are a number of psychological skills that can differentiate between positive and negative experiences, or indeed rehabilitation success. In van Vleuten's case, we can get a glimpse of this in her comments after one of her subsequent injuries. In 2020, she fractured her wrist in a crash at the Giro Rosa, forcing her to abandon the race while in the lead. Given the proximity to the World Championships just a week later, it seemed unlikely that she'd make a comeback in time to compete. Nevertheless, after a successful surgery and clearance from team medical staff, she was given the green light. She then went on to finish second in the race, wearing a protective brace on the injured arm. In a quote to Cyclingnews, she stated, *"I don't want to be a role model, or for people to think that it's cool to race with a broken wrist. I don't think this would be possible with every broken wrist … No, it's not cool, it's [expletive], but I was very lucky that I don't have pain. I have also had good advice from doctors."*[8] Here we can pick out a few key indicators of what allowed her to bounce back so quickly: (1) she had a clear recovery goal; (2) she acknowledged that rehabilitation is not one-size-fits-all; and (3) she found a means of coping with the impacts of the injury. We can break these down in more detail to see why they're so important.

When an athlete is injured, they often feel as though they're at the mercy of their body's healing process and there isn't much they can do to speed that up in the early days. An aspect of regaining a sense of personal control over the situation is developing a series of meaningful and achievable goals for the rehabilitation period. It might seem like this should be an automatic process – isn't returning to sport the end target? In a lot of cases it will be, though sometimes an injury is so severe that sport is a long way off and there are more immediate things to work toward. In these circumstances, or when the nature of the injury requires a lengthy rehabilitation, it's really important to have some short-term goals as well. These can help keep motivation high and give the athlete something to focus on while they're progressing toward a longer-term objective.[9,10] Figuring out what kind of goals to set can be a little tricky, though. For van Vleuten, the clear focus was racing in the World Championships, but there isn't always an immediate event for an athlete to aim for. Instead, they might be hoping to return by the end of the year, before the next season, or possibly just hoping they can return at all. Sustaining effort and motivation over that length of time can be really challenging and we would expect to see ebbs and flows. Choosing the right balance of short- and long-term goals can help to hold athletes accountable for their work ethic over the duration and is generally effective for boosting adherence to rehabilitation programs.[10–12]

Of course, in order to set realistic and achievable goals, the athlete needs to know what to expect during their recovery. Working in tandem with a medic or therapist who can provide those details is therefore really helpful. Setting goals collaboratively with them is even better. When athletes are left to set rehabilitation goals on their own, they tend to focus mostly on performance (e.g., lifting a set weight) instead of the process (e.g., time spent doing exercises), but research shows us that both are important.[10] When the emphasis is on performance, there's a risk that when setbacks occur, the athlete may become discouraged and demotivated. Failure to meet a goal, particularly when there's an expected timeline for reaching a milestone, can really undermine someone's self-confidence and lead to intense frustration. Luckily, gaining a sense of satisfaction from achieving process goals along the way can buffer against these negative emotions, as can keeping some flexibility in the plan. When athletes and medics regularly review their goals together, adjustment can be made based on clinical assessment and/or how the athlete feels to ensure that progress keeps ticking along on an appropriate time scale. That brings us to the issue of how goals are framed. Setting objectives for what we want to achieve ("I want to increase my range of motion") rather than things we'd prefer to avoid ("I don't want to feel pain") promotes more successful rehabilitation outcomes in the long run.[13] This is likely because it highlights progress, however modest that might be, and is more robust against setbacks.

Ultimately, the purpose of goal setting is to help athletes regulate their emotional responses and solve problems as they arise, which are key indicators of successful *coping*. We toss that term around a lot, but when we say someone is "coping well," what do we mean by that? Simply, coping is an attempt to overcome problems or difficulties one encounters in life by deploying a variety of strategies to either master, tolerate, or minimize the stress of said problems. These approaches can be broadly categorized as *active coping*, where we behave in ways to change the nature of the stressor or the way we respond to it, or *avoidance coping*, where we dodge the issue so we don't have to deal with it. Typically, those who cope well during injury rehabilitation use more active approaches,[14] though the specific ways in which they do this are nearly limitless. Gross and Thompson[15] suggested that we categorize all of the various coping strategies that athletes use according to five key descriptors: (1) *Situation Selection* – putting themselves into a particular situation instead of others; (2) *Situation Modification* – changing external aspects of the environment; (3) *Attention Deployment* – focusing on something or distracting ourselves to keep emotions in check; (4) *Cognitive Change* – reappraising a situation and changing its meaning or significance; and (5) *Response Modulation* – regulating our emotions and behaviors in response to a stressor. We can further subdivide this into *problem focused coping strategies* (finding solutions to a current problem) and *emotion focused coping strategies* (managing stress reactions). Okay, that's a little abstract. Let's put it into a more concrete framework.

First off, situation selection is largely off the table in the context of injury rehabilitation. It's not like the athlete can choose not to be injured, so there isn't really any way to put themselves into more preferable circumstances. The best they can hope for is situation modification, where they might decide to join a rehabilitation group or continue attending team functions to reduce feelings of isolation while they're recovering. Attention deployment is particularly relevant, and we see it all the time when athletes watch tv or listen to music as they're doing painful exercises. Staying focused on a goal can also help with this as a problem focused strategy. Cognitive change and response modulation are more about emotion focused coping and include strategies like reframing an injury as an opportunity to become healthier instead of it being a hugely negative event or using relaxation techniques to keep anxiety under control. These are all just examples and are nowhere near an exhaustive list, but we can begin to see how some athletes have really strong coping skills that make their rehabilitation experiences much more positive than others'. In our cycling vignette, it would have been very easy for Annemiek van Vleuten to withdraw and avoid engaging with the media or her fans in order to manage the stress of her injuries (e.g., situation modification through emotion focused avoidance coping). Instead, she got back on her bike despite the pain (attention deployment through active problem focused coping) and was able to appraise the situation as being a bump in the road instead of a catastrophe.

Getting by with a Little Help from My Friends

So, we've considered an example of a very quick rehabilitation process, but what about a more protracted one? Mason Raymond was a professional ice hockey player who sustained a number of injuries through his 10-year National Hockey League (NHL) career, but the worst occurred in 2011 in the Stanley Cup finals.[i] In his own words:

> *"It was game six of a best-of-seven series. We were leading the series 3-2, one win away from winning the cup! Game 6 was in Boston and my family was on hand in hopes of a celebration. Twenty seconds into the game I found myself in an awkward position with my butt against the boards and my head being pushed between my legs by an opposing player. I found myself laying on the ice in more pain that I had ever experienced before. The pain was instant. As a kid I was taught by my dad to always get up off the ice unless unable to. I remember trying to scramble to my knees and struggling to do so. Two of my line mates helped me get to my feet and held me up to get off the ice to the trainers' room, where I was looked over by team doctors. It was decided that I needed to go to the hospital by ambulance. I soon found out that I had broken two vertebrae in my back as well as having serious ligament damage. I was told by doctors that the next 6–12 months could be a long haul, but I should expect to make a full recovery.*
>
> *I was unable to get up off the bed without assistance. I had a full custom back brace made to keep me stable for the next 2–3 months. During that time, I was very limited. All daily activities one takes for granted were insurmountable tasks for me, even walking had its challenges. Going to the bathroom, walking upstairs and putting clothes on were huge obstacles. My wife and family were strong supporters and could not have done it without them. I met with a spine specialist, and he referred me to a clinician who specializes in sports therapy, osteopathy and acupuncture. He changed my life. I worked with him extensively every day for six months and have continued to see him intermittently to this day. I remember him looking me in the eyes and saying "this injury will heal as fast as you want it to. I will treat you and put you through the necessary steps to get you better, but if you don't put in the work away from when I'm with you then this program won't work." I had doubt I would ever play again right after the injury. This guy helped me believe that it was possible to come back and be better than I was before. This injury was more of a mental battle than a physical one, believe it or not. Negative thoughts and doubt entered my mind often but staying the course and following the set "map" I had for my rehabilitation was essential. Getting back to daily life and health was my initial priority, but the ultimate goal was progressing enough to be in hockey shape and play the game like I did before the injury. I returned to play hockey seven months after the injury and went on to play 5 more years. At the time I didn't think that was possible, but I know today that I am stronger than I was then. Not only physically, but mentally. It's still hard to say that I am stronger both physically and mentally. I would not wish this*

injury on any player, but I can honestly say the obstacles I had to overcome made me better hockey player and person. Without support from family, friends, doctors this journey may not have had the same outcome."

Aside from being incredibly inspirational, this story introduces several important elements of successful rehabilitation, and social support is the one ringing through loud and clear. The kind of support that injured athletes receive from family and friends can be broken down into four different types: *emotional support* (listening, comforting), *esteem support* (encouragement), *informational support* (providing guidance), and *tangible support* (helping with tasks).[16] Each of these has its place and might be useful at different moments during the recovery process. In Mason's experience, his family was a clear source of emotional and tangible support, whereas the specialists he worked with provided informational support when he needed it most. Interestingly, evidence suggests that *perceived support* (an athlete's belief that assistance is there if they need it) is more consistently and strongly related to physical and mental health[17] than *received support* (the supportive resources an athlete actually utilizes). Moreover, perceived support has been found to buffer the effect of stress on psychological responses to injury for athletes at lower competitive levels but not for elite groups.[18] This all seems very counter-intuitive and comes with the caveat that there isn't much dedicated research on the topic, though a possible explanation is that athletes who possess better coping skills don't need to rely on social support quite as much (though they still like knowing it's there). There will be personal variability in this, of course, but it's easy to see how some people may prefer more or less independence through the process. On occasion, social support can end up going awry as well – anyone who's felt smothered by well-meaning attention can probably relate. Having too much support, or the wrong kind of support at the wrong time, can end up exacerbating negative injury responses, so that's something to be careful of when helping someone out.[19,20]

Mason also highlighted *self-talk* as he spoke about the doubts and beliefs he held about his ability to recover. Most of us have a little voice in our heads[ii] that provides a running dialogue through our day, whether or not we're always aware of it. Sometimes that internal voice is kind and other times it can be really critical (in cartoons this duality is often depicted as an angel and devil sitting on someone's shoulders), and that has implications for rehabilitation. The *valence* of our self-talk (i.e., whether it's positive or negative) can either promote better mood and greater confidence or prolong negative emotional states.[10] It's not unusual for an athlete to experience ups and downs with this, often corresponding to progress and setbacks in recovery, but the very limited research in this area suggests that fast healers tend to use more positive self-talk while their slow healing counterparts produce more negative messaging.[22] This is likely due to the behavior brought about by the messages (e.g., positive comments might encourage more effort), but there's a reciprocal relationship between rehabilitation progress and self-talk that must be accounted for as well (slow healing may lead to negative talk, which in turn might decrease motivation). It's unclear to what extent message valence affects recovery or vice versa, but that little voice can perform a number of functions that could alter rehabilitation outcomes. *Motivational self-talk* hasn't been well studied in injury contexts, though it typically helps people progress toward their goals. The next time you feel pleased with yourself for a job well done, have a listen for the little message of self-encouragement that'll probably come with it. That's your motivational self-talk voice and it's a good one to keep around.

Instructional self-talk is where we give ourselves directions about what to do or how to do it. It's also responsible for the feedback we give ourselves when evaluating our own performance. This voice might be more salient for injury recovery than motivational self-talk because it helps us retain information (e.g., remembering cues for specific exercises) and triggers specific actions. It can also help us refocus our attention onto active coping when we stray into emotional tailspins, and as the voice of reason, it's also excellent at stopping negative thoughts. Having that internal mechanism for pointing out irrational ideas is incredibly useful after an injury[23] and there's some evidence that athletes with developed self-talk skills show greater performance improvement during rehabilitation sessions.[24] The good news is that this can be trained, and it's something that athletes can practice on their own or with the guidance of a mental skills consultant.

Closely related to self-talk is *imagery*. This refers to the visualization of an object, scene, or sensation, though it isn't restricted to "seeing" a mental picture – it can involve imagining feelings, smells, sounds, or tastes as well.[iii] In injury rehabilitation, imagery can be used for a number of different purposes. These include *cognitive imagery*, which can help an athlete learn how to perform exercises properly, regain sport-specific technique, or even keep their strategic abilities sharp by mentally rehearsing set plays while they're unable to practice.[10] *Motivational imagery*, which is arguably the most important function during rehabilitation, is often used alongside goal setting to maintain concentration and either calm the athlete or get them fired up, as the situation requires.[26] Two other forms of imagery unique to treatment settings are *healing imagery*, which involves the athlete imagining the internal repair of their tissues or their muscles physically getting stronger, and *pain management imagery* to distract the athlete during uncomfortable moments (e.g., thinking about more pleasant things or imagining their pain dissipating).[26] Though there's a lot of uncertainty about how it actually works, there is some evidence that imagery use can promote faster recovery (see Gledhill and Forsdyke[27] for an overview if you're keen). Healing imagery in particular has shown medium to large treatment effects in studies of pain, edema, muscular endurance, muscular strength, and re-injury anxiety.[10] There are some purported benefits for treatment adherence as well, though the effects seem to be smaller.[28,29] Despite a number of limitations to the research in this area, including small samples and a lack of replication, imagery at the very least has a solid track record of helping athletes manage stress and regulate emotion.[30] As these are influential factors in determining recovery trajectories, incorporating self-determined or practitioner-guided imagery into an athlete's recovery plan may be a low-risk opportunity to help them regain a sense of control and improve their overall outlook.

The Importance of Perspective

Regardless of how long the rehabilitation process takes, the key to success lies in managing the highs and lows of emotion and promoting adaptive behavioral responses. Some of this comes down to the athlete's personal characteristics and skills, and some is facilitated by the environmental resources they're able to draw upon. For many athletes, achieving a positive outcome depends upon how well they navigate these complexities and for those who get the balance right, injury can actually be a transformative process that leads to personal growth. For instance, Mason Raymond came out of his rehabilitation as a *"better hockey player and person."* After decades of focus on the negative effects of injury, researchers and practitioners are becoming increasingly interested in these kinds of positive changes that emerge from injury experiences. Though there isn't a whole lot of evidence to work with just yet, a compelling narrative is forming to help us understand why some injured athletes seem to excel.

To set the scene, take a moment to think about a challenge you took on at some point in your life where, at the time, it seemed unbelievably difficult, but afterward you were glad you'd done it. It might be going to school, learning a new skill, participating in a walking or running event, or something entirely personal to you. The setting doesn't matter, but the feeling it left you with does. Often, once we've set aside the initial rush of accomplishment for having done whatever it was, there's also a sense that we're fundamentally changed in some way. Our perspective on life might be slightly different, or maybe we learned something about ourselves along the way. Well, as it happens, athletes sometimes get these feelings after rehabilitating from injury. This is known as *Sport Injury-Related Growth (SIRG).*[31]

There's an important distinction to be made between athletes who do well during rehabilitation and those who experience genuine growth. The former group is typically characterized as being *resilient*, meaning that they're able to bounce back and excel after overcoming a significant obstacle. In modern workplace culture, 'resilience' has become a bit of a dirty word, used as a catch phrase to describe expectations that staff will simply buck up and endure whatever unrelenting demands are heaped upon them. That's not what we're talking about here. When used properly, it really refers to someone's positive adaptation to stressful conditions through awareness and acceptance of their emotions, finding meaning in the situation, being engaged in solutions, and staying open to experience. In other words, it's about seeing adversity as a challenge and not a threat.[32,33] Resilient individuals are able to rely on key coping skills that are built through practice (and some that develop with maturity) to become more confident in their stress responses and form optimistic future outlooks. They ask themselves "where's the opportunity" in the situation[34] and work toward it, though they might not emerge with a better level of functioning than they had before they were injured.

When true SIRG occurs, athletes report meaningful positive changes that cross physical, psychological, social, and/or behavioral domains.[35,36] These changes often extend beyond sport and into the broader context of their lives, leaving them with a sense of having become a better version of themselves. Whether or not these changes are outwardly visible, it's the athlete's perception of them that matters.[31] Based on this premise, Kylie Roy-Davis and colleagues[31] have developed a theory to explain the processes that lead to SIRG. Through a series of in-depth interviews with 37 British athletes (14 women, 23 men) from a variety of sports, they determined that personal development emerges from the ongoing stress caused by injury, though not in a linear way as we might expect. It isn't simply the injury event that triggers the process, it's the continuous demands of rehabilitation that prompt deployment and re-deployment of internal and external coping resources. So, stress is an essential catalyst in the process as it requires the athlete to adapt their cognitive appraisals and respond appropriately as the situation evolves. This might help to explain why some athletes experience growth and others do not – their perceptions of stress and the way they manage it are key determining factors.

This leads to the two core concepts of The Theory of Sport Injury-Related Growth: *metacognition/positive reappraisal* and *positive emotions/facilitative responses*.[31] Metacognition is all about how athletes recognize and take control of their own thoughts. Instead of allowing negative ideas to take over, athletes on the path to SIRG reflect on not only what they're thinking, but also why they're thinking it. This might be facilitated through self-talk or conversation with someone in their social support network, but ultimately it provides the opportunity to shut down unproductive thought patterns and reappraise the impact of the injury. For instance, it might at first seem like a major blow to the athlete's aspirations of winning an event, but after putting it into perspective with other negative life events (e.g., losing a loved one), they might decide that it's not the worst thing that's ever happened and so it becomes less threatening. Once these thoughts have been rationalized and the situation is positively reappraised, more adaptive emotional responses tend to emerge. Feelings of optimism, confidence, gratitude, and curiosity are often reported, and these in turn inspire active coping strategies like seeking out information about the injury, investing time in rehabilitation as well as non-sport interests, and nurturing valued social relationships (i.e., responses that enable personal growth).[31]

The theory also identifies a number of internal and external resources that facilitate the SIRG process. Internal resources include the athlete's personality (e.g., resilience), their coping style, their knowledge and prior experience, and perceived social support. Not all athletes will mobilize all four of these resources, nor are they likely to be used all at the same time, but they can influence metacognition and positive reappraisal, with clear effects on emotional and coping responses.[31] To illustrate, someone with a history of injury may be able to use their previous experience to appraise the significance of a new injury, whereas another athlete might rely more heavily on active coping (e.g., stress management techniques) to regulate their emotional responses. These might look like very different approaches, but both may be equally effective. Similarly, the four external factors identified in the theory can also affect cognitive and emotional responses differently at an individual level. These factors are cultural scripts (i.e., narratives within the sport culture about triumph over adversity), physical resources, received social support, and time (e.g., free time arising due to the injury that can be invested in personal development).[31] Early research suggests that these resources are context-dependent and, as with internal resources, some athletes will rely on certain ones more heavily than others.[31] Altogether, the likelihood than an athlete will experience SIRG depends on how internal and external resources interact to produce positive injury appraisals and emotions, and how they trigger adaptive responses.

At the end of the day, "growth" means different things to different people. To some, it'll be expressed in terms of being healthier or better equipped to manage stress, and for others it might be more about having a new perspective on how sport fits into their lives. In the development of The Theory of Sport Injury-Related Growth, Roy-Davis et al.[31] found that athletes experienced positive changes across a number of personally defined areas such as prosocial behaviors (helping others), health behaviors, physical improvements (strength and conditioning), emotional/social intelligence, social relationships, body-self relationship, self-acceptance, and appreciation of life. Interestingly, a number of these dimensions have also been mentioned by coaches when asked about their perceptions of athletes' stress-related growth.[36] So, although the way SIRG is conceptualized will be different for everyone, there are some common elements that we can focus on as we deepen our understanding of this phenomenon. Research on the topic is at a very early stage and much more work needs to be done to validate current theory, but things are off to a promising start.

Where the Mind Goes, the Body Will Follow?[37]

When discussing SIRG, people can generally wrap their heads around abstract ideas of personal development and changed worldviews, but inevitably the question arises: "what about performance?" Without a doubt, in the currency of wins and losses, knowing whether someone is fit and ready to compete is foremost in everyone's mind when they return to play. Yes, it's nice if they've had an enlightening experience through their recovery, but at the end of the day does it make them a better athlete? This is actually a fascinating topic, though it hasn't gotten much direct attention in the research literature so far.

There's plenty of evidence to show that physical capabilities are often diminished after various kinds of surgery,[38–40] yet the pervasive myth that a broken bone grows back stronger (spoiler: it doesn't[41]) has evolved into a false analogy for injury rehabilitation more generally. Take the improbable case of Tommy John surgery. Reconstruction of the elbow ulnar collateral ligament, primarily undertaken to repair damage associated with throwing sports, has been performed with increasing frequency over recent years. Since 1999, there has been an exponential rise in the number of procedures annually in Major League Baseball.[42] Somehow, despite medical evidence to the contrary,[43] a lot of people think that it will improve pitching speed. For instance, in a survey of 516 sports reporters, 25% thought that a primary reason for the surgery was performance enhancement and 20% thought it would lead to better pitching.[44] Even more concerning, another study (n = 260) found that a significant proportion of baseball coaches (30%), parents (37%), and young players (51% high school, 26% collegiate) believed that Tommy John surgery should be performed on healthy players to give them an advantage.[45] The idea of inflicting injury and forcing a lengthy rehabilitation in the hopes of SIRG – albeit in a very literal, physical sense – is a frightening application of the concept.

These kinds of misperceptions about the relationship between injury and performance highlight how little we really know about the complexities of injury recovery. We can pretty well bust the myth that an injury itself is going to make someone stronger or faster, but rehabilitation might do just that. Dedicated time and focus on building fitness can indeed help athletes return to sport in better shape than when they left, especially if they'd been nursing an injury for some time before they sought treatment. So, perhaps we can forgive the casual spectator for making an incorrect attribution for the source of physical improvement. But could there be other performance benefits to the overall injury experience? This is where we start to push the boundaries of what we know and consider some exciting possibilities. When injuries cause athletes to reflect on their motivations, the value of sport, and their willingness to take risks, it's conceivable that they might adapt their strategic approach to competition. Using time away from training to develop tactical skills through video analysis and imagery, for instance, might be a particularly facilitative response to emerge during that period. Sort of like a coach sitting a player in the press box to get a different perspective on the game, an injury might provide the opportunity for athletes to develop their game sense and become better students of the sport. Of course, this is all speculation, but it presents an interesting way forward for those seeking silver linings to unfortunate events.

Finding More Ups than Downs

Clearly, there are some things that set apart the athletes who excel through injury rehabilitation from those who have more difficulties. There are plenty of questions yet to be answered about why this is the case and how best to give people a nudge in that direction, but in the meantime we can learn from cases like Annemiek van Vleuten's and Mason Raymond's. Taking inspiration from their stories and picking out the strategies that they've used to good effect gives us a starting point, at least. From there, it's a matter of managing the highs and lows of the recovery process and remembering that it won't be an easy road for everyone. Although striving for personal growth is an admirable goal, and one we will hopefully one day be able to facilitate more regularly, simply finding some positives in the experience is still a win.

Notes

i The Stanley Cup is the trophy awarded annually to the winner of the NHL playoffs. It's the oldest existing trophy in North American professional sport, having been won for the first time in 1893. The authors also happen to think it's the best looking of all the trophies, but they're likely biased.

ii Not all of us, as it turns out. Though there aren't any prevalence estimates, a proportion of people don't have an internal monologue, so forming explicit self-talk messages may be challenging.[21]

iii Again, not everyone can do this. It's thought that around 2% of people are aphantasic, meaning they cannot conjure up mental images.[25]

References

1 Wiese-Bjornstal DM, Smith AM, Shaffer SM, et al. An integrated model of response to sport injury: psychological and sociological dynamics. *J Appl Sport Psychol* 1998;10(1):46–69; doi: 10.1080/10413209808406377.

2 Gledhill A. The downside of sports injury: poor mental health in injured athletes. In: A Gledhill, D Forsdyke (eds.). *The psychology of sports injury*. New York: Routledge 2021.

3 Kirshner A. Annemiek van Vleuten crashes horrifically while leading women's Olympic cycling road race. Available at: https://www.sbnation.com/2016/8/7/12398456/annemiek-van-vleuten-road-race-crash-olympics Accessed May 14, 2021.

4 Robinson J. One year after a horrific crash in Rio, Annemiek van Vleuten is back on top. Available at: https://www.wsj.com/articles/one-year-after-a-horrific-crash-in-rio-annemiek-van-vleuten-is-back-on-top-1502120253 Accessed May 14, 2021.

5 Westby, M. Annemiek van Vleuten suffers horror crash in Olympic road race. Available at: https://www.skysports.com/more-sports/cycling/news/15234/10527401/annemiek-van-vleuten-suffers-horror-crash-in-olympic-road-race Accessed May14, 2021.

6 Gaston MS, Simpson AH. Inhibition of fracture healing. *J Bone Joint Surg Br* 2007;89(12):1553–1560; doi:10.1302/0301-620X.89B12.19671.

7 Guo S, DiPietrro LA. Factors affecting wound healing. *J Dent Res* 2010;89(3):219–229; doi:10.1177/0022034509359125.

8 Frattini K. Annemiek van Vleuten: "I want to start, I feel ready to start Worlds." Available at: https://www.cyclingnews.com/news/annemiek-van-vleuten-i-want-to-start-i-feel-ready-to-start-worlds/ Accessed May 14, 2021.

9 Worrell TW. The use of behavioural and cognitive techniques to facilitate achievement of rehabilitation goals. *J Sport Rehabil* 1992;1:69–75; doi: 10.1123/jsr.1.1.69.

10 Hall C, Duncan L, McKay C. *Psychological interventions in sport, exercise & injury rehabilitation*. Dubuque, IA: Kendall Hunt 2014.

11 Evans L, Hardy L. Injury rehabilitation: a goal-setting intervention study. *Res Q Exerc Sport* 2002;73:310–319; doi: 10.1080/02701367.2002.10609025.

12 Gennarelli SM, Brown SM, Mulcahey MK. Psychosocial interventions help facilitate recovery following musculoskeletal sports injuries: a systematic review. *Phys Sportsmed* 2020;48:370–377; doi:10.1080/00913847.2020.1744486.

13 Danish SJ, Petitpas AJ, Hale BD. A developmental-educational intervention model of sport psychology. *Sport Psychol* 1992;6:403–415; doi: 10.1123/tsp.6.4.403.

14 Albinson CB, Petrie TA. Cognitive appraisals, stress and coping: preinjury and post-injury factors influencing psychological adjustment to sport injury. *J Sport Rehabil* 2003;12:306–322; doi: 10.1123/jsr.12.4.306.

15 Gross JJ, Thompson RA. Emotion regulation: conceptual foundations. In: JJ Gross (ed.). *Handbook of emotion regulation*. London: Guilford Press 2007.

16 Rees T, Hardy L. An investigation of the social support experiences of high-level sports performers. *Sport Psychol* 2000;14:327–347; doi:10.1123/tsp.14.4.327.

17 Lakey B, Orehek E. Relational regulation theory: a new approach to explain the link between perceived social support and mental health. *Psychol Rev* 2011;118:482–495; doi:10.1037/a0023477.

18 Rees T, Mitchell I, Evans L. Stressors, social support and psychological responses to sport injury in high and low-performance standard participants. *Psychol Sport Exerc* 2010;11:505–512; doi:10.1016/j.psychsport.2010.07.002.

19 Udry E, Gould D, Bridges D, et al. People helping people? Examining the social ties of athletes coping with burnout and injury stress. *J Sport Exerc Psychol* 1997;19:368–395; doi: 10.1123/jsep.19.4.368.

20 Freeman P. Social support. In: Arnold R, Fletcher D (eds.). *Stress, well-being, and performance in sport*. New York: Routledge 2021; doi:10.4324/9780429295874.

21 Felton J. People are weirded out to discover that some people don't have an internal monologue. Available at: https://www.iflscience.com/brain/people-are-weirded-out-to-discover-that-some-people-dont-have-an-internal-monologue/ Accessed May 14, 2021.

22 Ievleva L, Orlick T. Mental links to enhanced healing: an exploratory study. *Sport Psychol* 1991;5:25–40; doi: 10.1123/tsp.5.1.25.

23 Nippert AH, Smith AM. Psychologic stress related to injury and impact on sport performance. *Phys Med Rehabil Clin N Am* 2008;19:399–418; doi: 10.1016/j.pmr.2007.12.003.

24 Theodorakis Y, Beneca A, Goudas M, et al. The effect of self-talk on injury rehabilitation. *Eur Yearbook Sport Psychol* 1998;2:124–135.

25 Keogh R, Pearson J. The blind mind: no sensory visual imagery in aphantasia. *Cortex* 2018;105:53–60; doi: 10.1016/j.cortex.2017.10.012.

26 Driediger M, Hall C, Callow N. Imagery use by injured athletes: a qualitative analysis. *J Sports Sci* 2006;24:261–271; doi: 10.1080/02640410500128221.

27 Gledhill A, Forsdyke D. Seeing is believing: the role of imagery in sports injury rehabilitation. In: A Gledhill, D Forsdyke (eds.). *The psychology of sports injury*. New York: Routledge 2021.

28 Scherzer CB, Brewer BW, Cornelius AE, et al. Psychological skills and adherence to rehabilitation after reconstruction of the anterior cruciate ligament. *J Sport Rehabl* 2001;10:165–172; doi: 10.1123/jsr.10.3.165.

29 Wesch N, Hall C, Prapavessis H, et al. Self-efficacy, imagery use and adherence during injury rehabilitation. *Scand J Med Sci Sports* 2011 doi: 10.1111/j.1600-0838.2011.01304.x.

30 Munroe-Chandler KJ, Guerrero MD. Psychological imagery in sport and performance. In: *Oxford Research Encyclopedia of Psychology* 2017; doi: 10.1093/acrefore/9780190236557.013.228.

31 Roy-Davis K, Wadey R, Evans L. A grounded theory of sport injury-related growth. *Sport Exerc Perform Psychol* 2017;6:35–52; doi:10.1037/spy0000080

32 Luthar SS. Resilience in development: a synthesis of research across five decades. In: D Cicchetti, DJ Cohen (eds.). *Developmental psychopathology: risk, disorder, and adaptation* (Vol. 3, 2nd ed.). New York, NY: Wiley 2006.

33 Fletcher D, Sarkar M. A grounded theory of psychological resilience in Olympic champions. *Psychol Sport Exerc* 2012;13:669–678; doi:10.1016/j.psychsport.2012.04.007.

34 Gonzalez SP, Detling N, Galli NA. Case studies of developing resilience in elite sport: applying theory to guide interventions. *J Sport Psychol Action* 2016;7:158–169; doi: 10.1080/21520704.2016.1236050.

35 Podlog L, Eklund R. High-level athletes' perceptions of success in returning to sport following injury. *Psychol Sport Exerc* 2009;10:535–544; 10.1016/j.psychsport.2009.02.003.

36 Wadey R, Clark S, Podlog L, et al. Coaches' perceptions of athletes' stress related growth following sport injury. *Psychol Sport Exerc* 2013;14:125–135; 10.1016/j.psychsport.2012.08.004.

37 Schwarzenegger A. *The new encyclopedia of modern bodybuilding: the bible of bodybuilding.* New York: Simon and Schuster 2012.

38 Lizee C, Lepley AS, Birchmeier T, et al. Quadriceps strength and volitional activation after anterior cruciate ligament reconstruction: a systematic review and meta-analysis. *Sports Health* 2019;11(2):163–179; doi:10.1177/1941738118822739.

39 Wilson KW, Popchak A, Li RT, et al. Return to sport testing at 6 months after arthroscopic shoulder stabilization reveals residual strength and functional deficits. *J Shoulder Elbow Surg* 2020;29(7):S107–S114; 10.1016/j.jse.2020.04.035.

40 Jack II RA, Burn MB, Sochacki KR, et al. Performance and return to sport after Tommy John surgery among Major League Baseball position players. *Am J Sports Med* 2018;46:1720–1726; doi:10.1177/0363546518762397.

41 O'Connor A. The claim: after being broken, bones can become stronger. Available at: https://www.nytimes.com/2010/10/19/health/19really.html Accessed May 14, 2021.

42 Liu JN, Garcia GH, Conte S, et al. Outcomes in revision Tommy John surgery in Major League Baseball pitchers. *J Shoulder Elbow Surg* 2016;25:90–97; doi: 10.1016/j.jse.2015.08.040.

43 Makhni EC, Lee RW, Morrow ZS, et al. Performance, return to competition, and reinjury after Tommy John surgery in Major League Baseball pitchers: a review of 147 cases. *Am J Sports Med* 2014;42:1323–1332; doi: 10.1177/0363546514528864.

44 Conte SA, Hodgins JL, El Attrache NS, et al. Media perceptions of Tommy John surgery. *Phys Sportsmed* 2015;43:375–380; doi:10.1080/00913847.2015.1077098.

45 Ahmad CS, Grantham WJ, Greiwe RM. Public perceptions of Tommy John surgery. *Phys Sportsmed* 2012;40:64–72; doi: 10.3810/psm.2012.05.1966.

8

WHY INJURY ISN'T GENERALLY A POSITIVE THING: MOST PEOPLE HAVE TO PLAY THE CARDS THEY'RE DEALT

Carly McKay

We occasionally come across athletes who excel through their injuries but it's far more common to hear about the ones who don't. Contemporary media coverage is full of stories about athletes whose struggles with injury have impacted their performance, their ongoing health, or their mental wellbeing. At the amateur level there's less overt attention than for professionals, to be sure, but when an injury happens the same concerns arise regardless of the setting – will the athlete come back, and will they be the same player as before?

Although it's easy to think of injured athletes as either recovering well or not, it's not exactly an all-or-nothing distinction. The truth is that most people will fall somewhere in between, and their experiences will include both highs and lows, with day-to-day or even moment-to-moment fluctuations in thoughts, feelings, and actions. Yes, we know that variables like their injury history and personality can affect the way they appraise the situation, and that positive appraisals generally lead to positive emotions (e.g., hopefulness, confidence) and proactive behaviors (e.g., treatment adherence). We also know that negative appraisals can trigger emotional difficulties (e.g., fear, fatigue, sadness, guilt) and ineffective coping strategies (e.g., risk-taking).[1,2] Most of the research in this area has focused on the latter pathway, describing the difficult journey of destructive thoughts, anxiety, and frustration, and diminishing motivation that some athletes go through.[3,4] With considerable attention paid to extreme responses which are altogether too frequent, including cases of depression and self-harm,[5] the narrative around sport injury has shifted toward the dark end of the spectrum.[i]

There's plenty of nuance in the way people respond to injury, though, and this hasn't really been explored all that well. For instance, some athletes battle through negativity immediately after their injury and gradually become more positive as they improve, while others follow a U-shaped trajectory where immediate distress dissipates through rehabilitation only to re-emerge as a return to sport draws

DOI: 10.4324/9781003088936-8

nearer.[7] Yet others find the entire process to be difficult, but eventually manage to put it all behind them and move on with varying degrees of success. Supporting athletes through all of this can be a challenge, and for the majority who simply have to roll with the ups and downs as best they can, there isn't a ton of evidence to say what the best approach might be. So, for now at least, there's a certain amount of art in the science of psychological recovery and in order to limit negative effects on health and performance, we need to rely on a combination of theory and lived experience for guidance.

Developing a Game Plan

Any time a sport injury happens, whether it be at amateur or professional level, it begins a cascade of events that have the potential to affect the athlete's ultimate outcome. Our understanding of these events and how they influence recovery is still developing, though nearly every theoretical model is explicit that post-injury personal and situational factors are dynamic and don't operate in a linear fashion.[1] So, just as injury susceptibility is driven by context-dependent interactions between intrinsic and extrinsic risk factors (see chapter 3), responses to injury are formed by a complex web of determinants that produce different effects depending on the individual athlete and their particular circumstances. This makes predicting how an athlete will respond a little bit challenging but, based on research evidence and common threads in athletes' accounts, we're starting to see some stable patterns emerging. These suggest that if we want to come up with a plan for how to manage post-injury responses, we first need to consider the injury event itself.

The first parameter of interest is how the injury happened. Did it occur in training or competition, with or without an audience? Was the mechanism particularly traumatic or were there warning signs of a problem? The circumstances surrounding the injury can immediately affect an athlete's cognitive appraisals and have lasting effects on their coping responses. Though there hasn't been much research into the psychological effects of the inciting event itself, it's not unreasonable to expect that injuries caused by someone else (e.g., in a tackle) might prompt different thought processes than non-contact or overuse injuries. It's tough to know whether feeling as though the injury was someone else's fault would be better or worse than believing your own body let you down, but either way there's a possibility of heightened stress reactions. A sense of having little personal control over the injury contributes to poor outcomes,[8,9] and this can be extreme in some cases. Take for example college gymnast Samantha Cerio, who dislocated both of her knees at a competition in 2019 during a blind landing. It was enough for her to live through it in real time, but video of the event was shared repeatedly over social media to the point that she had to plead for people to stop forcing her to relive it over and over again.[10] Imagine having to cope with one of the worst experiences of your life in the public eye, with constant reminders of how gruesome it was and how much you have to overcome. For many athletes, that kind of stress would be overwhelming, and the early phases of rehabilitation might be especially difficult as a result.

Similarly, injury type can color perceptions, so that's the second parameter to consider. Minor injuries or those that are common in a given sport context may be viewed as less threatening than severe or rare injuries,[9,11,12] though we can't always count on that. For some athletes, even the smallest injury might be devastating if it happens at the wrong time, and major injuries don't elicit overly negative responses from everyone. Plus, certain injury types, like concussions or the dreaded anterior cruciate ligament (ACL) rupture, come with certain expectations about their consequences which can make some athletes worry about their ability to recover.[13] The way other people speak about the injury might affect these perceptions, too – if members of the athlete's social support network are anxious, that's likely to rub off. Yet another factor adding to the complexity of these issues is the recovery timeframe of different injury types. Staring down a lengthy rehabilitation can be daunting to even the most seasoned performer and managing dynamic interactions between personal and situational factors over an extended period presents its own unique challenges.

Where does that leave us? Although there isn't a tried-and-true method of determining which athletes are likely to have a rough time, anticipating what might happen based on the circumstances of their injuries is a good starting place. The way they describe the event and what they think caused it might help us figure out whether or not they feel a sense of control over the situation, which may be an early indicator of distress. From there, we can focus on how other personal and environmental factors might combine to nudge them toward a positive or negative outlook. Let's take a look at a couple of examples of how this has turned out in practice, to get a sense of what we might be looking for.

Restacking the Deck

Cory Sarich was a professional ice hockey player in the National Hockey League (NHL). About two-thirds of the way into his 15-year career, he had what he describes as "*a very intensive battle with osteitis pubis.*" This condition is characterized by pain and deterioration in the cartilage where the pelvic bones meet at the base of the abdomen. He recalls that he first began experiencing a dull ache and, after months of playing with the injury, it became "*excruciatingly painful*" every time he skated with any intensity. He managed to make it through the end of the season but noted that he was only functioning at "*about 85%*" of his ability and could no longer continue playing in that condition. Although his injury didn't have an acute, traumatic mechanism, there were still some key events that started his rehabilitation down a difficult path. The first of these was seeking advice from the team doctor:

> "*His suggestion for treatment after a 20-minute exam was for me to have my pelvis fused together with surgery, and my career would most likely be over! This came as*

quite a shock. I remember driving home from his office with tears in my eyes as I spoke to my wife on the phone. I was rattled."

Here's an example of how communication and the interpersonal climate within a particular sport context can trigger negative responses after an injury event.[1] Even in cases where the injury itself doesn't initially seem too daunting, the reaction of those in the athlete's support network can dramatically affect how they perceive its severity and likely outcome. And it's not just the information itself, but the way in which it's delivered that can impact how it's received and processed. Panic among immediate care providers or teammates can obviously heighten stress responses, for example, but this can play out in more subtle ways as well. When someone in a position of authority is dismissive or condescending in the way they speak about the injury, feelings of mistrust, anxiety, and anger can emerge. In Cory's case, his negative interaction with the doctor prompted him to get a second opinion, which turned out to be a good idea. He ended up working with another doctor who provided an alternative treatment plan over the next several months, with the possibility of saving his career.

> *"The workouts were the most intense and difficult training I did throughout my career. [The doctor] broke me down and built me back up. He told me when we first met that if I wasn't willing to do the work, then I could piss off. He wasn't going to magically fix me. It was going to take total dedication. It was all worth it. I ended up playing for five more years with no residual pain or issues with my pelvis."*

This was a turning point in the story, and it illustrates perfectly the up and down nature of most rehabilitation experiences. After an initially negative cognitive appraisal and emotional response, the situation improved considerably through the interaction of Cory's personal characteristics (e.g., coping style) and a change in the rehabilitation environment. The story also highlights the fact that negative emotions can actually be facilitative. Some athletes channel anger and feelings of diminished physical capacity into active coping strategies like help-seeking and rehabilitation engagement, like getting a second opinion and committing to an intensive treatment plan.[14] This doesn't happen in every case, and it probably depends on the source of one's frustration,[ii] but it goes to show that just because someone is dealt a bad hand, it doesn't mean they can't turn it around. Helping athletes develop the skills to take stock of their thoughts and emotions, reframe them, and use problem-focused coping approaches can help with this. Part of that process might involve addressing who/what the athlete holds responsible for the injury and its outcomes. As Cory explains:

> *"Reflecting back on the injury several years later it dawned on me that it was more than likely a direct result of three other broken bones in my career. In the two seasons prior to the pelvic issues, I suffered a broken right ankle. I wore an air cast for three*

weeks while it healed. I continued with normal off-ice training which involved being on the stationary bike in the air cast every day."

He had two metatarsal fractures the following year, which required additional time in an air cast. Looking back on it, he says, *"I believe it was spending the better part of half a year walking and riding every day in that air cast that messed up my movement patterns and caused my pelvis to deteriorate."*

This raises an interesting discussion about how athletes form causal attributions. *Internal attributions* are when they see the outcome of a situation as being something under their control and caused primarily by their own characteristics or actions. Anything they see as being caused by the situation or factors outside of their control are *external attributions*. We don't know a whole lot about how attributions for the source of an injury affect coping responses, though we can see from Cory's description that it might play a role in coming to terms with their experiences and moving past them. Being able to form a coherent narrative about why and how something has happened can help to dispel uncertainty, which in turn can ease negative emotions.[16] The concept of attribution has also popped up in the rehabilitation literature. There's some evidence that athletes who perceive themselves as recovering rapidly make more internal attributions, or see external factors as being under their control, compared to those who recover more slowly.[17,18] This seems to suggest that internal attributions might prompt more positive injury outcomes, but we need to be careful with that interpretation.

When people make causal attributions for their successes and failures, or indeed anything that happens in their lives, there are a set of cognitive biases that come into play. These are known as *attribution errors*, and we're all prone to making them from time to time. In an injury rehabilitation setting, a few of these in particular might have meaningful influences on athletes' perceptions (or those of their support network). One of these is the *fundamental attribution error*, which describes how we often chalk someone else's behavior up to their personal characteristics, overlooking the input of situational factors.[19] Related to this is the *actor-observer bias*, which is our tendency to attribute others' behavior to their personal characteristics but see our own behavior as a product of our circumstances.[19] Together, these might affect how athletes see injury-inciting events, possibly leading to unhelpful responses (e.g., calling out an opponent for being a "dirty" player without considering how the situation might have driven their actions). There's also evidence that coaches sometimes attribute rehabilitation success – or lack thereof – to an athlete's personal qualities without acknowledging external factors that are also involved.[20] This has clear implications for return to sport and the ongoing coach-athlete relationship. *Self-serving biases* might be a big part of the injury experience, too. These happen when we attribute our personal successes to things under our own control but blame other people or the environment for our failures.[19] Although this could be a helpful short-term way for athletes to maintain emotional control during rehabilitation (e.g., preserving self-image and self-confidence), over time an abdication of responsibility may lead to poor treatment adherence, diminished motivation, and a poor outlook for return to sport.

Managing a Bad Turn

Right, we've considered an injury vignette that showed how initially negative responses might ultimately be turned around for a positive outcome. But what about cases where things end differently? Let's take a look at the experiences of one of Cory's peers as another example. Jason Wiemer played 11 seasons in the NHL and in the 2005–2006 season was playing in the first round of the playoffs. His team was set to win 4–0 in their best of seven series. In the second period of game four, Jason was skating up the ice and took a relatively innocent bump (bearing in mind this is hockey, where "innocent" is a relative term) and he awkwardly twisted his knee. He felt a *"pop"* and significant pain but made it to the bench and headed straight to the locker room for medical assessment. The team doctor examined his knee and determined there was no structural damage, so it was taped up and he played the third period. They won the game, completing the series sweep and earning a week's rest before the next playoff round. During this time Jason recalls that his knee was *"extremely sore"* and made it difficult for him to train, so he asked for an MRI referral. He was told that he had a contusion at the top of his tibia which would cause pain when his knee moved, but he was given clearance to play. In the second round of the playoffs, Jason played five games in his team's six-game series defeat. He remembers that *"the pain was intense, but I didn't want to miss any games."* With the season over, he took three weeks off to recover before beginning off-season training.

Over the summer, workouts proved to be incredibly difficult. The initial pain had subsided, but Jason began to experience concerning instability around the joint; whenever he would jump or run, he could feel his knee wobble. Taking matters into his own hands, he scheduled a private MRI and received drastically different results. The scan showed a complete ACL tear, additional ligament damage, and a severely torn meniscus. He was also told that skating with these injuries (including the bone contusion, which was still visible) could result in lasting damage. When he contacted his team, they *"didn't seem too surprised with the news, they just simply asked where I was going to have the surgery done."* This represents a common scenario across many sports, where an athlete is injured at a crucial moment in the season and there's pressure – both internal and external – to keep playing despite pain and potential longer-term consequences. Whether this occurs at a professional level or in a purely recreational setting, athletes must often rely on medical advice to determine whether or not it's safe to continue, and as we also saw in Cory's case, trust becomes a significant factor. The *therapeutic alliance*, or the working relationship between a patient and their medical care provider, has been shown to affect treatment adherence and outcomes in a number of clinical populations.[21] Although sport-specific evidence is lacking, collaboration, clear communication, therapist empathy, and mutual respect are the cornerstones of an effective alliance in other healthcare settings. Personal bonds between medic and athlete are likely to promote more positive cognitive appraisals, emotional responses, and coping behaviors.[8] In Jason's situation, we can clearly see how the therapeutic alliance eroded almost immediately and set him along a negative path from the start.

Rehabilitation from a significant knee ligament injury is a long, arduous process that typically takes 8–12 months.[22,23] Quite notably, only 55% of patients who undergo ACL reconstruction actually return to competitive sport,[24] often due to lingering performance deficits and concerns about immediate and/or long-term consequences. A key factor in whether or not an athlete is able to return to sport successfully is their adherence to rehabilitation, and there are a number of salient barriers and facilitators that can affect this.[25] In a review of 71 research articles, Walker and colleagues[25] identified patients' perceptions of their relationship with the medical team, the social support they receive from family and friends, interactions with their coach/team, their personal motivation, reinjury fear, and interpersonal comparisons as key factors in rehabilitation success. This matches with Jason's experience. His recovery stretched over a period of eight months and for him, the most difficult things to handle were the countless hours of therapy and the mental strain of staying focused and motivated during that time.

His story also highlights how poor relationships with the medical team and insufficient support from the club can shape the rehabilitation environment. Specifically, Jason returned to a situation where the business of sport played a bigger part in his return than his health or fitness:

> *"It wasn't until January the following year that I was fully rehabbed and ready to play. The only issue was the salary cap – we were right up against it. In order for me to come off Long Term Injured Reserve we would have had to shed my salary and that would have meant taking two guys that had played all year and were contributing players on the team and putting them on waivers, where the team would have surely lost them. All to replace them with me, a 32 year-old winger who hadn't played since May the previous year. I completely understand the reasoning they let me sit [and not be cleared to return to the roster]. The issue I had, and still have, was in the communication. They just pushed me aside, out of sight out of mind. At the end of the season, I had had it. I was frustrated with the game and with the way I had been handled, so I decided to pack it in."*

We'll get into the implications of injuries that force retirement in chapter 12, but Jason's story really brings home the idea that both internal and external factors play a role in shaping injury experiences. As the Integrated Model of Response to Sport Injury points out, personal factors like the athlete's age, sport experience, pain tolerance, and motivation can influence their perceptions of what an injury means and how they respond to it.[1] We can see clearly how each of these factors influenced Jason's recovery (e.g., his ability to play through pain and motivation to return to hockey) and the overall outcome (e.g., his age and experience, which fed into his contract situation). The overarching effect of his external environment certainly speaks for itself, and we can begin to understand how complex the interactions between all of these variables can truly be.

Recognizing a Losing Streak

As common as Jason's story might be, particularly in professional sport, it obviously doesn't represent everyone's pathway through the injury process. There are countless personal and situational factors that might be involved, depending on the sport setting and the athlete's individual circumstances. As just one example, another characteristic that's gaining more attention in the research literature is *athletic identity*. This is defined as the degree to which someone holds their role as an athlete central to who they are as a person.[26] For instance, when we meet someone for the first time, they often ask what we do for a living. Someone with a strong athletic identity might say, "I'm a hockey player." Notice the language – it's not a reference to the fact they play hockey, it's a personal statement about how they see themselves ("I am") and how they'd like to be seen by others. When something challenges this identity, such as an injury forcing them to be away from sport or even causing them to contemplate their future as an athlete, significant emotional distress can emerge.[27] This is consistent with anecdotal accounts of athletes' negative injury experiences that often describe struggles with anxiety or depression, but research in this area has actually been contradictory – some studies have found that athletic identity is positively associated with mood disturbances after injury[28,29] and others haven't.[30] This might be because of two complementary processes that occur when we attempt to maintain a positive self-image: *self-enhancement* and *self-protection*.

Self-enhancement involves trying to promote our good qualities to project a positive self- or public image, whereas self-protection is all about diminishing what we see as our negative features or failures.[31,32] We do this through a number of cognitive processes (e.g., selectively remembering things that make us look good, being careful about who we compare ourselves to) and behaviors (e.g., making excuses for poor performance). We sometimes see this play out when kids try out for a team; if they don't make it, they might say "I didn't really want to play anyway." Well, this same protective mechanism can be activated after a sport injury, when people decrease their identification with the athlete role if the injury itself or rehabilitation difficulties start to threaten their self-image.[33–35] For others, a drive for self-enhancement can renew focus and energize rehabilitation efforts in a bid to get back to the lineup as quickly as possible. Those with strong athletic identity are actually more likely to return to sport after a significant injury;[30] however, over-adherence to treatment or cutting corners in an attempt to return faster can be maladaptive byproducts.[36,37] Unfortunately, such actions put physical health at risk and relapses or reinjuries can be particularly crushing for athletes who are desperate to recover.

A threat to someone's self-perception is obviously only one factor that might affect post-injury responses, but it's important to remember that individual variables like this don't operate in isolation. If we imagine a scenario where an athlete with a strong athletic identity has an injury with a long rehabilitation timeframe, during which they're following a strictly regimented program away from their usual team environment, it's not hard to see how they might fare poorly. That same athlete might not have such a bad time of it in a different environment, with access to a better support network or a more flexible recovery plan. When athletes feel a low sense of *autonomy* – in other words, when they have no control over the injury and have limited decision-making power about their treatment – motivation can really suffer and unhelpful emotional or behavioral coping strategies often emerge.[8,38] Because the rehabilitation environment is so dynamic, though, oftentimes something will change quickly (e.g., swelling might come down) and set that athlete onto a more positive trajectory because they feel as though they've regained the upper hand. But what about cases where a negative spiral, perhaps gradual to begin with, seems to be getting worse and worse? Some athletes end up in a loop of negative cognitive appraisals and worsening emotional problems, no matter what changes in their surroundings. It's like once they've lost control over the situation, they can't seem to get it back. This is where it becomes so important to recognize the signs of an athlete in distress and to intervene early to prevent an extreme outcome.

A number of indicators might emerge when an athlete is in distress. Things like low mood, emotional outbursts, or interpersonal conflicts are simple to spot, but other signs can be more subtle. Stalled rehabilitation progress without a clear physiological cause, for example, can be a warning sign that psychological recovery isn't going well. One contributor to this is *catastrophizing*, which is a bias toward the negative aspects of a situation and a tendency to exaggerate their importance or think they're more influential on the outcome than they really are. For instance, an athlete might dwell on their inability to cope and imagine they'll be unable to recover because of it, or they might anticipate all the things that could go wrong and behave in a way that increases the likelihood that they will (almost like a self-fulfilling prophecy).[39,40] For example, they might believe that intense strengthening exercises will cause damage, so they avoid doing their rehabilitation routine to protect themselves, but this actually slows their recovery progress. Pain catastrophizing in particular, where the athlete interprets pain as an indicator that the situation is worse than it really is, can have some nasty knock-on effects. It can cause an excessive fear of movement because the athlete worries that pain is an indicator that they're vulnerable to re-injury (e.g., "my knee hurts when I bend it, so it mustn't be healed and if I bend too much, I'll hurt myself again"). This fear is also known as *kinesiophobia* and in severe cases, it can cause people to avoid specific movements to the point that they're hypervigilant about pain, have reduced pain tolerance, and ultimately end up with physiological problems from disuse.[41] This is a vicious cycle where fear leads to less movement, which actually promotes pain sensitivity, thereby increasing fear. Chronic pain and depression are known results of this process, not to mention its impact on physical function and sport participation.[39,42,43]

Kinesiophobia isn't the only kind of fear with relevance to the rehabilitation process. Research has shown that athletes often report concerns as they get close to returning to sport, too. These typically involve a fear of re-injury and of not being able to perform to pre-injury levels.[44] This seems to be more pronounced for athletes recovering from their first major injury, those who have a chronic injury with a high likelihood of recurrence, and those with strong athletic identity,[40] but it's certainly not an exclusive phenomenon. And these kinds of fears manifest in different ways. For some athletes, it causes impaired performance in rehabilitation or in training/competition settings after they've returned, because they're hesitant or they hold back effort so as not to put themselves at risk. Others engage in *malingering* behaviors (exaggerating, fabricating, prolonging symptom reports, or intentionally underperforming on return to play tests) to avoid having to go back to sport at all.[45] Now, avoidance coping – which malingering certainly qualifies as – is often seen as debilitating, but contemporary perspectives suggest that it might be facilitative in some cases.[46] When people feel like they have limited control over the outcome of a situation, disengagement can diminish feelings of help-lessness[46] For example, athletes who are under significant pressure may find that being injured provides an excuse to take some time away from training.[1] Staying in the rehabilitation environment for a bit longer than strictly necessary may therefore be beneficial for their mental wellbeing and help them to marshal their coping resources before going back. So, avoidance coping isn't necessarily a bad thing when it comes to managing distress, but in the longer term it's likely to inhibit recovery and malingering in particular could end up preventing athletes from returning to sport at all.

Of course, there's an underlying assumption here that athletes' top priority is recovering and returning to play as quickly and completely as possible. We have to bear in mind that this isn't always the case. People may decide that they no longer wish to pursue sport for various reasons including changing interests or family pressures, or they may become burned out and lose the drive to continue at their current level. Particularly in elite contexts, it can be difficult to exit sport in a graceful way, and injuries are sometimes used as an escape hatch. They can allow someone to retire while maintaining a public image (self-protection), or they can represent a natural transition period to new endeavors. It's important that we don't automatically think of a "failure" to return to sport as a sign of distress, but rather as a viable alternative that athletes might choose in their own best interests.

Shortening the Odds

Don't you hate it when books give meandering descriptions about things that may or may not happen without providing any tangible suggestions for what to do about it? Us, too. In this chapter there's been a lot of talk about how personal and situational factors may lead to negative sport injury outcomes, but the key message is that we don't always know which athletes are going to have problems. From looking at the research and listening to athletes' stories, we find some patterns in the way that certain factors interact with each other to produce unfavorable conditions. That's really helpful, though how strongly an athlete reacts to these, or how long a negative response might last, is much tougher to predict. So, we have two options for managing risk: we can either take a reactive approach and intervene as and when we recognize the signs of distress, or we can proactively help athletes develop cognitive appraisal and coping skills to buffer the stressful effects of an injury if and when one occurs. A combination of both tactics is probably best, though intervention research in this area has been limited so we don't know how effective either might be in practice. The good news is that many of the skills we'd use for injury prevention are appropriate during rehabilitation as well. Activities like journaling or cognitive behavioral therapy can help with reframing situational appraisals in a more positive direction, while stress management techniques (imagery, guided relaxation, self-talk) and problem-focused coping strategies (help-seeking, goal setting) can be useful for steering athletes toward more positive behaviors.[40] Even the best prepared can find themselves overwhelmed, mind you, and even for athletes with strong psychological skills there's a fair chance of difficulties emerging at some point. When signs of anxiety or depression do start to crop up, referring for professional support is typically the best course of action before things get out of hand.

It's important to remember that injuries always come with challenges and eliminating all negativity is an unreasonable aim. Most athletes just have to ride out the ups and downs of the experience and work hard to gain back their confidence, protect their sense of self, and overcome their fears in order to be psychologically ready to return to sport (or move on to whatever their next interest might be).[7] This can take time, in a lot of cases longer than physical recovery does. As we seek to minimize the impact of injury on health and performance, it's important to keep in mind that return to sport isn't the end of the process, and there are often lasting effects on an athlete's mental wellbeing that need to be addressed as well. How best to do that is the next big frontier in this area of research and practice.

Notes

i Bet you thought we were going for a Star Wars reference there, didn't you? Actually, that line brought to mind a quote from Harry Potter and the Order of Phoenix: *"… the world isn't split into good people and Death Eaters."*[6] Injury experiences aren't black and white either, even though we often think of them that way. Not to get too philosophical, of course.
ii Spite and an "I'll show you" mentality are actually very effective motivators for some folks, with some healthy and adaptive behavioral upsides.[15]

References

1 Wiese-Bjornstal DM, Smith AM, Shaffer SM, et al. An integrated model of response to sport injury: psychological and sociological dynamics. *J Appl Sport Psychol* 1998;10(1):46–69; doi:10.1080/10413209808406377.

2 Wiese-Bjornstal DM. Psychology and socioculture affect injury risk, response, and recovery in high-intensity athletes: a consensus statement. *Scand J Med Sci Sports* 2010;20(s2):103–111; doi:10.1111/j.1600-0838.2010.01195.x.

3 von Rosen P, Kottorp A, Friden C, et al. Young, talented and injured: injury perceptions, experiences and consequences in adolescent elite athletes. *Eur J Sport Sci* 2018;8:731–740; doi:10.1080/17461391.2018.1440009.

4 Arvinen-Barrow M, Clement D. Role of emotions in sport injury. In: MC Ruiz, C Robazza. *Feelings in sport: theory, research, and practical implications for performance and well-being.* New York: Routledge 2020; doi:10.4324/9781003052012.

5 Wiese-Bjornstal DM, Wood KN, Kronzer JR. Sport injuries and psychological sequelae. In: G Tenenbaum, RC Eklund (eds.). *Handbook of sport psychology* (4th ed.). Hoboken, NJ: John Wiley & Sons, Inc 2020.

6 Rowling JK. *Harry Potter and the order of the Phoenix.* London: Bloomsbury Publishing Plc 2003.

7 Forsdyke D, Smith A, Jones M, et al. Psychosocial factors associated with outcomes of sports injury rehabilitation in competitive athletes: a mixed studies systematic review. *Br J Sports Med* 2016;50:537–544; doi:10.1136/bjsports-2015-094850.

8 Truong LK, Mosewich AD, Holt CJ, et al. Psychological, social and contextual factors across recovery stages following a sport-related knee injury: a scoping review. *Br J Sports Med* 2020;54:1149–1156; doi:10.1136/bjsports-2019-101206.

9 Clement D, Arvinen-Barrow M, Fetty T. Psychosocial responses during different phases of sport-injury rehabilitation: a qualitative study. *J Athl Train* 2015;50:95–104; doi:10.4085/1062-6050-49.3.52.

10 Bieler D. 'My pain is not your entertainment': gymnast who broke both legs wants people to stop sharing video. Available at: https://nationalpost.com/news/world/my-pain-is-not-your-entertainment-gymnast-who-broke-both-legs-wants-people-to-stop-sharing-injury-video Accessed May 20, 2021.

11 Smith AM, Stuart MJ, Wiese-Bjornstal DM, et al. Competitive athletes: preinjury and postinjury mood state and self-esteem. *Mayo Clin Proc* 1993;68:939–947; doi:10.1016/s0025-6196(12)62265-4.

12 Smith AM, Scott SG, O'Fallon WM, et al. (1990). The emotional responses of athletes to injury. *Mayo Clin Proc* 1990;65:38–50; doi:10.1016/s0025-6196(12)62108-9.

13 Kuhn AW, Yengo-Kahn AM, Kerr ZY, et al. Sports concussion research, chronic traumatic encephalopathy and the media: repairing the disconnect. *Br J Sports Med* 2017;51:1732–1733; doi:10.1136/bjsports-2016-096508.

14 Roy-Davis K, Wadey R, Evans L. A grounded theory of sport injury-related growth. *Sport Exerc Perform Psychol* 2017;6:35–52; doi:10.1037/spy0000080.

15 McCarthy-Jones S. *Spite and the upside of your dark side.* London: Oneworld Publications 2020.

16 Tracey J. The emotional response to the injury and rehabilitation process. *J Appl Sport Psychol* 2003;15:279–293; doi:10.1080/714044197.

17 Laubach WJ, Brewer BW, Van Raalte JL, et al. Attributions for recovery and adherence to sport injury rehabilitation. *Aust J Sci Med Sport* 1996;28:30–34.

18 Brewer BW, Cornelius AE, Van Raalt JL, et al. Attributions for recovery and adherence to rehabilitation following anterior cruciate ligament reconstruction: a prospective analysis. *Psychol Health* 2000;15:283–291; doi:10.1080/08870440008400307.

19 Jhangiani R, Tarry H. Principles of social psychology – 1st International Edition. Creative commons attribution-noncommercial-ShareAlike 4.0 International License. Available at: https://opentextbc.ca/socialpsychology/chapter/biases-in-attribution/. Accessed May 20, 2021.

20 Lewis DK. *Personal and situational bases for coaches' causal attributions for the recovery outcome of injured athletes.* Michigan State University 2004.

21 Babatunde F, MacDermid J, MacIntyre N. Characteristics of the therapeutic alliance in musculoskeletal physiotherapy and occupational therapy practice: a scoping review of the literature. *BMC Health Serv Res* 2017;17:375; doi:doi.org/10.1186/s12913-017-2311-3.

22 Dekker TJ, Godin JA, Dale KM, et al. Return to sport after pediatric anterior cruciate ligament reconstruction and its effect on subsequent anterior cruciate ligament injury. *J Bone Joint Surg* 2017;99:897–904; doi:10.2016/JBJS.16.00758.

23 Myklebust G, Bahr R. Return to play guidelines after anterior cruciate ligament surgery. *Br J Sports Med* 2005;39:127–131; doi:10.1136/bjsm.2004.010900.

24 Ardern CL, Taylor NF, Feller JA, et al. Fifty-five per cent return to competitive sport following anterior cruciate ligament reconstruction surgery: an updated systematic review and meta-analysis including aspects of physical functioning and contextual factors. *Br J Sports Med* 2014;48(21):1543–1552; doi:10.1136/bjsports-2013-093398.

25 Walker A, Hing W, Lorimer A. The influence, barriers to and facilitators of anterior cruciate ligament rehabilitation adherence and participation: a scoping review. *Sports Med Open* 2020;6:32; doi:10.1186/s40798-020-00258-7.

26 Brewer BW, Van Raalte JL, Linder DE. Athletic identity: Hercules' muscles or Achilles heel? *Int J Sport Psychol* 1993;24:237–254.

27 von Rosen P, Heijne, A. Subjective well-being is associated with injury risk in adolescent elite athletes. *Physiother Theory Prac* 2019 2021;37:748–754; doi:10.1080/09593985.2019.1641869.

28 Brewer B. Self-identity and specific vulnerability to depressed mood. *J Pers* 1993;61:343–364; doi:10.1111/j.1467-6494.1993.tb00284.x.

29 Christino MA, Fantry AJ, Vopat BG. Psychological aspects of recovery following anterior cruciate ligament reconstruction. *J Am Acad Orthop Surg* 2015;23:501–509; doi:10.5435/JAAOS-D-14-00173.

30 Green SL, Weinberg RS. Relationships among athletic identity, coping skills, social support, and the psychological impact of injury in recreational participants. *J Appl Sport Psychol* 2001;13:40–59; doi:10.1080/10413200109339003.

31 Grove JR, Fish M, Eklund RC. Changes in athletic identity following team selection self-protection versus self-enhancement. *J Appl Sport Psychol* 2004;16:75–81; doi:10.1080/10413200490260062.

32 Alicke MD, Sedikides C. Self-enhancement and self-protection: what they are and what they do. *Eur Rev Social Psychol* 2009;20:1–48; doi:10.1080/10463280802613866.

33 Brewer BW, Cornelius AE, Stephan Y, et al. Self-protective changes in athletic identity following anterior cruciate ligament reconstruction. *Psychol Sport Exerc* 2010;11:1–5; doi:10.1016/j.psychsport.2009.09.005.

34 Scolnik M, Nakamura Y, Howard A, et al. A qualitative analysis of the psychosocial effects of injury in female athletes. *Graduate J Sport, Exerc Physical Educat Res* 2018;6:29–43.

35 Branstrom H, Fahlstrom M. Kinesiophobia in patients with chronic musculoskeletal pain: differences between men and women. *J Rehabil Med* 2008;40:375–380; doi:10.2340/16501977-0186.

36 Murphy P, Waddington I. Are elite athletes exploited? *Sport Soc* 2007;10(2):239–255; doi:10.1080/17430430601147096.

37 Bianco T. Social support and recovery from sport injury: elite skiers share their experiences. *Res Q Exerc Sport* 2001;72(4):376–388; doi:10.1080/02701367.2001.10608974.

38 Podlog L, Dimmock J, Miller J. A review of return to sport concerns following injury rehabilitation: practitioner strategies for enhancing recovery outcomes. *Phys Ther Sport* 2011;12(1):36–42; doi:10.1016/j.ptsp.2010.07.005.

39 Vlaeyen JWS, Kole-Snijders AMJ, Rotteveel AM, et al. The role of fear of movement/(re)injury in pain disability. *J Occup Rehabil* 1995;5:235–252; doi:10.1007/BF02109988.

40 Hall C, Duncan L, McKay C. *Psychological interventions in sport, exercise & injury rehabilitation.* Dubuque, IA: Kendall Hunt 2014.

41 Miller RP, Kori SH, Todd DD. The Tampa Scale: a measure of kinesiophobia. *Clin J Pain* 1991;7(1):51–52.

42 Flanigan DC, Everhart JS, Pedroza A, et al. Fear of reinjury (kinesiophobia) and persistent knee symptoms are common factors for lack of return to sport after anterior cruciate ligament reconstruction. *Arthroscopy* 2013;29:1322–1329; doi:10.1016/j.arthro.2013.05.015.

43 Watkins R, Young G, Western M, et al. Nobody says to you "come back in six months and we'll see how you're doing": a qualitative interview study exploring young adults' experiences of sport-related knee injury. *BMC Musculoskelet Disord* 2020;21(1):419; doi:10.1186/s12891-020-03428-6.

44 Podlog L, Eklund RC. Return to sport after serious injury: a retrospective examination of motivation and psychological outcomes. *J Sport Rehabil* 2005;14:20–34.

45 Bloom GA, Trbovich AM, Carron JG, et al. Psychological aspects of sport-related concussion: an evidence-based position paper. *J Appl Sport Psychol* 2020; doi:10.1080/10413200.2020.1843200.

46 Carson F, Polman RCJ. The facilitative nature of avoidance coping within sports injury rehabilitation. *Scand J Med Sci Sports* 2010;20:235–240; doi:10.1111/j.1600-0838.2009.00890.x.

9

TECHNOLOGY AND INJURY: LIVING IN THE IRON(MAN) AGE

Carly McKay and Nicol van Dyk

The Rise of Digital Monitoring

Every weekend, billions of fans across the globe enjoy the thrill of watching live sport. We feel the excitement of victory, the disappointment of defeat, cheer for our favorite players and complain about umpiring decisions that don't go our way. Whether it's your favorite football team playing in the final, a new young golf protégé demonstrating skills you can only dream of, or a seasoned race car driver completing the final lap, we participate in every moment. And through the use of technology, these experiences are becoming completely immersive. In real time we get to see the team statistics: metres gained, passes completed, tackles made, possession, territory, the works. The athlete's heart rate, power output, and even their swing dynamics are now on display. These features are captured digitally, allowing fans a much deeper insight into what's happening. But all this represents just the tip of the proverbial data iceberg. For the athlete, the data dive goes much deeper.

We've touched on this already with respect to training load (see Chapter 5), but athlete monitoring in a broader sense aims to capture information in three areas: 1) physiological output and performance, 2) workload, and 3) metabolic changes. Physiological measures such as heart rate and VO_2 max are used to understand performance – how strong is the athlete's "engine"? Workload measures the athlete's exposure to training and competition, and can be as simple as counting playing minutes or as complex as analysing global positioning system (GPS) tracking of sprint metrics. Metabolic changes are measured to understand the effect of training and to inform recovery strategies and schedules for individuals or teams. Only recently has the importance of psychological monitoring been emphasized across all three domains, although we're still not sure how best to integrate this with other metrics to provide actionable insight for performance or health.

DOI: 10.4324/9781003088936-9

In principle, the overall concept here isn't new. Athletes and coaches have long kept logbooks and training diaries to understand exactly what they're doing and how they're improving. With every leap forward in technology, though, their ability to quantify training and performance takes a commensurate step forward. Not too long ago, heart rate was measured by finding a radial pulse and counting. Now they can strap on a monitor for continuous recording during a session. These kinds of advances in modern technology (wireless data capture through wearable devices in particular), has changed the landscape significantly. Professional athletes have become accustomed to wearing sensors when they train and play, and even the average recreational athlete (or fitness buff) is used to their smartphone acting as a GPS device or their watch measuring their vital signs. CCS Insight, a research firm that studies the wearable technology market, has projected that sales of smart wearables for fitness will double between 2020 and 2025, approaching 1.2 billion devices in use by the end of that period.[1] There's no sign of the trend slowing, either. This booming market has given rise to digital platforms such as Strava™ and Garmin™, to enable real time data sharing. And there are a host of companies vying for a slice of this pie in professional sport as well, all hoping to capture data that provide insights to give athletes a competitive edge.

Although advances and development in this space are exciting, we have to understand the potential benefits and harms of such technologies. While they might lead to better performances, this may come at a price. Let's take a look at how digital monitoring influences athlete behavior and wellbeing, and how these practices are shaping injury rehabilitation.

Harder, Better, Faster, Stronger[i]

Given the unbelievable popularity of superhero films over the last decade or so (and the comic books well before them), it's impossible to ignore the parallels between the origin stories of some of their characters and modern-day athletes. Whether your preferences run to DC Comics or Marvel, one of the most common backstories involves an average person who, through the use of advanced technology and cutting-edge science, has transformed into a powerful avenger (pun intended). This might be the result of intentional experimentation (e.g., Steve Rogers, the Bionic Woman) or simply the development and use of advanced technology (e.g., Batman). Either way, it exposes our human limitations and subsequent desire to overcome them. In a sense, the current drive to quantify every aspect of human performance through wearables and monitoring devices tells a similar tale – we're figuring out where the limits are and using technology to push beyond.

For elite athletes, this approach totally makes sense. As the saying goes, there's no prize for second place and the margins for victory have become increasingly small. In fact, when we look at how close the gold medal races were at the 2016 Rio Olympics, the values are startling. In the women's cycling time trial, Kristin Armstrong beat Olga Zabelinskaya by just 0.21% (<6 seconds over 44 minutes of racing). Usain Bolt beat Justin Gatlin in the men's 100m sprint by 0.09 seconds.[2] Of course, winning is one thing, but many athletes are well aware that they might never crack the top three and often just staying competitive at the highest level is difficult. For example, F1 driver Chris Amon started 96 grand prix during his career and despite leading for a total of 183 laps across this span, he didn't win a single race (he lost one by just 1.1 second). In such a competitive landscape, the motivation to find that extra edge has become relentless.

Enter the age of athlete monitoring and the high-tech sport approach. Coaches and training staff, and in many cases athletes themselves, now rely on quantifiable data to find those smallest of improvements that might make a difference on the goal line. Table 9.1 lists a number of technological applications in the performance context, all of which are common across different sports. Primarily, these monitoring techniques aim to determine athletes' responses to training and evaluate their physical outputs. For instance, with GPS tracking devices, we now know how much high-speed running an athlete does compared to the total distance covered and we're able to determine their work rate (often described as training

TABLE 9.1 Technological applications in the performance context (reprinted with permission from the Aspetar Sports Medicine Journal)[7]

Technology and Performance Context		
Contexts for technology application	*Purpose of technological application*	*Examples*
Determining characteristics of elite performers	To provide evidence-based determination of the characteristics of an elite athlete	VO_2 max testing; genotyping; mathematical modeling of performance; force plates; GPS
Identifying talent	To assist in the process of recognizing high-quality raw materials (i.e., talented athletes)	Dynamometers; ergometers; strain gauges; angle sensors; communications technology to enable fast transmission of information about talent
Testing and refining performance	To develop skill; to improve decision making to improve physiological capacity; to analyze individual and team performance; to diagnose, prevent, and manage injury and illness; to complement quality coaching	Technologies to rapidly assess immunological status; athlete tracking devices; Dartfish in individual sports; Sportscode; cooling vests; highly engineered equipment; scientifically advanced race wear
Monitoring competition performance outcomes	To objectively analyze individual and team performance and monitor outcomes in training and competition	Video analysis and software programs

zone) in any activity. These data can be compared to previous sessions or plotted against targets they're hoping to achieve, allowing training programs to be developed and adjusted with greater effectiveness. And it's working, too. Advances in training practices have led to dramatic shifts in athlete fitness and strength, as well as playing intensity in some sports.[3,4,ii] Of course, not all of this can be attributed to athlete monitoring – a better understanding of human physiology and biomechanics certainly plays a big part – but real time feedback and various metrics have allowed athletes and coaches to get a much more granular perspective on where their competitive advantages lie, and where a little more gain can be found.

On top of the apparent physical performance benefits of athlete monitoring, having access to a steady stream of information can support the implementation of some psychological skills as well. Performance statistics and physiological feedback often indicate an athlete's progress toward a set goal[8] and may help when identifying performance targets. As evidence suggests hitting the right combination of appropriate goal difficulty and specificity seems to improve performance outcomes, monitoring data is proving quite useful in forming these parameters during goal setting exercises.[9] For instance, identifying a particular indicator to work on (e.g., relative peak power output during a countermovement jump) and estimating what would be an attainable improvement in that value can be informed by an athlete's existing data. Furthermore, it's been suggested that self-set, participatory, and assigned goals may all be facilitative in sport – after all, personal and team outcomes are equally important – so keeping tabs on individual and collective metrics may be valuable to all stakeholders involved.[9]

There's risk in this level of monitoring that needs to be acknowledged, though. Every day, athletes are asked about their wellbeing, training status, recovery, and readiness to participate or compete. They're strapped in, wired up, and assessed on every parameter imaginable. Aside from the tedium and burden of this routine, the act of measurement itself can lead to a bunch of unintended consequences. Specifically, when people know they're being watched (either actively or passively), they often change their behavior. During the 1920s, employees at the Western Electric company in Hawthorne, near Chicago, were assessed for their productivity.[10] The best performance was observed among a selected group of workers who were supervised intensively by their managers, and thus the *Hawthorne effect* was born. This is a well-known bias in research (sometimes called a *demand effect*) whereby the awareness of being studied leads people to adapt their actions, often to match the expectations of the researcher or to model "good" behavior. So, what they do in the context of a study (or while being monitored) may not represent what happens the rest of the time.

The rabbit hole goes much deeper than that, too. It seems only natural that someone would alter their behavior when being monitored, but once they become accustomed to the scrutiny, return to their regular patterns. When once again made aware of the observers, the cycle repeats itself. Think of an athlete catching a glimpse of themselves on the big screen at a live match. They might quickly pat down the disheveled hair that didn't seem to matter a few seconds ago in the heat of competition, and once the play begins again that vanity is soon forgotten. This underlying, oscillating awareness of being watched can affect an athlete's psychological wellbeing; constantly thinking of the image they portray can trigger *self-presentation anxiety*. Athletes don't like to appear unfit compared to their teammates or opponents, or even against a coach's expectations.[11] Unfortunately, when every aspect of their sporting life is being quantified, it's very difficult to manage others' perceptions. This is of particular concern after injury, when physical self-perception might be impaired and objective markers of fitness are likely to be below the athlete's previous standard. When returning to the training environment, external evaluation is inevitable when the numbers are being tracked on a daily basis. If this information is made public, as is increasingly the case, social anxieties can become pronounced and potentially debilitating. For instance, preliminary research has shown that self-presentation anxiety is associated with choking and the yips, not to mention problems with rehabilitation adherence.[12,13]

So, what's an athlete to do? Impression management can be approached in a lot of different ways, but the easiest solution is to lie. That's right, some athletes don't provide accurate responses when asked for monitoring data. Take rate of perceived exertion (RPE) for example, which captures the subjective intensity of a training session or match. Given how often they're asked that question, athletes often end up defaulting to their "regular" score. But, if an athlete wants to appear fitter, they'll say the session wasn't that difficult (or if they want a day off, they might go the other way). Athletes have also been known to "sandbag" pre-season assessments so that decrements in performance (or the occurrence of an injury) goes undetected later on.[14] Of course, these are overt and deliberate actions that in reality are probably less widespread than we might think; however, repetitive subjective measurements and a culture of constant query may lead athletes to devalue the process. In turn, they may only complete questionnaires for the sake of the task or their responses might be affected by *self-report* or *social desirability biases*.[15] These occur when athletes don't disclose information (e.g., under-reporting negative wellbeing) or they answer in a way they think others expect or want them to. Not only will this affect data quality, it can also mask important health and wellbeing issues. Self-handicapping[iii] is also not out of the question as a strategy for athletes to manage others' expectations, though this has not yet been investigated in the context of athlete monitoring.

Altogether, there are some potentially unfavorable side effects of current monitoring practices, psychologically speaking. There's also a "Big Brother" feeling about the whole thing.[iv] Jeremy Bentham, an 18th century English philosopher, wrote about the *Panopticon*, a hypothetical building design that would enable a single observer (e.g., a prison guard) to see everyone in the institution (e.g., prisoners) from a tower in the centre of a rotunda.[17] In this scenario, it would be impossible for the observer to see everyone simultaneously, but because the subjects wouldn't be able to tell who was being watched at any particular moment, they would all be compelled to regulate their behavior. This very literal application has since been extended as a metaphor for power structures and the modern ability to accumulate surveillance data to shape peoples' actions.[18] And now the lens has turned to digital monitoring tools in sport. Jones and colleagues[19] explored GPS tracking in professional rugby and found that wearing a GPS vest caused players to feel constantly under observation, even if the coach wasn't systematically collecting and using the data. Some of this was related to anxiety around how the data could be deployed, such as sanctioning certain behaviors, affecting selection, or influencing contract negotiations.[19] This raises concerns about the long-term mental strain placed on athletes in these situations and prompts some important ethical questions about power relations and the future of such practices.

The (Super)Man in the Mirror

It's one thing to be worried about the consequences inflicted by external digital monitoring, but another thing entirely when we do it to ourselves. Tracking mood, sleeping patterns, nutrition, and fitness is now commonplace in recreational sport and exercise and this is generally seen as empowering, a means by which individuals can control the determinants of their own performance and quality of life.[20] Much like Tony Stark constantly working to adapt and improve his Iron Man suit, people are now able to use technology to maximize their personal training, plot their daily routines, and learn about their own responses to various challenges. But what motivates this level of self-assessment?

Self-determination theory is the most well-developed macro-theory of human motivation, comprising six mini-theories to describe different sources of motivation and their role in cognitive and social development, individual differences, wellbeing, and performance.[21] Entire volumes have covered its development in detail[21] and we won't summarize all of that here. Instead, let's focus on how it applies to behavioral regulation with respect to digital self-monitoring.

In brief, self-determination theory suggests that motivation exists along a continuum (Figure 9.1).[22] At the one end, people can be *amotivated*, meaning they have zero intention of engaging in a given behavior. Forms of *controlled motivation* come next, where behaviors are largely directed by external factors like reward/punishment. As one progresses toward the autonomous end of the spectrum, behaviors are increasingly driven by personal values and a desire to seek opportunities for growth. *Intrinsic motivation*, as the extreme end of the scale, describes those situations where we engage in a behavior simply for the joy or inherent value of the behavior itself (like dancing when nobody's watching).

There are three basic needs that underpin movement along the continuum: autonomy, competence, and relatedness. *Autonomy* is the desire to be a causal agent in one's own life, a sense of having free will when choosing how to act. *Competence* speaks to feelings of mastery and *relatedness* is borne from the human imperative to interact with and be accepted by others. If the environment satisfies these needs, motivation becomes increasingly autonomous, whereas need-thwarting environments have the opposite effect.[23] Bear in mind that this is a very simple overview and in reality, motivation is a lot messier than that; however, it

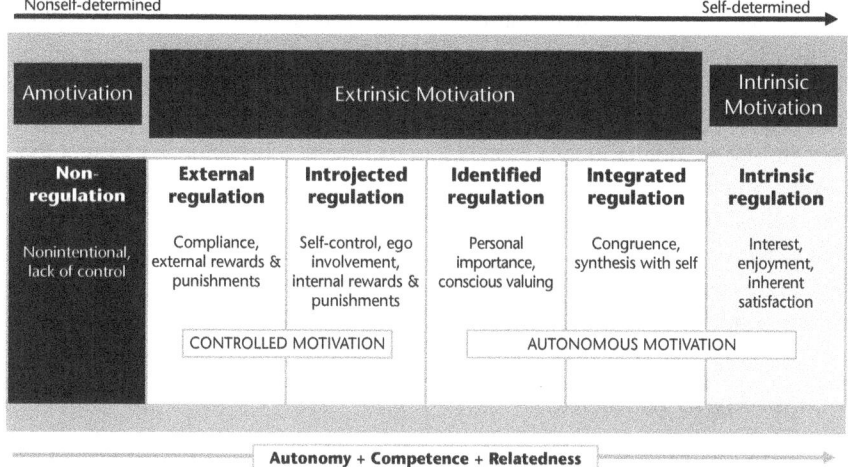

FIGURE 9.1   A composite representation of Self-Determination Theory.

provides a foundation to see how digital monitoring can shape – or be shaped – by one's motivational climate.

In elite sport, athletes who only comply with monitoring under the terms of their contract or in response to team norms likely sit at the controlled end of the continuum (they're doing it because they have to). When athletes see value in monitoring and attach personal importance to what it provides, they start to become more autonomously motivated. People who self-monitor likely sit toward the right-hand side of our diagram, particularly if they're doing it out of pure interest rather than having a defined performance goal. What's more, if monitoring is congruent with one's basic needs, say by being self-directed (autonomy) and helping them track improvement or goal achievement (competence), then the behavior will be reinforced. And achievement satisfaction is one thing, but a lot of athletes also happen to be competitive. Platforms allowing data sharing and social comparison (e.g., Strava, where people post their workout metrics) or which are gamified (e.g., apps that allow users to run from virtual zombies[v]) can satisfy the need for relatedness as well. So can being part of a social group/team of other self-monitoring people.

Self-monitoring is generally seen as adaptive, though for some it can be problematic. There's a risk that digital feedback can undermine competence, particularly if athletes are unable to reach their goals or experience performance setbacks. This starts to tip motivational processes toward amotivation.[24,25] For users of interactive or data sharing platforms, constant comparison with others can have the same effect when those comparisons are unfavorable.[24] Furthermore, there's emergent evidence that wearable fitness trackers can be associated with *exercise dependence* (a pattern of exercise that leads to impairment or distress, often with a loss of control over exercise volume and symptoms of withdrawal if stopped).

Wearables can exacerbate harmful compulsions and emotional distress in young people who exercise.[26] This increases the likelihood of overuse injury and other health problems like disordered eating and relative energy deficiency in sport (RED-S).[26,27] These issues obviously diminish physical and mental health, but there are also reports of people engaging in maladaptive behaviors when wearing trackers. Much like motorists who drive their cars into lakes at the instruction of their navigation systems, athletes are sometimes prompted to ignore environmental cues in pursuit of competitive records. Anecdotes abound of STRAVA™ users ignoring traffic light signals to achieve personal bests, for example, and a lot of these people end up severely injured.[28]

Technology as Medicine

In terms of the digital revolution in sport, it's important to remember that the primary driver has been performance enhancement. Applications in injury rehabilitation and prevention have had much less fanfare. Functional and efficient digital health tools really are in their infancy, yet their scope for improving athlete care is extensive. Although we're still a way off from some of the fanciful medical interventions we see in futuristic films, technology in healthcare is experiencing a rapid period of development. In addition to the smartwatches and hearing aids we've grown accustomed to, we're now seeing electronic/optical tattoos, head-mounted displays, subcutaneous sensors, smart footwear, and electronic textiles popping up in clinical settings to provide medical alerts or measure physical and biochemical information.[29] In the near future, there's hope that these might even be used for drug delivery. Technology isn't just for passive monitoring anymore, it's becoming an active intervention in its own right. This means that athletes, their care providers, and coaches/trainers/sport scientists now have unprecedented access to monitoring data with the ability to use that information in real-time during treatment.

The key to all of this is *biofeedback*, a process that uses physiological or biomechanical assessments to enhance athletes' awareness of emotions, thoughts, or behaviors. Basically, a device measures a particular indicator like heart rate or foot pressure and then emits a signal to the athlete to trigger an immediate response. It's been used very successfully to enhance sport performance by reducing anxiety, decreasing sympathetic arousal, and promoting self-regulation skills (e.g., breathing techniques).[30] Similar benefits can be seen in rehabilitation settings. Using heart rate variability as biofeedback has a small effect on symptom management and emotional health for people with pain, depression, and anxiety.[31] Neurofeedback (e.g., brain wave information) appears to be promising in the treatment of post-concussion syndrome,[32] and real-time gait or movement biofeedback can reliably improve high-risk biomechanics when running, squatting, or performing other rehabilitation exercises.[33,34] So, what the best form of biofeedback? Some modern systems provide visual information to athletes using independent screens or watches, others emit an auditory signal to alert the user to a particular threshold in their metrics, and newer devices can deliver vibro-tactile feedback. Research is ongoing to determine which of these prompts the most effective and sustained behavioral adaptation, but for now all of them seem to work.

In addition to its immediate benefits, the overall success of biofeedback, and indeed simpler approaches like using activity trackers to support clinical decision-making, lies in its ability to facilitate goal-directed actions and promote adherence to rehabilitation programs. As in a sport performance context, digital monitoring during treatment can help athletes and their caregivers form salient, appropriate goals and assess their progress toward them. As we know, goal attainment can be particularly important in this setting for sustained motivation and emotional regulation. For athletes, objective data can provide reassurance to athletes that the improvements they observe are real. This can help with expectation management by informing realistic perceptions about recovery speed and thresholds for return to play clearance.

Monitoring data can also bring richness to guided imagery exercises. By giving athletes a tangible appreciation for their physiological responses, it can help them to form multisensory imagery, enhancing the effects of that technique. Together, these may instill athletes with a greater sense of control over their recovery (e.g., boosting autonomy and competence), thereby contributing to greater engagement with the rehabilitation process. After all, rehab programs only work if people do them. Early evidence suggests that digital tools can improve adherence to traditional physiotherapy when used as alternative or adjunct interventions (e.g., gamifying exercise goals[35]) and this is likely to be an area of considerable research interest in the coming years.

The Downside to Technology as Medicine

Aside from similar consequences to monitoring for performance (e.g., controlled motivation, anxiety, fatigue), there are some unique issues that bear more dedicated attention than they've had up to this point. *Over-adherence*, for example, sometimes occurs when athletes do too much in the hopes of speeding up their recovery. As an analogue to exercise dependence, digital feedback can trigger an unhealthy fixation on specific treatment milestones and cause athletes to push themselves beyond safe or reasonable limits to achieve (or exceed) them. Obviously, this can lead to setbacks and/or subsequent injury, not only putting the athlete's mental wellbeing at risk but also reducing their confidence in the value of the rehabilitation approach.[36] Furthermore, we have to be aware that some athletes thrive on information and want to know everything about their condition and how they're healing. Others find that overwhelming.

The *Paradox of Choice* refers to the idea that people often put off acting or making a decision when they've got too many options to select from.[37] Extending this to a rehabilitation setting, a simultaneous focus on lots of different metrics might make it difficult to decide which should be targeted at what point. Trying to interpret a whole bunch of data can become very confusing and, conceivably, athletes who find it all a bit too much may end up with so-called *analysis paralysis* – not doing anything because they don't know where to start.

The accumulation of datasets isn't just a concern for athletes, either. One of the biggest unknowns in this developing topic area is how data might shape practitioner or coach behavior. It's an interesting phenomenon that when people have more data, they tend to be more confident in their decisions, but they aren't always more accurate. An oft-quoted Central Intelligence Agency (CIA) report detailed an exercise they conducted with a group of oddsmakers using a collection of horse races where the outcome was already known (though not to the bookies themselves). They were given increasingly more information about the races and were asked to pick a winner and assign a confidence level to that bet. Amazingly, with each additional piece of information, confidence rose dramatically though the accuracy of their predictions didn't change.[38] We might encounter the same thing during sport injury rehabilitation. With more and more data available on which to make treatment and/or return to play decisions, it's likely that confidence will increase but we don't know if any of that information will make meaningful changes in rehabilitation outcomes. Moreover, when the clinimetric properties of the digital tools (i.e., reliability, minimal clinically important difference, diagnostic sensitivity and specificity) aren't well established for the population in which they're being used, there's the double whammy of having imprecise information to work from as well.

Based on the work of Daniel Kahneman and Amos Tversky,[39] the CIA experiment nicely illustrated the *anchoring and adjustment heuristic*. When we need to estimate the value of something, we generally make an initial guess (anchoring) and then adjust it up or down based on available information. Confidence increases with every adjustment, but it turns out that whatever the final estimate ends up being, it's usually biased toward the original anchor. Contract negotiations work on this principle – players are offered an amount (the anchor) and it's adjusted up or down based on contextual details like their performance in the previous season. If the team manager sets the initial anchor low, the final contract is likely to be skewed in that direction (assuming the athlete doesn't walk away and sign someplace else).

By the same token, this heuristic can change our interpretation of values we're presented with. If you're shopping for a sweater and the first one you see costs $1200, then the second one for $200 will seem cheap by comparison, even though it's still objectively expensive. The exact same problem might arise when interpreting monitoring data in rehabilitation. If there's a particular metric or threshold set as an a-priori criterion for a return to play decision, it anchors the interpretation of subsequently collected data to that value and assessment of the athlete's progress may be biased relative to that target. Obviously, the athlete needs to have healed and be medically safe to resume training. But if criteria are based on either an "average" indicator of recovery or an assumption about a sufficient level of performance to rejoin the team, then the decision might fail to account for the athlete's individual context. Not everyone regains their pre-injury performance levels, and a "successful" rehabilitation might be defined differently depending on the athlete's role, career stage, and skillset, not to mention the type and seriousness of the injury. Using group-derived metrics is therefore a reductionist approach which might artificially raise or lower the bar for a return to play decision.

Probability judgments are also affected by the *representativeness heuristic*.[39] This means that we tend to categorize objects or events based on their similarity to things we've come across before. Stereotypes are a good example – we've got a prototype in our mind and if someone comes along who seems to fit it, we categorize them as such without too much thought. This mental shortcut is efficient, cognitively speaking, but it often causes us to overestimate the similarity between things we're comparing. Ultimately, we can end up seeing correlations that aren't really there. Take a group of athletes who've experienced the same injury in their careers. We might have a concept of how long their rehabilitation took and what the outcome was, so when someone else has a similar diagnosis, there's a tendency for us to lump them into the same category. It doesn't matter that every athlete responds to injury differently and plenty of variables can affect recovery, our expectations will usually be the same. So, when it comes to return to play decisions, there's a risk that monitoring data might be assessed through this heuristic. If an athlete's recovery metrics are similar to those of other athletes with the same injury, assumptions might be made about their ability to return even if they aren't psychologically ready.

Superhero or Supervillain?

While treatment and medical return to play decisions are largely based on clinical reasoning, and rightfully so, there's a danger in slipping toward a reliance on objective markers of fitness in coaching. It's easy to imagine how the interpretation of various metrics might be colored by a heuristic lens, with potential effects on player availability, allocation of playing time/team roles, or even contract negotiations. Now, there's a big difference between being data-driven and data-informed (Figure 9.2), and the former is akin to operating on autopilot. Blindly trusting the values, or the output of an algorithm or data-driven neural network (i.e., machine learning or artificial intelligence), removes the context-sensitive interpretation of what the information means for individual athletes. Instead, objective data should be used to inform shared decision-making processes, appreciating the experiences, beliefs, and social influences that may lead to very different decisions for different people, even when the objective data might look the same.

The truth is, technology development is far outpacing research and, as a result, the implications of digital monitoring for mental wellbeing is poorly understood. What we need first is a better appreciation for the value of the data being captured so we can concentrate on the minimum number of variables necessary to facilitate physical and psychological recovery. There's no sense in collecting information that isn't practically useful, so for now the imperative is to minimize athlete

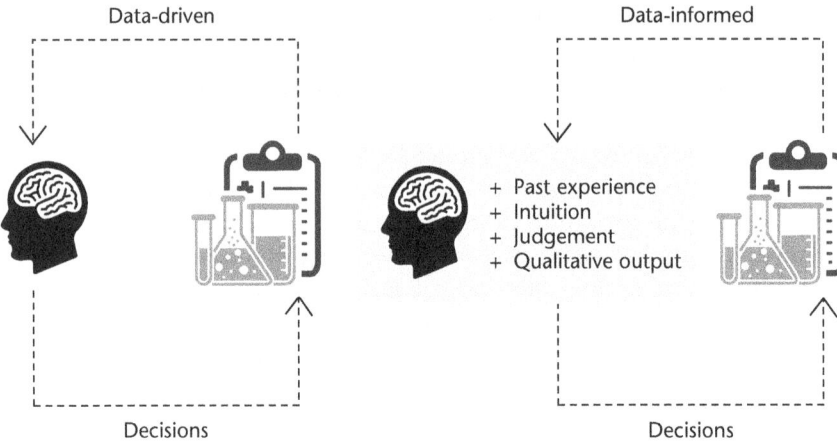

FIGURE 9.2 The difference between decision making that is data-driven versus data-informed.

burden, but greater consideration is needed around how the possible pressures of surveillance affect sport/injury experiences. Therefore, the second priority needs to be unpicking the relationships between information delivery and behavior. If we can determine how athletes, practitioners, and coaches respond to monitoring as a process, we can establish guidelines for beneficial (rather than detrimental) use.

The Peter Parker Principle

Even if you're not Spider-man, you'll recognize the popularized phrase, *"with great power comes great responsibility."* The advantages we may gain from greater monitoring and surveillance need to be balanced with what's good for the individual (and the group). Consider the implications if clubs allow an athlete to compete when they're deemed "at risk" of injury based on their metrics, for instance. And might athletes reconsider their willingness to accept injury risks if the data used to make coaching decisions is also made available to them? These murky ethical and/ or legal areas have been largely unexplored but have great potential to affect the sport landscape moving forward. A certain amount of respect therefore needs to be given to the power of technology in the sport injury space because, given the healthy dose of moral ambiguity around its application, it could easily become the Ozymandias[vi] of the story – incredible potential to support athletes, but possibly at the cost of their welfare.

The future success of technology in sport largely relies on our ability to integrate objective measures with our subjective clinical reasoning skills. Developing both these areas is important and, to this end, a number of questions remain. What's the best way to provide digital feedback to users? How do we create autonomy-supportive digital tools? What's the most effective way to integrate monitoring into regular sport and clinical practice? In the evolving landscape of technological advances, it is imperative that we continue to ask these questions because we know that many of our modern-day monitoring practices influence behavior and psychological wellbeing. Understanding how to make these practices safe, unintrusive, and meaningful to the athlete should be our primary goal. We want to provide all athletes with the greatest chance of participation and ultimate performance, but not at any cost.

Notes

i Good luck getting that song out of your head. If you have no idea what we're referring to, it's an iconic single from Daft Punk's 2001 *Discovery* album that went on to win a Grammy in 2009 for its live version recording. Check it out.

ii Importantly, increases in sport performance follow a non-linear trend as we approach physiological limits. World records are being broken at a slower rate than in recent decades,[5] although it may not seem like it because instant media access lets us know about them much more often these days. Equipment/rule changes are likely to be a greater source of improvement than training methods moving forward (e.g., rapidly falling marathon times with the advent of a particular shoe[6]), but a notable exception is in team sport. Where performance is not simply a product of speed, endurance, or strength, tactical, and open skill development are areas where there may yet be considerable gains.

iii *Claimed self-handicaps* are excuses athletes make ahead of time, just in case they perform poorly (like saying they're tired or injured). *Behavioral self-handicaps* are things like not practising, which provide tangible explanations for poor outcomes. For a nice review on the topic, see Coudevylle et al.[16]

iv If you don't know where the Big Brother metaphor originally came from, go read Nineteen Eighty-Four by George Orwell. Now. Put this book down and find a copy of that one (we won't be mad about it, and you can pick us up again when you're done).

v Yes, these exist. No, we haven't tried them.

vi Ozymandias is a principal character in the celebrated graphic novel series *Watchmen* by Alan Moore, Dave Gibbons, and John Higgins. He tried to save the world from impending nuclear doom by engineering an alien attack to unite everyone against a common foe – a true hero turned villain.

References

1 CCS Insight. Healthy outlook for wearables as users focus on fitness and wellbeing. Available at: https://www.ccsinsight.com/press/company-news/healthy-outlook-for-wearables-as-users-focus-on-fitness-and-well-being/ Accessed May 28, 2021.

2 Armstrong M. Rio 2016 vs. the world: percentage margin of victory. Available at: https://www.statista.com/chart/5597/rio-2016-vs-the-world_-percentage-margin-of-victory/ Accessed May 28, 2021.

3 Hill NE, Rilstone S, Stacey MJ, et al. Changes in northern hemisphere male international rugby union players' body mass and height between 1955 and 2015. *BMJ Open Sport Exerc Med* 2018;4:e000459; doi:10.1136/bmjsem-2018-000459

4 Eaves S, Hughes M. Patterns of play of international rugby union teams before and after the introduction of professional status. *Int J Perform Anal Sport* 2003;3(2):103–111; doi: 10.1080/24748668.2003.11868281.

5 Berthelot G, Sedeaud A, Marck A, et al. Has athletic performance reached its peak? *Sports Med* 2015;45:1263–1271; doi:doi.org/10.1007/s40279-015-0347-2.

6 Reuters. Factbox: Nike's Vaporfly running shoes and tumbling records. Available at: https://www.reuters.com/article/athletics-shoe-idINKBN1ZN0NN. Accessed May 28, 2021.

7 Ringuet-Riot C, James A. How innovative are you? High performance sport training centres. Available at: https://www.aspetar.com/Journal/viewarticle.aspx?id=19#.YK92SflKhPY Accessed May 28, 2021. Permission requested from Publisher.

8 Kingston KM, Wilson KM. The application of goal setting in sport. In: S Mellalieu, S Hanton (eds.). *Advances in applied sport psychology: a review*. Abingdon, Oxon: Routledge 2009.

9 Jeong YH, Healy LC, McEwan D. The application of Goal Setting Theory to goal setting interventions in sport: a systematic review. *Int Rev Sport Exerc Psychol* 2021; doi: 10.1080/1750984X.2021.1901298.

10 McCambridge J, Witton J, Elbourne DR. Systematic review of the Hawthorne effect: new concepts are needed to study research participation effects. *J Clin Epidemiol* 2014;67:267–277; doi:10.1016/jclinepi.2013.08.015.

11 Podlog L, Dimmock J, Miller J. A review of return to sport concerns following injury rehabilitation: practitioner strategies for enhancing recovery outcomes. *Phys Ther Sport* 2011;12:36–42; doi:10.1016/j.ptsp.2010.07.005.

12 Clarke P, Sheffield D, Akehurst S. Personality predictors of yips and choking susceptibility. *Front Psychol* 2020;10:2784; doi:10.3389/fpsyg.2019.02784.

13 Gledhill A, Ivarsson A. Believe in your ability to create change: psychosocial factors influencing sports injury rehabilitation adherence. In: A Gledhill, Forsdyke A (eds.). *The psychology of sports injury*. Abingdale, Oxon: Routledge 2021.

14 Higgins KL, Denney RL, Maerlender A. Sandbagging on the Immediate Post-Concussion Assessment and Cognitive Testing (ImPACT) in a high school athlete population. *Arch Clin Neuropsychol* 2017;32:259–266; doi:10.1093/arclin/acw108.

15 Delgado-Rodriguez M, Llorca J. Bias. *J Epidemiol Community Health* 2004;58:635–641; doi:10.1136/jech.2003.008466.

16 Coudevylle G, Martin Ginis K, Famose JP. Determinants of self-handicapping strategies in sport and their effects on athletic performance. *Soc Behav Pers: Int J* 2008;36:391–398; doi:10.2224/sbp.2008.36.3.391.

17 Bentham J. *Panopticon or the inspection house (1791)*. Montana: Kessinger Publishing 2009.

18 Foucault M. *Discipline and punish: the birth of the prison*. London: Penguin Books Ltd. 1977.

19 Jones L, Marshall P, Denison J. (2016). Health and well-being implications surrounding the use of wearable GPS devices in professional rugby league: a Foucauldian disciplinary analysis of the normalized use of a common surveillance aid. *Perform Enhance Health* 2016;5:38–46; doi:10.1016/j.peh.2016.09.001.

20 De Moya JF, Pallud J. From panopticon to heautopticon: a new form of surveillance introduced by quantified-self practices. *Inf Syst J* 2020;30:940–976; doi: 10.1111/isj.12284.

21 Ryan RM, Deci EL. *Self-determination theory: basic psychological needs in motivation, development, and wellness*. New York: Guilford Press 2017.

22 Deci EL, Ryan RM. Self-determination theory: a macrotheory of human motivation, development, and health. *Can Psychol* 2008;49:182–185; doi:10.1037/a0012801.

23 Bartholomew KJ, Ntoumanis N, Ryan RM, et al. Psychological need thwarting in the sport context: assessing the darker side of athletic experience. *J Sport Exerc Psychol* 2011;33(1):75–102; doi:10.1123/jsep.33.1.75.

24 Kerner C, Goodyear VA. The motivational impact of wearable healthy lifestyle technologies: a self-determination perspective on Fitbits with adolescents. *Am J Health Ed* 2017;48:287–297; doi:10.1080/19325037.2017.1343161.

25 Gowin M, Cheney M, Gwin S, et al. Health and fitness app use in college students: a qualitative study. *Am J Health Ed* 2015;46(4):223–230; doi:10.1080/19325037.2015.1044140.

26 Blackstone SR, Herrmann LK. Fitness wearables and exercize dependence in college women: considerations for university health education specialists. *American Journal of Health Education* 2020;51:225–233; doi:10.1080/19325037.2020.1767004.

27 Mountjoy M, Sundgot-Borgen J, Burke L, et al. The IOC consensus statement: beyond the female athlete triad—relative energy deficiency in sport (RED-S). *Br J Sports Med* 2014;48:491–497; doi:10.1136/bjsports-2014-093502.

28 Hill K. A quantified self fatality? Family says cyclist's death is fault of ride-tracking company. Available at: https://www.forbes.com/sites/kashmirhill/2012/06/20/a-quantified-self-fatality-family-says-cyclists-death-is-fault-of-ride-tracking-company-strava/ Accessed May 28, 2021.

29 Yetizen AK, Martinez-Hurtado JL, Ünal B, et al. Wearables in medicine. *Adv Mater* 2018;30(33):1706910; doi:10.1002/adma.201706910.

30 Ferguson KN, Hall C. Sport biofeedback: exploring implications and limitations of its use. *Sport Psychol* 2020;34:232–241; doi:10.1123/tsp.2019-0109.

31 Lehrer P, Kaur K, Sharma A, et al. Heart rate variability biofeedback improves emotional and physical health and performance: a systematic review and meta-analysis. *Appl Psychophysiol Biofeedback* 2020;45:109–129; doi:10.1007/s10484-020-09466-z.

32 Bonn M. *The effectiveness of neurofeedback and heart rate variability biofeedback for individuals with long-term post-concussive symptoms.* Western University 2018.

33 Napier C, MacLean CL, Maurer J, et al. Real-time biofeedback of performance to reduce braking forces associated with running-related injury: an exploratory study. *J Orthop Sports Phys Ther* 2019;49:136–144; doi:10.2519/jospt.2019.8587.

34 Diekfuss JA, Grooms DR, Bonnette S, et al. Real-time biofeedback integrated into neuromuscular training reduces high-risk knee biomechanics and increases functional brain connectivity: a preliminary longitudinal investigation. *Psychophysiology* 2020;57:e13545; doi:10.1111/psyp.13545.

35 Meijer HA, Graafland M, Goslings JC, et al. Systematic review on the effects of serious games and wearable technology used in rehabilitation of patients with traumatic bone and soft tissue injuries. *Arch Phys Med Rehabil* 2018;99(9):1890–1899; doi:10.1016/j.apmr.2017.10.018.

36 MacWilliam K. *Sport perfectionism and risk factors of sport injury rehabilitation overadherence.* Lakehead University 2018.

37 Schwartz B. *The paradox of choice: why more is less.* New York: Ecco 2004.

38 Heuer RJ. Psychology of intelligence analysis. Available at: https://www.cia.gov/static/9a5f1162fd0932c29bfed1c030edf4ae/Pyschology-of-Intelligence-Analysis.pdf Accessed May 28, 2021.

39 Tversky A, Kahneman D. Judgment under uncertainty: heuristics and biases. *Science* 1974;185:1124–1131; doi:10.1126/science.185.4157.1124.

10

NAVIGATING TEAM DYNAMICS THROUGHOUT THE INJURY PROCESS: "FAMILY" VALUES IN A SPORT ENVIRONMENT

Carly McKay, Jordan D. Herbison, and Luc J. Martin

As we've seen over the past few chapters, a lot of academic literature and practical guidelines have been dedicated to promoting processes for adaptive rehabilitation and re-entry to sport. We've also highlighted the inherent complexity of athletic injuries, and what is becoming increasingly evident across the injury process is that athletes rarely experience an injury, rehabilitate, and return to sport in isolation. Rather, they're surrounded by significant others, medical staff, teammates, and coaches. An injury is clearly not only an individual experience, but one that is shaped by – and has consequences for – an entire *social context*. So, let's take a look at the salient features of the sport environment within the injury process, and consider how to take a team dynamics-informed approach to assisting injured athletes through their journeys.

Beginning with a Narrow View

What becomes apparent rather quickly when combing through the sport injury literature is that until recently, the emphasis has been on factors that influence risk and rehabilitation at a personal level. Of course, it has. An injury obviously happens to an individual and we need to understand things from that athlete's point of view. This narrow approach has yielded a treasure trove of information and has laid the foundations for the most influential models in the field, including Diane Wiese-Bjornstal and colleagues' Integrated Model of Response to Sport Injury[1] and the Biopsychosocial Model.[2] Although these frameworks pre-dominantly focus on individual characteristics, cognitive appraisals, and emotional responses, there has always been a strong acknowledgement that such factors interact dynamically with the athlete's environment. This environment is comprised of both the physical and social elements of the athlete' surroundings. Now, whether or not you put stock into the value of models for informing research or

DOI: 10.4324/9781003088936-10

practice, they all highlight the central role of these social factors in the injury process. So, what does this mean in practical terms?

Consider the following contrasting situations. In one, we have a 20-year-old university tennis player who has sprained her wrist and is unable to compete for several weeks as she undergoes treatment. The other involves a 20-year-old university netball player who has a similar wrist injury, and her prognosis and expected rehabilitation timeline are the same as the tennis player's. On the surface, these appear to be nearly identical injury scenarios. Yet, the rehabilitation environments are likely to be quite different for each athlete due to the nature of their sports and the social contexts that come along with them. For example, the tennis player may be able to work one-on-one with her coach on a regular basis during the rehabilitation period and adjust her personal competition calendar to accommodate her recovery. The netball player, on the other hand, is likely to be left at home while her team travels to compete, and she will need to fit her personal rehabilitation needs around the team's ongoing schedule. Thus, the amount and quality of social support these athletes receive on a daily basis is likely to differ and may ultimately have implications for their injury outcomes.

Evidence can be drawn from sport injury research to demonstrate the important role that "others" play through the rehabilitation process, but this is still very much an emerging area of enquiry. Let's take a look at what we know so far, and which big questions still need to be answered.

Expanding Our Horizons

An all-encompassing review of the injury literature is beyond the scope of this chapter (you can breathe a sigh of relief), but it is important to demonstrate *why* a chapter like this one is worthwhile. If we consider a general overview of research from the past 10 years, we can clearly see that across age ranges, competition levels, and stakeholder roles (i.e., athletes, parents, and coaches), social support is a key component of successful injury recovery. So, instead of promoting a narrow view of injury rehabilitation, where we focus only on the athlete's individual responses and behaviors, we need to take a wider view where athlete-centred approaches account for the social structures in which injuries occur. For those who are interested, complete reviews of social support and injury rehabilitation can be found elsewhere,[3] but for now, let's describe the big concepts as they relate to athlete, parent, and coach perspectives.

Athletes

The majority of recent research examining psychosocial factors in athlete injury rehabilitation has focused on elite level sport (i.e., university, national, and/or international athletes) through the lens of athlete experiences. For instance, Clement and colleagues conducted semi-structured interviews with eight NCAA Division II athletes to better understand their psychosocial responses after injury.[4]

The athletes described family members, teammates, coaches, and sports medicine practitioners (e.g., physiotherapists, athletic trainers) as key sources of social support at different stages of their rehabilitation. Early on in the recovery process, when athletes reported experiencing more negative emotions and cognitive appraisals, they valued support from family, teammates, and coaches. As recovery progressed and they were closer to returning to play, the informational and emotional support received from sports medicine practitioners became more important. This suggests that elite athletes' cognitive appraisals, emotions, and behaviors may be influenced by both personal (e.g., demographics) and situational (e.g., social support) factors. Importantly, these factors have received additional support in a systematic review of psychological factors that promote adherence to injury rehabilitation,[5] reinforcing the idea that social factors can have both direct and indirect effects on injury outcomes.

This evidence has been replicated in a professional sport context, where Conti et al. explored Italian professional male basketball players' perceptions of the psychosocial and behavioral factors that helped them to return to or exceed their pre-injury performance levels.[6] Ten players were interviewed at three-time points: between commencement of rehabilitation and their return to sport, at the time of their first competition, and during the six months following their return. These athletes recognized social support as a key factor across all three phases of their rehabilitation, indicating that family, friends, and especially teammates with similar injury experiences provided valuable emotional and motivational support. As with the NCAA athletes, informational support from sports medicine practitioners as they neared return to play improved their knowledge about what to expect and increased their perceptions of control. Most notably, the information that athletes received from coaches and sports medicine practitioners in the latter part of their recovery helped formulate realistic expectations that facilitated their return to pre-injury levels of performance.

These example studies provide a decent picture of how social support can be, well, *supportive*. It doesn't always turn out that way, though. In another example from collegiate sport, Iñigo et al. used the Sport Commitment Model (SCM[7])[i] to examine athletes' reasons for staying committed to sport following injury.[8] Collegiate athletes from the University of Philippines Diliman who had recently missed at least one month of competition due to injury participated in semi-structured interviews. Participants discussed five of the six dimensions from the SCM, including sport enjoyment, personal investments, valuable opportunities, social constraints, and social support. These authors reported that helping injured players stay connected with teammates and coaches during recovery can foster intrinsic motivation to remain committed to sport (i.e., valuable opportunities) and provide a conduit for social support. That's all well and good, but this study also indicated the potential for teammates, coaches, and parents to be sources of external pressure (i.e., social constraint), contributing to a sense of obligation to return to sport too soon. This probably rings true for a lot of people who have been involved in sport (or any other performance domain, for that matter). Those in our close social circles often manage to exert pressure whether they intend to or not. Sometimes it's overt, like a coach circling a return date on the team calendar. Other times, it can be more subtle, for instance a parent saying they are "disappointed" that their child will miss a big game. Either way, feelings of letting others down or not fulfilling one's own potential can become overwhelming for athletes if the influence of their social networks trends toward "pushing" them rather than "supporting" them.[8-10]

It's clear that the social context can influence injury experiences, but on the flip side, an individual athlete's injury can also have group-level effects on the social context. Surya and colleagues interviewed 10 collegiate male basketball players to explore (1) the team- and individual-level adjustments needed following injury, (2) how an athletes' injury affects other team members, and (3) how the group environment influences an athlete's rehabilitation process.[11] These athletes described how even a single injury event can have broad implications for a team, specifically in the areas of strategy and individual athlete roles. The loss of a core player necessitates a collective shift in team strategy and a cascade of role adjustments that may have negative consequences for interpersonal relationships and the emotional climate within the team.

Professional sport headlines are rife with examples of star players being injured and their team underperforming in their absence, despite the talent and capability of their teammates (e.g., the WNBA's Washington Mystics' unsuccessful 2020 defence of their championship without star Elena Delle Donne). Some of this is down to missing the particular skillset of that individual, but contemporary theories also suggest that the blow to collective morale can be equally detrimental. *Social contagion*, defined as the spread of a mood state, attitude or behavior from one person to another in a group setting, might be particularly relevant when discussing how the loss of a "glue" player can be harmful.[12] *Emotional contagion*, which specifically refers to the spread of mood states, is affected by the membership stability of a group (e.g., turnover rates and how long they've been together), task interdependence (e.g., how much group members rely on each other to do their jobs), and social interdependence (e.g., the extent to which one person's actions affect the ability of others to complete their tasks).[13-15] Any adjustment made to team members' roles and responsibilities in the wake of an injury may indeed influence these factors and set the scene for negative emotional states to affect team performance. It is therefore incumbent on the coach and others within the team leadership structure to ensure that such changes are addressed early and clearly to avoid role ambiguity and maintain team functioning.

So far, research has supported a number of intuitive assumptions about social support during injury rehabilitation and many of us can imagine how the process would play out in our own sport(s) of choice. What we may not stop to think about is what this might look like for younger athletes. After all, kids aren't just mini adults – no matter how much they might act like it sometimes – and it seems silly to assume that the function of interpersonal relationships during injury rehabilitation will be the same across age groups. This may be especially poignant during adolescence, when social dynamics can be volatile and take on extra-ordinary significance under the best of circumstances. And yet, the scant evidence we have so far suggests that it might not be all that different. Podlog and colleagues provided rare insight into adolescent athletes' perceptions of injury rehabilitation and return to sport by interviewing 11 young sportspeople who competed for regional academies or state/national teams in New South Wales, Australia.[10] These athletes reported similar concerns and supports to those from adult athletes, recognizing family, teammates, coaches, and sports medicine practitioners as key contributors to their successful injury rehabilitation. There were a few features that stood out prominently in this age group, however, and warrant additional investigation as potential make-or-break factors for successful return to sport for young athletes.

Podlog et al. found that competence-related perceptions seemed to be integral to successful return from injury amongst their interviewees.[10] In other words, building a young athlete's self-efficacy is a crucial part of the recovery process. This suggests that the support provided by coaches and sport medicine practitioners needs to be structured in a way that includes gradual progression focusing on challenging, self-referenced goals. Coordination between coaches and sports medicine practitioners therefore becomes particularly critical, as young athletes have reported that receiving conflicting information about the return to sport process (e.g., differing feedback on milestones or achievements) causes confusion and distress.[10] Perhaps most importantly, young athletes desire adapted role assignments so they can stay connected with their teammates during rehabilitation and they particularly benefit from leaning on others who are experiencing similar challenges.[10] This means that support from peers and maintaining social connections within the team should be a priority. So, as it turns out, asking an injured player to sit on the bench and keep game statistics for their teammates may not be such a bad idea after all.

Parents

Parents occupy an interesting niche in the sport injury process. Their influence is naturally more pertinent for younger athletes, but not much research has been devoted to understanding their perspectives so we cannot say for certain where they are in the social support structure of older groups. For instance, there are several well-known examples of parents who remained involved with their children as coaches and mentors through to adulthood (e.g., Earl and Tiger Woods, Judy and Andy Murray, Richard, and Venus and Serena Williams), and many athletes credit their parents as invaluable sources of support throughout their careers. It's reasonable to suggest that they're important figures during injury rehabilitation as well, though research hasn't specifically addressed this issue.

In one of the few investigations to include parents, Podlog and colleagues interviewed 10 ($n_{mothers} = 7$, $n_{fathers} = 3$) with adolescent children who played on state or institute squads in Australia, and who had incurred an injury requiring a minimum of one month's absence from participation.[9] Parents referenced their adolescents' strong negative emotional responses to injury, rooted in competence-based perceptions that they were falling behind their peers. Exacerbating these perceptions were adolescents' self-referenced beliefs that their injuries had caused physical deficits that would be difficult to overcome (e.g., loss of stamina and strength, pain and mobility difficulties). Parents indicated that they felt coaches and sports medicine practitioners should coordinate the injury rehabilitation process based on individualized factors such as graduated physical tests, simulated training, and one-on-one goal-setting meetings. Parents also felt that a decrease in their child's interactions with their teammates negatively influenced feelings of connection and identity. This study thereby reinforced the perspectives of the athletes themselves and provided further support for ensuring they are provided meaningful opportunities to be involved with their teams during the rehabilitation process.

Interestingly, there is some evidence that parents can be stressors during the rehabilitation process, with young athletes identifying situations where their parents exerted pressure on them to play through pain and injury.[10] Parental pressure has been extensively documented in the sport performance and youth development literature, and understanding the dynamics of parent-child relationships during recovery and return to sport is an area for future focus.[16]

Coaches

As perhaps the most maligned stakeholder group in the injury rehabilitation setting, coaches have a bad rap as people who put performance above health. Enough anecdotal accounts exist to suggest that this is probably (sadly) true in a number of cases, but research in the area indicates that they aren't all cut from the win-at-all-costs cloth. Podlog and Doinigi examined coach strategies for addressing athletes' psychological challenges in returning from injury.[17] Coaches with experience at senior international competitions (e.g., Olympics and World championship) and/or national level juniors (i.e., 18–20 years old) identified several strategies for facilitating athletes' successful return to sport. These involved (1) coordinating a "team approach" with sports medicine practitioners, (2) fostering open communication with athletes and sports medicine practitioners, (3) providing social support, (4) reinforcing positive thinking and goal setting, and (5) coordinating interactions with role models. Efforts to foster a team approach and effective communication with athletes and sports medicine practitioners was seen to protect athletes from returning to sport too soon, but also to promote their perceived internal locus of causality over the rehabilitation process. In other words, they want athletes to feel like they have control over their recovery. Further, coaches articulated the importance of keeping injured athletes involved with the day-to-day activities of the team (e.g., training, meetings) to offset the potentially isolating effects of injury and facilitate re-integration when returning to sport. This aligns with what athletes and parents have highlighted as key factors, so at least everyone seems to be on the same page with what *should* happen.

What *actually* happens might be a different story. Van Woezik and colleagues explored how coaches manage team dynamics following an injury event.[18] Ten Canadian university head basketball coaches perceived injury events as potentially destabilizing and disruptive to existing group dynamics and saw themselves as vital stewards in managing the process. For example, an injury to a core player may result in a series of adjustments that encourage other athletes to "step-up" but not necessarily "replace" injured teammates. This might be required to maintain team performance, but it could clearly cause role confusion or conflict when the injured player returns and wants (or is given) their spot back. Coaches also recognized the need to ensure that injured athletes felt socially connected to their team and de-scribed purposefully increasing the amount of interaction with them, checking in on them periodically. To prevent things from going off the rails, coaches identified deliberate strategies to manage their team during a period of injury, including addressing the situation immediately, having open communication with the entire team and the medical staff, and keeping consistent contact with the injured athlete.

Why Aren't We Talking About Team Dynamics?

Right, now that we have a picture of the social context around injury re-habilitation, it's time to think about it a little more critically. Even a cursory look at the literature shows that the types and timing of interactions that an injured athlete has are critical, regardless of their age and competition level; however, most of this has been framed as "social support." That's all well and good, but it's a very narrow way of looking at it. Research has essentially focused on the effects of the environment on the athlete without accounting for the fact that the athlete is only one part of a complex network and the effects of social interactions are not unidirectional. It's a bit like measuring how hard a billiard cue hits the cue ball without accounting for which balls end up in the pocket. In sports where social interactions are ever changing and injuries can have all kinds of consequences for individuals and teams, it makes sense to consider the bigger picture. Maybe it's time to start thinking about this from a team dynamics perspective.

Wait, what do we mean by *team dynamics*? Also known as group dynamics, this describes the processes that shape the direction of a team's behavior and perfor-mance, including the relationships between its members and how their interac-tions influence decision-making and goal attainment.[19] Applying a team dynamics approach to sport has spawned some fascinating theoretical and practical work toward improving performance and sustaining participation across a number of settings.[20] Yet, despite what we understand about the significance of the social climate during injury rehabilitation and return to sport, it hasn't really been ap-plied in this context.

There are several reasons to contemplate a team dynamics approach to sport injuries. For starters, regardless of whether you are an individual or team sport athlete, sport is inherently comprised of group situations. On top of this, by nature, humans exhibit a fundamental need to belong and sport is an ideal context to satisfy the desire for membership.[21,22] Indeed, athletes consistently reference social motives for sport participation, so removal due to injury is understandably a difficult experience and is often reflected when injured athletes reference feelings of isolation during rehabilitation. Other experiences of being deprived involvement, such as deselection or receiving limited playing exposure (e.g., "benching" or being a substitute) are rife with struggles and are often part of the injury process as well.[23,24] So, based on established team dynamics research, we might be able to guide coaches or practitioners working with injured athletes to minimize disruption and promote both individual and team performance.

Traditional team dynamics frameworks have been grounded in "input-process-output" approaches,[25] whereby certain antecedents (e.g., member characteristics) are thought to influence the way that people interact (e.g., communication), and by extension, how a group functions (e.g., performance). Researchers have adopted this type of thinking with innovations tailored to sport.[19,20,26] Figure 10.1 provides a version of such frameworks that could be applied to an injury rehabilitation scenario. Specifically, it highlights the value of considering member attributes (both those of the injured athlete and their teammates) and the context within which the team competes. It is also necessary to understand the structural features inherent in all sports, including accepted hierarchies and individual roles (e.g., rookies vs. veterans; captains). Important team processes such as leadership and competition will also inevitably influence how athletes experience the injury process. Lastly, emergent states like team cohesion and social identity will impact how athletes think about their immediate environment.

Every Team is Different

In line with research specific to the injury process,[5] both member attributes and the team environment are principal input factors that need to be accounted for.

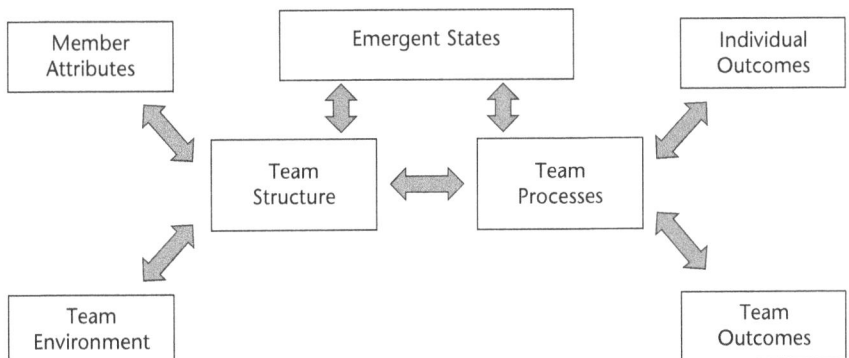

FIGURE 10.1 Summary framework for team dynamics in sport.

Clearly, a recreational athlete is likely to have a very different experience to someone in an elite or professional setting, in the same way that coaches and teammates are likely to respond differently in these groups. Team size and sport type are likely to be significant factors as well, which we can explore with a few examples. To start with, let's look back to the university netball and tennis players we introduced earlier. Injuries in the netball team create opportunities for reserve players to step into starting roles, but injured players may still attend training and competition where they can contribute by providing encouragement from the bench. Further, in larger teams, an athlete is likely to encounter a teammate who has gone through the injury process and can provide social support during recovery. Alternatively, in a smaller group like the tennis team, there may be fewer opportunities to connect because teammates may not all train or compete at the same time and finding someone with a similar injury history may be more difficult.

So, how big should a team be? This question has been asked in relation to outcomes like performance,[27] player satisfaction,[28] and cohesion,[29] but it hasn't been explicitly examined with respect to injuries. We can extrapolate from previous research, though, which suggests that the ideal number of athletes is typically less than the traditional roster size for a sport.[30] This is largely because smaller teams provide more opportunities for individual participation; however, one identified disadvantage of smaller teams is a lack of roster depth. Indeed, seminal research shows that team productivity can improve as team size increases, but individual member performance typically decreases.[27,31] So, it seems that from a team perspective, having more athletes is better for overcoming the loss of an injured teammate, but for the injured athlete it can mean a diminished chance of cracking the line-up when they return. To be clear, having an injured athlete on a curling team (composed of 5 or 6 athletes) will present different challenges than for an American football team (composed of approximately 70 athletes).

Well, it will unless all of your injuries (or in this case, illnesses) happen within a single positional group. In 2020, at the start of the COVID-19 pandemic, The Denver Broncos of the NFL were faced with a ridiculous situation where every one of their quarterbacks had either tested positive for COVID-19 or had been deemed "close contacts" of a player who had. With all four quarterbacks in medical isolation and unable to play, the team was on the verge of forfeiting a game against the New Orleans Saints until two hours before kick-off when they activated their emergency quarterback, rookie wide receiver Kendall Hinton (who until that point had been on the practice roster). The Broncos lost the game 31-3, to nobody's surprise, but it was a brilliant case study of how player absence can cause systemic changes within a team. Although the players rallied around Hinton emotionally, they were unable to do so on the field – Hinton threw for just 13 yards, with a sack and two interceptions. Clearly, even within a large team, roster depth can be a problem when health concerns arise.

This highlights another environmental feature that coaches or practitioners should be aware of: the type of sport they're involved with. That's kind of an odd statement – of course people know their sport! But a feature that's not always explicitly discussed is the interdependence the sport requires. Sport type has traditionally been thought of as individual versus team, but there is actually an *interdependence typology* that specifies the degree to which teammates must interact for either task (i.e., performing the sport itself) or outcome (i.e., final standings, scoring) purposes.[32] Relevant examples include team sports that are integrated (e.g., soccer, volleyball) or segregated (e.g., cricket, baseball) and individual sports that are collective (e.g., cross country running where teammates compete for both individual and team medals in the same race), cooperative (e.g., intercollegiate wrestling where teammates compete in different weight classes but contribute to a team title), or contrient (e.g., a national team of trampolinists who compete against each other with no group-level goal). Having an injured athlete within an integrated sport, where their absence is felt by teammates and requires adaptive strategy decisions is quite a bit different than in a contrient environment where there is no team-level outcome.[11] Understanding the need within a particular sport for athletes to interact to achieve common superordinate objectives will influence the ways that they experience an injury-related absence, and by extension, the way it should be approached by a coach or other members of the support network.

Teams Have Structure (Which May or May Not be Conducive to Rehabilitation)

Although every team is different, there are consistencies that researchers and practitioners can turn to when attempting to understand the complex interactions between group members. In sport, we call these *structural features* of teams, and they involve *roles* and *norms*. When talking about injured athletes, a third relevant structural feature is what might be termed *subgroups/faultlines*.[33]

Roles represent behaviors that are expected of an individual within a particular social context. These often involve specific functions such as responsibility for a given task or social purpose and/or can be formally specified (e.g., team captain). They can also develop informally, as individuals can distinguish themselves as an "energy player" or team comedian, for example.[34,35] How well athletes understand their roles and how committed they are to satisfying their obligations have great implications for sport experiences and team functioning.[20,36] This is clear from the injury-specific literature where athletes describe the desire for realistic and adapted role expectations post-injury.[6,11] To illustrate, Eoin Morgan, who captained England's 2019 Cricket World Cup winning team, experienced a back injury during the tournament. When asked if he intended to captain the England T20 World Cup team the following year, he said he wanted to lead but didn't *"want to let anybody down"* and was considering relinquishing his role if he could not regain his pre-injury form.[37] Coaches have noted role management as a priority for helping athletes successfully return from injury without any detriment to overall team chemistry,[18] though this is only now gaining research attention and best practice recommendations are yet to be established.

Norms refer to assumptions concerning behaviors that are expected of group members. These are essential to effective group functioning, with clear implications for athlete effort,[38] moral behaviors,[39] and team performance.[40] However, when behaviors expected within a team are not adaptive in nature, norms still influence member behavior, but not in ways that are desirable (e.g., alcohol use, drinking and driving).[41–43] The same goes for injuries, where there is evidence that athletes will underreport or "power through" based on expectations felt within their team.[41] A superficial glance through the sports media pages on any given day returns some sort of glorifying statement of an athlete playing through injury to benefit the team, so we don't need to look too far to see how pervasive this can be. It's fairly evident how expectations within a group to quickly return to play after injury could impact the recovery process and add additional pressure to athletes.

Whereas team roles and norms can be easy for outsiders to recognize, the third major structural feature, *subgroups/faultlines*, is sometimes only apparent to those in the team's inner circle. Any observable grouping of team members, whether it be the leadership group, athletes of a similar age/cohort, or from different positions (e.g., offense vs. defence) can be classified as a subgroup, and these form somewhat inevitably.[44] Although traditionally positioned as problematic, emerging research provides a more nuanced understanding whereby smaller groupings of teammates are a natural occurrence and can be adaptive in relation to both individuals (e.g., support, belonging) and a team as a whole (e.g., establishing normative expectations).[45,46] Injured athletes are likely to spend time with other injured athletes or those on training rosters, so understanding how these individuals are interacting and what discourses emerge within the group can be crucial for coaches to keep on top of.[46] Ensuring that athletes receive support and can interact with other athletes in similar situations is important, but emphasis must be placed on establishing connections with the entire team to prevent a grouping that alienates itself from everyone else.[ii]

The Importance of Team Processes

The way teams operate can dramatically shape injury experiences. For example, coaches obviously play a significant role, from communicating expectations and discussing role assignments, to providing support throughout rehabilitation.[17] Therefore, deliberately demonstrating individual consideration and making injured athletes feel as though they are important members of the group are just some strategies that coaches should prioritize.[18] Coaches aren't the only leaders within the team, though. Emerging evidence reinforces the range of roles and functions undertaken by athlete leaders,[47,48] and coaches use a range of strategies to encourage shared leadership emergence in their teams, ranging from rotating formal leaders, to purposefully not having designated leaders, to clearly describing leadership roles.[49] Considering the importance of peer support during injury rehabilitation, explicitly empowering athlete leaders to be involved in their teammates' rehabilitation could be an interesting means of leveraging their influence.

This would need to be managed carefully, though. Some of the major issues described by athletes during the return to sport process are lack of clarity about roles and having to fight their way back into the line-up. This often stems from *positional competition*, a social comparison process that occurs when teammates vie for the same limited playing time at a particular position.[50] Though some level of competition can promote athletes to excel, social comparison, negative or ambiguous coach feedback, and pressure from teammates can cause a number of problems including anxiety, loss of self-efficacy, and conflict.[51] This can apply to the injured athlete or the teammate they are competing with, or both. After all, it's easy to imagine that someone who stepped up to fill a role, and has been doing a good job, would be reluctant to relinquish it. Indeed, communicating why playing time changes occur and how they relate to injury is recognized as an important point of emphasis by coaches.[52] For those who work with injured athletes, being aware of where they are on the teams' depth-chart and how an injury may affect their playing time is a critical prerequisite to understanding how they might experience the return process and how to go about clarifying role expectations and being transparent with decision making. It is also incumbent upon coaches to manage player expectations when absent teammates return to the roster, to prevent unintended negative consequences for their uninjured teammates.

Emergent States – The Result of the Rest

Although there are several emergent states relevant to the injury process, two have received a fair amount of attention in the research literature: cohesion and social identity.[19] *Cohesion* refers to the degree to which team members share common objectives and experience quality interpersonal relations.[53] Athletes describe the benefits of feeling as though they are contributing members of a group while injured, which means that considering the injury process through the lens of cohesion would be an informed approach. Specifically, research suggests that athletes sometimes experience stress and anxiety when attempting to return to sport, and an inverse relationship has been demonstrated with perceptions of cohesion and anxiety in sport.[54] Cohesion also has a positive association with coping ability, suggesting it may help to ease the return to sport transition.[14] There is also the potential for injured athletes to disengage and feel as though they have a diminished role in the team. When athletes perceive greater levels of cohesion, they tend to be on time for events and have greater attendance at games and practices,[55] and they are also more likely to return the following season.[56] Similarly, there is evidence that athletes are more willing to demonstrate sacrifice behavior (e.g., accept a diminished role) when they perceive high levels of cohesion.[57] Regularly using cohesion-boosting strategies, such as encouraging open communication and setting a shared team vision, may ultimately help athletes reintegrate into the line-up throughout the season.

It is, however, essential to emphasize the need for relatively equal levels of task (performance-based) and social (relationship-based) cohesion. Further, the values within the team must prioritize athlete well-being above performance, because if not, high levels of task cohesion could lead to increased pressure to conform to group norms and return from injury too soon.[58] Ensuring that an injured athlete's individual objectives and plans for recovery align with the task objectives of the group should be a priority, while also providing ample opportunity to interact with team members to maintain the connections that satisfy perceptions of social cohesion.

This relates to the other important emergent state, *social identity*, which refers to the identity that people cultivate as a result of group membership. Perceptions of social identity are based on (1) quality relations and interactions with members (ingroup ties), (2) the importance that one attributes to the group (cognitive centrality), and (3) the positive feelings associated with membership (ingroup affect).[59] There is a large and growing body of evidence that demonstrates a range of correlates of social identity in sport, many of which are relevant to injury. For instance, we've discussed the importance of teammate support during the injury process. Across several studies, Bruner and colleagues have demonstrated links between prosocial teammate behaviors and perceptions of social identity.[60] Further, in youth populations, ingroup affect is related to youth development in the form of personal and social skills, goal setting, and commitment, and ingroup ties to athletes' initiative and perceived effort.[61,62] These are all components of healthy return to sport and can be maximized by promoting team identity through things like intra-team rituals (e.g., pre-game routines) or distinctive team kit.

But, as with cohesion, we must be mindful of the impact social identity can have on athletes. Normative behaviors are likely to become more salient during a vulnerable time like injury, so it's important to ensure that these remain adaptive in nature and promote the values agreed upon by the group. Otherwise, there's a chance that people will reinforce problematic behaviors. To illustrate, Benson et al. noted a positive relationship between antisocial norms and antisocial actions within a team, and this relationship was strengthened with high perceptions of social identity.[39] Extending this work, Graupensberger et al. demonstrated highly identifying athletes to be more susceptible to peer influence for risky behaviors.[41,iii] Although not a perfect example, one could surmise that peer influence could instigate early return to sport when an athlete is not ready, or any number of other maladaptive behaviors. Accordingly, social identity is a factor that has not been well investigated in the sport injury literature, but probably should be.

Bringing It All Together

The big message from all of this is that the social environment in which injuries happen is as central a factor in rehabilitation outcome as any other, but it has received far less attention than cognitions or emotions. Why? That's tough to say, but it might have to do with a historical focus on the athlete as an independent unit rather than taking a network view of their position within a complex and interactive social structure. With an ongoing shift toward systems-level thinking in sport injury research,[63] considering team dynamics is a logical next step for research and practice in this area. Hopefully the framework presented within the chapter can provide a starting point for anyone interested in learning more about how team dynamics relate to the injury process. As a coach or athlete, it can provide a sort of "map" to help navigate what is undeniably a complex process. From a researcher's perspective, maybe it can provide some potential avenues for future enquiry—there is certainly a lot to be learned!

Notes

i   Oh boy, another model. We know we've argued that models may not be all that helpful in everyday practice, but this one is fairly simple and is based on a whole lot of common sense. Basically, it states that there are five direct predictors that increase/decrease people's commitment to their sport: (1) **sport enjoyment** – you have to like it to keep doing it; (2) **involvement alternatives** – if there's something you'd rather be doing, you'll go do it instead; (3) **personal investment** – if you've put in a lot of time/money/energy, you're likely to keep doing it; (4) **social constraints** – if you feel obligated, you'll keep turning up; (5) **involvement opportunities** – if there are benefits from participating, like friendships and fitness, you'll stay involved. Most research also includes a 6th predictor, **social support** – if significant others encourage you, you're more likely to participate.

ii The analogy that comes to mind here is when members of a band go off to do a solo project then come back – sometimes they rejoin seamlessly and sometimes, not so much. For instance, all four members of U2 have done numerous side projects since 1985, with or without ~~you~~ their bandmates, with no detriment to their collective work. For other bands, creative differences and loss of shared vision cause tension and ultimately, irreparable rifts break up the group (e.g., The Beatles).

iii These also happen to be common features of gangs. They promote social identity and cohesion by adopting group colors or other distinctive physical signifiers, members conform to specific normative behaviors, and group goals come to supersede those of the individual (e.g., valuing "we" before "me"). Peer influence within this context is also linked to risky and/or antisocial behaviors, which tends to be self-perpetuating. Actually, the same could be said for stereotypical high school cliques… This is obviously not to say that sport teams are like gangs (or awful Hollywood tropes), but the point is illustrative all the same.

References

1 Wiese-Bjornstal DM, Smith AM, Shaffer SM, et al. An integrated model of response to sport injury: psychological and sociological dynamics. *J Appl Sport Psychol* 1998;10(1):46–69; doi:10.1080/10413209808406377.

2 Brewer B. The role of psychological factors in sport injury rehabilitation outcomes. *Int Rev Sport Exerc Psychol* 2010;3(1):40–61; doi:10.1080/17509840903301207.

3 Fernandes HM, Reis VM, Vilaça-Alves J, et al. Social support and sport injury recovery: an overview of empirical findings and practical implications. *Revista de Psicología del Deporte* 2014;23(2):445–449.

4 Clement D, Arvinen-Barrow M, Fetty T. Psychosocial responses during different phases of sport-injury rehabilitation: a qualitative study. *J Athl Train* 2015;50(1):95–104; doi: 10.4085/1062-6050-49.3.52.

5 Goddard K, Roberts CM, Byron-Daniel J, et al. Psychological factors involved in adherence to sport injury rehabilitation: a systematic review. *Int Rev Sport Exerc Psychol* 2020;1–23; doi:10.1080/1750984X.2020.1744179

6 Conti C, di Fronso S, Pivetti M, et al. Well-come back! Professional basketball players perceptions of psychosocial and behavioral factors influencing a return to pre-injury levels. *Front Psychol* 2019;10:222;doi:10.3389/fpsyg.2019.00222.

7 Scanlan TK, Carpenter PJ, Schmidt GW, et al. An introduction to the Sport Commitment Model. *J Sport Exerc Psychol* 1993;15:1–15.

8 Iñigo MM, Podlog L, Hall M. Why do athletes remain committed to sport after severe injury? An examination of the Sport Commitment Model. *Sport Psychol* 2015;29(2):143–155; doi: 10.1123/tsp.2014-0086.

9 Podlog L, Kleinert J, Dimmock J, et al. A parental perspective on adolescent injury rehabilitation and return to sport experiences. *J Appl Sport Psychol* 2012;24(2):175–190; doi:10.1080/10413200.2011.608102.

10 Podlog L, Wadey R, Stark A, et al. An adolescent perspective on injury recovery and the return to sport. *Psychol Sport Exerc* 2013;14(4):437–446; doi:10.1016/j.psychsport. 2012.12.005

11 Surya M, Benson AJ, Balish SM, et al. The influence of injury on group interaction processes. *J Appl Sport Psychol* 2015;27(1):52–66; doi:10.1080/10413200. 2014.941512.

12 Hurley OA. Impact of players' injuries on teams' mental states, and subsequent performances, at the Rugby World Cup 2015. *Front Psychol* 2016;7:807; doi:10.3389/psyg.2016.00807

13 Wolf SA, Eys MA, Kleinert J. Predictors of the precompetitive anxiety response: relative impact and prospects for anxiety regulation. *In J Sport Exerc Psychol* 2015;13:344–358; doi:10.1080/1612197X.2014.982676.

14 Wolf SA, Eys MA, Sadler P, et al. Appraisal in a team context: perceptions of cohesion predict competition importance and prospects for coping. *J Sport Exerc Psychol* 2015;37(5):489–499; doi:10.1123/jsep.2014-0276.

15 Wolf SA, Harenberg S, Tamminen K. et al. "Cause You Can't Play This by Yourself": athletes' Perceptions of Team Influence on Their Precompetitive Psychological States. *J Appl Sport Psychol* 2018;30(2):185–203; doi:10.1080/10413200.2017.1347965.

16 Knight CJ, Dorsch TE, Osai KV, et al. Influences on parental involvement in youth sport. *Sport Exerc Perform Psychol* 2016;5(2):161; doi:10.1037/spy0000053.

17 Podlog L, Doinigi R. Coach strategies for addressing psychosocial challenges during the return to sport from injury. *J Sports Sci* 2010;28(11):1197–1208; doi:10.1080/02640414 .2010.487873.

18 Van Woezik RA, Benson AJ, Bruner MW. (2020). Next one up! Exploring how coaches manage team dynamics following injury. *Sport Psychol*, 34 (3), 198–208; doi: 10.1123/tsp.2019-0148.

19 Eys MA, Bruner MW, Martin LJ. The dynamic group environment in sport and exercise. *Psychol Sport Exerc*2019;42:40–47; doi:10.1016/j.psychsport.2018.11.001.

20 Eys MA, Evans MB, Benson AJ. *Group dynamics in sport* (5th ed.). Morgantown, WV: Fitness Information Technology 2020.

21 Baumeister RF, Leary MR. The need to belong: desire for interpersonal attachments as a fundamental human motivation. *Psychol Bull* 1995;117: 497–529; doi:10.1037/0033-2909.117.3.497.

22 Allen JB. Social motivation in youth sport. *J Sport Exerc Psychol* 2003;25(4):551–567; doi:10.1123/jsep.25.4.551.

23 Neely KC, McHugh TLF, Dunn JG, et al. Athletes and parents coping with deselection in competitive youth sport: a communal coping perspective. *Psychol Sport Exerc* 2017;30:1–9; doi:10.1016/j.psychsport.2017.01.004.

24 Battaglia A, Kerr G, Stirling A. (An outcast from the team: exploring youth ice hockey goalies' benching experiences. *Psychol Sport Exerc* 2018;38:39–46; doi:10.1016/j.psychsport.2018.05.010.

25 Mathieu JE, Hollenbeck JR, van Knippenberg D, et al. A century of work teams in the Journal of Applied Psychology. *J Appl Sport Psychol* 2017;102(3):452–467; doi:10.1037/apl0000128.

26 McEwan D, Beauchamp MR. Teamwork in sport: a theoretical and integrative review. *Int Rev Sport Exerc Psychol* 2014;7: 229–250; doi:10.1080/1750984X.2014.932423.

27 Steiner ID. *Group processes and group productivity.* New York: Academic 1972.

28 Widmeyer WN. *The size of sport groups with special implications for the triad.* Unpublished paper 1971; University of Illinois, Champaign, IL.

29 Widmeyer WN, Brawley LR, Carron AV. The effects of group size in sport. *J Sport Exerc Psychol* 1990;12:177–190; doi:10.1123/jsep.12.2.177.

30 Carron AV, Widmeyer WN, Brawley LR. Perceptions of ideal group size in sport team. *Percept Mot Skills* 1989;69:1368–1379; doi:10.1177/00315125890693-255.

31 Kravitz DA, Martin B. Ringelmann rediscovered: the original article. *J Pers Soc Psychol* 1986;50:936–941; doi:10.1037/0022-3514.50.5.936.

32 Evans MB, Eys MA, Bruner MW. Seeing the "we" in "me" sports: the need to consider individual sport team environments. *Can Psychol* 2012;53:301–308; doi:10.1037/a0030202.

33 McGrath JE. *Groups: interaction and performance.* Englewood Cliffs, NJ: Prentice-Hall 1984.

34 Benson AJ, Surya M, Eys MA. The nature and transmission of roles in sports teams. *Sport Exerc Perform Psychol* 2014;3(4):228–240; doi:10.1037/spy0000016

35 Cope CJ, Eys MA, Beauchamp MR, et al. Informal roles on sport teams. *Int J Sport Exerc Psychol* 2011;9:19–30; doi:10.1080/1612197X.2011.563124.

36 Beauchamp MR, Bray SR, Eys MA, et al. Multidimensional role ambiguity and role satisfaction: a prospective examination using interdependent sport teams. *J Appl Sport Psychol* 2005;35:2560–2576; doi:10.1111/j.1559-1816.2005.tb02114.x.

37 ESPNcricinfo staff. (2019, August 16). *Eoin Morgan admits back injury key to captaincy future.* https://www.espncricinfo.com/story/eoin-morgan-admits-back-injury-key-to-captaincy-decision-1197831. Accessed: March 4, 2021.

38 Crozier AJ, Spink KS. Coach and peer normative perceptions in relation to youth athlete effort. *Int J Sport Exerc Psychol* 2018;18(1):17–31; doi:10.1080/1612197X.2018.1478870.

39 Benson AJ, Bruner MW, Eys M. A social identity approach to understanding the conditions associated with antisocial behaviors among teammates in female teams. *Sport Exerc Perform Psychol* 2017;6:129–142; doi:10.1037/spy0000090.

40 Hodge K, Henry G, Smith W. A case study of excellence in elite sport: motivational climate in a world champion team. *Sport Psychol* 2014;28:60–74; doi:doi.org/10.1123/tsp.2013-0037

41 Graupensperger SA, Benson AJ, Evans MB. Everyone else is doing it: the association between social identity and susceptibility to peer influence in NCAA athletes. *J Sport Exerc Psychol* 2018;40:117–127; doi:10.1123/jsep.2017-0339.

42 Graupensperger S, Turrisi R, Jones D, et al. Longitudinal associations between perceptions of peer group drinking norms and students' alcohol use frequency within college sport teams. *Alcohol Clin Exp Res* 2020;44(2):541–552; doi:10.1111.acer.14270.

43 Cusimano MD, Topolovec-Vranic J, Zhang S, et al. Factors Influencing the underreporting of concussion in sports: a qualitative study of minor hockey participants. *Clin J Sports Med* 2017;27(4):375–380; doi:10.1097/JSM.0000000000000372.

44 Wagstaff CRD, Martin LJ, Thelwell RC. Subgroups and cliques in sport: a longitudinal case study of a rugby union team. *Psychol Sport Exerc* 2017;30:164–172; doi:10.1016/j.psychsport.2017.03.006.

45 Martin LJ, Wilson J, Evans MB, et al. Cliques in sport: perceptions of intercollegiate athletes. *Sport Psychol* 2015;29:82–95; doi:10.1123/tsp.2014-0003.

46 Martin LJ, Evans MB, Spink KS. Coach perspectives of "groups within the group": an analysis of subgroups and cliques in sport. *Sport Exerc Perform Psychol* 2016;5:52–66; doi:10.1037/spy.0000048.

47 Cotterill ST, Fransen K. Athlete leadership in sport teams: current understanding and future directions, *Int Rev Sport Exerc Psychol* 2016;9(1):116–133; doI:10.1080/1750984X.2015.1124443.

48 Fransen K, Van Puyenbroeck S, Loughead TM, et al. Who takes the lead? Social network analysis as a pioneering tool to investigate shared leadership within sports teams. *Soc Networks* 2015;43:28–38; doi:10.1016/j/socnet.2015.04.003.

49 Duguay AM, Loughead TM, Hoffmann MD, et al. Facilitating the Development of Shared Athlete Leadership: insights from Intercollegiate Coaches. *J Appl Sport Psychol* 2020; doi:doi.org/10.1080/10413200.2020.1773576.

50 Harenberg S, Riemer HA, Karreman E, et al. As iron sharpens iron? Athletes' perspectives of positional competition. *Sport Psychol* 2016;30:55–67; doi:10.1123/tsp.2014-0131.

51 Harenberg S, Riemer HA, Dorsch KD, et al. Advancement of a conceptual framework for positional competition in sport: development and validation of the positional competition in team sports questionnaire. *J Appl Sport Psychol* 2019; 1–22; doi:10.1080/10413200.2019.1631903.

52 Harenberg S, Riemer HA, Karreman E, et al. Coaches' perspectives of intrateam competition in high performance sport teams. *Int Sport Coach J* 2016;3(2):156–169; doi:10.1123/iscj.2016-0056.

53 Carron AV. *Group dynamics in sport: theoretical and practical issues.* London, Ontario: Spodym 1988.

54 Eys M, Hardy J, Carron AV, Beauchamp MR. The relationship between task cohesion and competitive state anxiety. *Journal of Sport & Exercize Psychology* 2003,25:66–76.

55 Carron AV, Widmeyer WN, Brawley LR. Group cohesion and individual adherence to physical activity. *J Sport Exerc Psychol* 1988;10:119–126; doi:10.1123/jsep.10.2.127.

56 Spink KS, Wilson KS, Odnokon P. Examining the relationship between cohesion and return to team in elite athletes. *Psychol Sport Exerc* 2010;11:6–11; doi:10.1016/j.psychsport.2009.06.002.

57 Prapavessis H, Carron AV. Sacrifice, cohesion, and conformity to norms in sport teams. *Group Dyn* 1997;1:231–240; doi:10.1037/1089-2699.1.3.231.

58 Rovio E, Eskola J, Kozub SA, et al. Can high group cohesion be harmful? A case study of a junior ice-hockey team. *Small Group Res* 2009;40:421–435; doi:10.1177/1046496409334359.

59 Cameron JE. A three-factor model of social identity. *Self Identity* 2004;3: 239–262; doi:10.1080/13576500444000047.

60 Benson AJ, Bruner MW. How teammate behaviors relate to athlete affect, cognition, and behaviors: a daily diary approach within youth sport. *Psychol Sport Exerc* 2018;34:119–127; doi:10.1016/j.psychsportr.2017.10.008.

61 Bruner MW, Balish S, Forrest C, et al. Ties that bond: youth sport as a vehicle for social identity and positive youth development. *Res Q Exerc Sport* 2017;88:209–214, doi:10.1080/02701367.2017.1296100.

62 Martin LJ, Balderson D, Hawkins M, et al. The influence of social identity on self-worth, commitment, and effort in school-based youth sport. *J Sport Sci* 2018;36(3):326–332; doi:10.1080/02640414.2017.1306091.

63 Bittencourt NF, Meeuwisse WH, Mendonca LD, et al. Complex systems approach for sports injuries: moving from risk factor identification to injury pattern recognition – narrative review and new concept. *Br J Sports Med* 2016;1309–1314; doi:10.1136/bjsports-2015-095850.

11

HOW SPORT CULTURE AND COMMODIFICATION INFLUENCE INJURY EXPERIENCES: ANOTHER ONE BITES THE DUST

Carly McKay and Caroline Bolling

Imagine someone offered you a job. You would need to work, or be preparing for work, 365 days of the year. The role would be physically, mentally and emotionally exhausting and it would require you to strictly control your diet, your sleeping patterns, your physical condition, and the way you behave in public. You would need to live in a specified city and because of the travel requirements you may be away from your family for days, weeks, or months at a time. The job does not observe ordinary holidays and you cannot request days off during the busy season. You would need to become comfortable with public speaking and engage with this often, and sometimes you'd be asked to defend your work or the work of your colleagues during interrogation. Your job performance would be publicly scrutinized, and you would be subjected to performance reviews from people who may or may not be qualified to assess your work. Observers would be present during most of your shifts, and they would be encouraged to judge your every move, vocalising their approval or disapproval the entire time. Daily assessments may be delivered in absentia through public channels and there may be policies that prevent you from responding to them directly. You may be required to partially fund your own position and you would be working on a fixed-term contract basis. You could be transferred at any moment and your career is only likely to last a few years. There are few, if any, personal or professional development programs to help you train for a new career or build additional marketable skills. Oh, and your medical records wouldn't be entirely confidential and though the work carries an inherent risk to your health, an injury or illness can be grounds for termination…

The Job of Being an Athlete

Let's start this chapter with a disclaimer. Every now and then we need to take a critical look at the things we engage with to recognize their limitations. How else

DOI: 10.4324/9781003088936-11

can we appreciate what we have and seek improvement for the future? This chapter takes a deep dive into the professional sport environment, and it might come across as overly negative; however, it's important to keep some perspective. This isn't meant as a condemnation, but an opportunity to assess the balance of effects that sport can have on the psychosocial wellbeing of its participants.

Now that's out of the way, let's get into it.

It's pretty safe to say that sports stars occupy a prominent place in our collective culture. Children run around with their favorite players' names on the backs of their branded jerseys (so do adults, to be fair), and many of us have imagined the glory of bringing home a trophy or medal at some point in our lives. People watch their heroes on television or follow them on social media, they manage them in fantasy leagues and video games, and they hunt for autographs and other memorabilia. We are bombarded by stories of athletes' brands, their contracts, their extravagance. In other words, the glitz and glamour of the professional sport lifestyle are in the public eye all the time. This creates a romanticized view of a life of fame, money, and influence. Is it any wonder that people often think that professional athletes have a dream job?

In the past few decades, the business of sport has become bigger and professionalized systems are now worth billions in the global economy. The total worth of the sports industry worldwide is estimated at $500 billion USD.[1] Just in North America for instance, the broadly-termed 'sports market' was worth $60 billion USD in 2014, reaching over $73 billion USD in 2019.[2] This growth is primarily derived from media rights agreements.[3] As sport has evolved into an entertainment business (connected with other economic drivers like marketing and mass media), grassroots organizations have developed into enormous multinational networks comprising more structure, more competitions, more money, more visibility, and also more demands for a competitive slice of the market. So, instead of being able to focus on the fun of playing sport every day, athletes are being increasingly subsumed by the industrialization of what was once a recreational pursuit. As The Notorious B.I.G. said, "mo' money, mo' problems."[i]

Of course, most athletes are well aware of this and still wouldn't trade their career for the world, but try to put yourself in their shoes for a moment. Imagine you have a contract worth millions, you're playing the most popular sport in your country, and you have legions of adoring fans. Not bad, right? On the other hand, you have to manage constant pressure and increasing demands, everything you do is highly visible, and in the midst of this you need to perform at the top of your game *every day* to keep your place and status. That's an intense and somewhat less attractive way to look at your daily grind. Throw an injury into the mix and, on top of everything else, your ability to work (and your job) is suddenly looking a lot less secure.

Professionalization and the Shift in Athlete Roles

Professionalization has affected athletes across the spectrum from recreational to elite levels, whether or not we realize it. For instance, where once the focus was on play and enjoyment, formalized developmental pathways now exist to recruit talented children into dedicated training environments where they can focus exclusively on a single sport. One factor driving this emphasis on early specialization is the increasingly common practice of talent identification, whereby coaches and scouts are on the lookout for promising young athletes in the hopes of finding the next superstar. In some sports, these pathways extend even within local clubs or schools, with children as young as nine appearing in sport-specific professional training systems.[4] This is most visible in soccer, where nearly every professional club around the world has a Youth Academy. Estimates in England suggest that, of the 1.5 million or so boys playing organized soccer, only about 180 will go on to play in the Premier League. This is a hit rate of 0.012%.[5] Academies fare only marginally better, with less than half of 1% ending up making a living as a player. This ultimately influences players both in and outside of the system, as it fosters competition and intensive sport focus in children even before they reach Academy entry age, whether or not they have aspirations of going on to a professional career.

Of course, early specialization can have benefits, such as access to quality coaching and better equipment. It can also be a requirement for early-entry sports like gymnastics. On the other hand, emerging research shows that it can be seriously detrimental in a lot of cases. To highlight, the International Olympic Committee published a consensus statement on youth athletic development, citing physical and mental health concerns including insufficient sleep, increased overuse injury rates, burnout, and eating disorders, not to mention the knock-on risks of poor general motor development and reduced/discontinued sport involvement later in life.[6] Yet, despite numerous position statements and a growing body of evidence advocating against the practice,[7,8] young athletes are being recruited onto professional pathways earlier and earlier.

A 2017 article in Time magazine illustrated how youth sports have become a huge industry worth more than $15.3 billion USD in the USA alone.[9] This revenue grew by 55% between 2010–2017, and the trend shows no signs of slowing. This has funneled vast amounts of resource into coaching, athlete support services, and facilities, creating unbelievable competition for access to a limited number of places within the developmental pathway. Particularly for those training in "the big sports" (e.g., soccer), there is a need to walk a tightrope between progressing fast enough to remain in this system while surviving the injury and burnout risk associated with high intensity training. These young athletes represent assets within a system that is designed to make money. We'll dig into that a bit more in a second, but first let's follow this thought through to its natural conclusion.

For those athletes who do make it to the elite level, there is a vital need to perform consistently at maximal capacity because the system is set up to ensure that there's always someone younger and fitter ready to take their place. It's kind of like an athlete conveyor belt. When performance cannot be maintained or begins to decay, it spells the end for a relatively short career. For example, the estimated peak performance age for explosive power or sprinting sports is around 20–27 years old, while for endurance events a lot of athletes can prolong success into their mid-late thirties.[10] It's common practice in a lot of professional sports to sign athletes to shorter contracts as they near these upper age limits, based on a belief that their abilities have begun to crest.[11] Of course, there are some athletes who completely ignore conventional limits and continue to dominate well into their later years, but elite sport is really a metaphorical *Logan's Run*.[ii] Importantly, similar contract restrictions can be imposed on athletes with previous or chronic injuries, meaning that concerns about career longevity can enter the picture well before age or performance is in question.

Balancing Form and Function

Right, so here's the part where we cycle back to the psychological issues associated with viewing athletes as assets. Without mincing words, professionalized sport systems are designed to support mass consumerism. That's harsh, but the interesting by-product is an unparalleled opportunity for athletes to excel in pursuit of their personal goals and to continually push the limits of performance within a resource-rich environment. On the surface, this presents a win-win scenario, providing a space for individuals to engage in autonomous, goal-directed behaviors (often with a healthy boost to self-efficacy, self-esteem, social connectedness, and ego satisfaction along the way).[12] Not a bad thing. But it also creates a complex set of tensions and interdependencies at the interface between those individuals and components of the system.[13] To illustrate, let's take the case of professional road cycling. Here we have athletes who are very clearly operating at or near the maximal threshold of endurance, and when they're healthy and winning, enormous resource is put into maximising their success through cutting edge training methods, bespoke nutritional strategies, tailored equipment design, etc. When the leader of the Tour de France can get a yellow bike shipped overnight from Italy to start the next morning in color-coordinated kit, we're talking about serious support structures! And this is the perfect recipe for excellence. Any rider who has goals of winning a race or setting a record finds themself in a system with aligned priorities.[14] In this way, it's a symbiotic relationship – what's good for the athlete is good for the bottom line. In an instant, however, this could all change off the back of a bad crash. Easy enough to do at speed or in bad weather conditions, but a rider who comes off the bike is suddenly at odds with the goals of the system. Their priorities shift to recovery, whereas the race must go on and a teammate suddenly becomes the group leader. Though the injured rider is looked after by the team and its sponsors, their primary resources are dedicated elsewhere, and it becomes a scramble to get back to fitness before that temporary replacement in the team hierarchy is made permanent. This relationship can become antagonistic and fraught with internal competition, contract disputes, and risky behaviors in an effort to retain position.[14]

Imagine being an "asset" in this environment. When your entire focus has been on carving out a sporting career and you're used to being the best in your team, your school, or your league, suddenly discovering that you're an average-sized fish in a large pond can cause feelings of frustration and diminished confidence, not to mention heightened sensitivity to social comparison.[15–17] A show of weakness or vulnerability can take on inflated importance, prompting athletes to take undue risks in training or competition, hide injuries or downplay their severity, or seek to accelerate injury rehabilitation timelines in any way they can in order to maintain their place in the system.[18,19] We'll talk about each of these issues, but first we need to appreciate exactly how common injuries are in high performance settings.

Injuries are an occupational hazard in sport and considering the physically demanding nature of the work, this is often accepted as part of the deal when people sign up. But even when compared to other high-risk occupations, the overall injury risk in sport is considerably higher. For instance, epidemiological studies have shown that the injury rate in professional soccer is 1000 times higher than in construction or mining.[20,21] So those who enter into a professional pathway with fierce competition for roster spots are in double jeopardy – the sport itself carries an inherent risk, plus a win-at-all-costs attitude has the potential to dramatically increase the likelihood of harm. There's a lot to unpack there. We're dealing with a situation where only those who are willing to accept such risks will remain in the system (either by choice or by selection), and then these athletes are driven to push even greater boundaries in order to meet both their own and their employers'/sponsors'/fans' expectations. Needless to say, this environment isn't for everyone.

If the average worker was asked to accept the fact that they would almost certainly be injured on the job once or more per year, there would be a mutiny at most workplaces. Yet, in the sport context, nobody bats an eye. We've encountered the term "risk-taking" before (see chapter 3) and have established that in sport it's broad and loosely defined. It comprises not only the notion that sport, by its nature, carries inherent risk of physical, psychological, and social harm, but also the idea that sport is imbued with a wide range of normative practices that can be detrimental (e.g., hazing, harassment). It's also a vehicle for cultural capital that can elevate or denigrate individuals and groups depending on their adherence to, or deviation from, what is deemed "acceptable" by those in positions of power. Take the very public example of Colin Kaepernick, whose social activism on the NFL field derailed his professional football career.[22]

One of the most well-researched aspects of risk-taking in sport is the normalization of injury and its lingering effects. This is related to the idea of "The Sports Ethic," which encompasses the core ideas of (1) making sacrifices for the game; (2) striving for distinction; (3) accepting risks and playing through pain; and (4) refusing to accept limits when pursuing possibilities.[23] A distinct, yet related concept is the "Culture of Risk," describing a set of socialized beliefs around the importance of playing through pain. This becomes most evident when comparing athletes who are glorified for persevering versus those who are mocked or stigmatized when they step out of competition after being injured.[24,25] As this culture has been perpetuated, the professional athlete identity has been attached to tough and heroic imagery.[26] Iconic stories of injured players competing or sacrificing their health in the name of their sport have become embedded in collective memory. The well-known footage of Gabriela Andersen-Schiess finishing the marathon in the 1984 Olympic games is a good example: the athlete with heat exhaustion limps around the track, clearly suffering, and is hailed as a heroine. The public gives audience to such stories as the media extol the virtues of strength and bravery in competition, reinforcing the value placed on athletic achievement over personal health.[iii]

These values have become prerequisites at the elite end of the sporting spectrum and have subsequently been systematized into all levels of competition (e.g., youth and recreational leagues).[27] As the culture of a particular sport begins to coalesce around a tacit agreement on acceptable risk, individual athletes must sublimate their own beliefs and values to conform with their social environment if they want to succeed. This inevitably leads to debate, as we're seeing now around whether or not it is reasonable to include tackling in school-level rugby in light of the consequent risk of concussion.[30] Yet, whether such controversies are escalated to context-wide adaptation (such as banning dangerous elements of play)[31] or individuals are left to make a value judgement for themselves, sport cultures tend to be robust, and some features persist through time.

Sometimes It Isn't about Pain

The most commonly held norm within sport is the "no pain, no gain" maxim. This goes hand-in-hand with the acceptance of injury risk as part of sport participation, and is prevalent in nearly all age groups, competitive levels, and settings to a certain extent. Interestingly, however, the way athletes define pain and its role in performance depends largely on the immediate context.

Research here coincides with widely held anecdotal impressions that the gravity of a particular performance can influence pain perception. Whether we think about it in terms of a championship match or an opening night solo, the importance an athlete places on a given outcome can manipulate their perception of what does or doesn't constitute an injury.[32] This is often mediated by the demands of the sport and the tolerance of that individual.[33] For example, a soccer player may perceive an ankle sprain as an injury, while a swimmer might not because of the discrepant demands of the sport or differences in pain tolerance. But the same soccer player may view the sprain as an injury if it happens during preseason, whereas during the league finals it might not be considered as such. For many of us, pain signals that something's wrong, that we should stop what we're doing or perhaps seek medical attention. Conversely, athletes often remark that "it's just pain," perceiving this as a normal component of their day.[34]

With qualitative research becoming more commonplace in sport medicine, we're starting to better understand how injury is defined differently by key stakeholders. For instance, while doctors and sport scientists might define injury according to diagnostic codes or an objective clinical assessment, professional athletes typically define injury based on the impact of symptoms on their ability to train or deliver an optimal performance.[34,35] In other words, what constitutes an "injury" will vary, depending on who you ask. This has implications for all sorts of things, including injury surveillance (e.g., how many injuries we pick up will depend on who is reporting and how they define an injury), medical management (e.g., should we treat the tissue or the impairment?), coaching decisions (e.g., who decides whether an athlete is fit to play?), and certainly not least, athletes' long-term health and wellbeing. But as we've seen, though an injury happens to an individual, it happens in a specific context and these two factors cannot be separated. Therefore, a sport injury is not simply a health condition in itself, but it reflects an interaction between the physical damage and the athlete's perceptions of the contextual factors that shape the injury experience.

Since high-level athletes mostly define injury based on its consequences, why don't we take a look at three examples to see how this might play out. To kick off, we'll consider an elite middle-distance runner. The competitive calendar for this person will be periodized with up and down changes in training load, dictated by their target events for that season or where they are in an Olympic cycle. Early in a training block, pain may be reported as an "injury," an obstacle to be overcome with rest, treatment, or adapted training; however, as races get closer, the same pain may be re-conceptualized as "background noise" to be battled through. When this happens, the cause of the pain often isn't addressed completely, so the symptoms can drag on for weeks or months. There's plenty of evidence for this in different sports, where high proportions of athletes are injured at the start of major competitions.[36,37] Therefore, for our runner, an injury can impact the full season, or have no major consequences, depending on how proximally it happens to competition.

As a second vignette, let's think about professional acrobats (e.g., Cirque du Soleil). These performers tend to have a relatively uniform show schedule through the year, with short breaks built in for each show. The main requirement for a circus artist is to deliver a consistent level of performance, night in and night out. This means that they don't have much room to adapt their routine or take it easy while an injury heals. If an injury is severe, they'll be out of show which may impact show quality and audience feedback. There are also knock-on effects for the rest of the show, as these are often composed such that artists must rely on each other to transition between performance elements. A reorganization of the show around a missing artist is usually only undertaken as a last resort. Pain or injury for these individuals must therefore be defined in terms of how it affects their ability to perform and its impact on safety (e.g., an artist cannot put themselves or others at risk by being unable to land or catch someone properly). In this case, pain is often something to be managed throughout the year in such a way that it does not become too debilitating to continue and "injuries" are only those conditions severe enough to warrant time off.

Our third example takes us into the world of professional dance, where individuals may have frequent changes in their repertoire, requiring them to manage the dynamic demands of different performing styles and choreographies. An additional feature of this context is the aesthetic element, where time off due to an injury may result in altered body composition, loss of flexibility, or constrained technique. Dance is in itself incredibly demanding and it's not uncommon for the majority of those in pre-professional training or performing companies to experience pain and other symptoms regularly.[38] These rarely result in time off, as an injury can cost a dancer a leading role or casting in a future production, meaning diminishing cache in an industry that is already geared to value younger, fitter, healthier bodies as part of the end product.[39] So, when dancers define "injury," it's not surprising that they often do so in terms of its impact on execution and expression during performance.[35]

So, what does all of this mean from a psychological point of view? The truth is, when we talk about how professionalized systems influence injury risk and rehabilitation, we may ultimately be comparing apples to oranges. An injury in one context may not be considered an injury in another. Some of that is down to individual motivations – you're hardly going to let a broken finger stop you from a shot at a World Cup, are you? – but a lot of it is driven by competition, job security, and marketability within a particular sport structure. Injury reporting is therefore a complex phenomenon influenced by subjective injury definitions, the Culture of Risk and its related social pressures, and fear of losing playing time and/ or career vulnerability.[40]

As we've seen in other chapters, athletes and performers must balance their personal health and wellbeing against the pressures of the environment, and this often results in trade-offs with lasting repercussions across psychological, social, and financial domains (Figure 11.1). The occurrence of burnout and mental health issues such as anxiety, depression, and substance misuse often arise under these

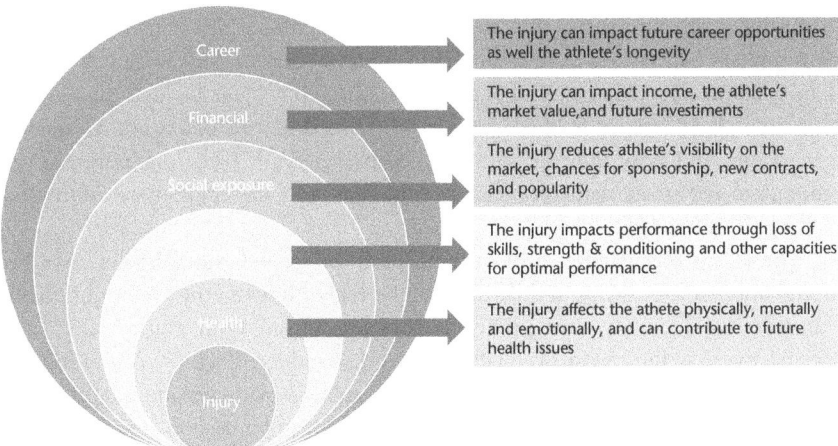

FIGURE 11.1 Potential consequences of injury (or injury-related absence) across the psychological, social, and career domains of the sport environment.

conditions, and they are increasingly well-documented within professional sport communities.[41] It's not just the athletes themselves who are vulnerable to such outcomes, either. Coaches, referees, and others working in the professional domain are also exposed to the pressures of a performance-driven environment and are subject to similar risks.[42,43] Perhaps not surprisingly, we're only beginning to understand how athletes are affected, and we know even less about the situation in these other groups. Much more research is needed here to give us a clearer picture of the prevalence and impact of such issues, followed swiftly by practical recommendations for managing them in practice.

The "Disposable" Body and Competition for Roster Places

Even though there's a standing expectation among athletes and their support staff that they will be injured at some point, there remains a tension around how injuries are managed in many cases. You don't end up at the elite end of your discipline without being highly familiar with the tools of your trade, and athletes are no exception. They're the experts when it comes to their own bodies and what is, or is not, normal for them. Consequently, they are always the first to recognize the warning signs of injury (whether they're paying attention to them is another question altogether), and the onus is on them to communicate health complaints to their coach or medical provider. This should ideally be a two-way street, where coaches and health teams are watching for changes in performance that could be related to an injury. This, unfortunately, is where communication can start to break down. Athletes may not want to talk about it in the hopes of keeping it off the coach's radar, and those around them may sometimes ignore the signs of injury when performance is on the line. This goes to show that within the professionalized system, athletes are increasingly viewed as commodities and there is a rich literature that chronicles the history of this accelerating shift over time.[44] Researchers have taken critical aim at this intersection of consumer culture, celebrity culture, race theory, and exploitation, though it's well beyond the scope of our immediate interest to delve into these. Indeed, entire books are devoted to such issues and how they fit within modern society.[45,46] For our purposes, it's enough to recognize that commodification shapes the way injuries are interpreted and acted upon.

The fact is that from a sport business perspective, individual bodies have become disposable in the sense that they can be replaced when they're not optimally functioning. This has emerged in the discourse from both athlete and coach perspectives, as illustrated by qualitative work conducted within American collegiate sport.[47] This research reinforces a view that, in many situations, athletes are not considered as persons but rather as bodies that can be used for the betterment of their team, club, or organization. The monetary worth attached to athletes and their scholarships or contracts is often seen by coaches and others in the management hierarchy – not to mention spectators and the media – as an entitlement to expect certain outputs. When an athlete cannot produce those outputs, they are no longer "valuable" and can therefore be discarded.[47] For athletes, this can begin a negative feedback loop where a diminished team role or inability to perform against expectations results in a loss of self-confidence, loss of identity, aggression or conflict in social relationships, and increasingly poorer performance.[48] This creates a tension between what's best for the athlete and what's best for the team.

At the organizational level, cost-benefit analyses are often undertaken in terms of whether it's worth rehabilitating an injured athlete or whether it would be better to replace them. If there are healthy and equally capable replacements waiting in the wings, the business decision is fairly straightforward. This obviously has implications for not only the athlete's career, but potentially their ability to continue accessing necessary medical care, too – if they are out of a contract, they may no longer have access to support resources unless there is a players' union or charity in place to help. Conversely, some athletes are "irreplaceable" because of their skill level, leadership qualities, or sometimes simply because there's nobody available to take their place. In this way, there is a duality in health care for professional athletes. The quality of care is often better than that delivered to the "average" person, but the system itself may serve other interests (eg, facilitating team performance). Here athletes may employ different coping strategies when navigating injury rehabilitation. Some attempt to return to the lineup as quickly as possible (either volitionally or under pressure from the organization they play for), whereas others adapt to bring different value to the team (eg, becoming a "role player" or excelling as a leader instead of a scorer).[49] In some instances, athletes survive in the system because older and wiser players are needed to mentor the next generation, in essence training their own eventual replacements. How's that for some heavy emotional lifting?

Different (Sport) Cultures and the System

There's a quote from David Foster Wallace that explains how culture is part of us: *"There are these two young fish swimming along and they happen to meet an older fish swimming the other way, who nods at them and says, 'Morning, boys. How's the water?' The two young fish swim on for a bit, and then eventually one of them looks over at the other and goes, 'What the hell is water?'"*[50] Culture is the water we swim in every day. It exists around us and shapes on our lives, though we may not recognize it.

The high-performance sport environment constitutes a very particular culture, but we must also acknowledge that different sports foster unique cultures that shape injury experiences. For instance, it's perfectly ordinary for ice hockey players to lose teeth and keep on playing, happily sporting a toothless grin for years to come. In another environment, dental trauma would be managed very differently. Similarly, ballerinas routinely dance through foot damage (think bruising, ulcers, stress fractures), which would be considered debilitating in other settings. So, some of the psychological response to injury is shaped by how it's contextualized within the culture of that particular domain. And there are other sociological elements that feed into injury responses as well. Athletes don't leave their heritage behind when they play sport, and there is a substantial body of evidence suggesting that norms around pain reporting and healthcare-seeking can vary between geographic and social communities.[51] It's therefore important that when interpreting an athlete's injury responses and behaviors, a sensitive lens is applied to understand the influence of their cultural milieu *within* the professional sport system. We have very little research to rely on for guiding practice in this regard, but open communication, strong leadership from coaching and medical staff, and shared decision making with athletes are key to minimizing the deleterious effects of injuries on individuals and teams.[52]

Where Do We Go From Here?

Right, so this has been a dense chapter with a lot of moving parts. How do we take this information and put it to good use? There is increasing momentum in the sport injury research sphere toward examining risk and rehabilitation using a *systems approach* that accounts for the complexity of the context.[53] After all, an injury involves an athlete who is characterized by many intra-individual features, as well as multiple extra-individual factors that take place across multiple levels of a particular cultural context (Figure 11.2). The aspiring or professional athlete therefore exists within a dynamic and rapidly evolving landscape which can exert direct and indirect effects on cognitive, emotional, and social factors that influence individual injury experiences.

We've discussed the multilevel structure of professional sport and how appreciation for its inherent pressures is instrumental in providing better care for athletes. Interventions should ideally focus on facilitating communication, building trustworthy

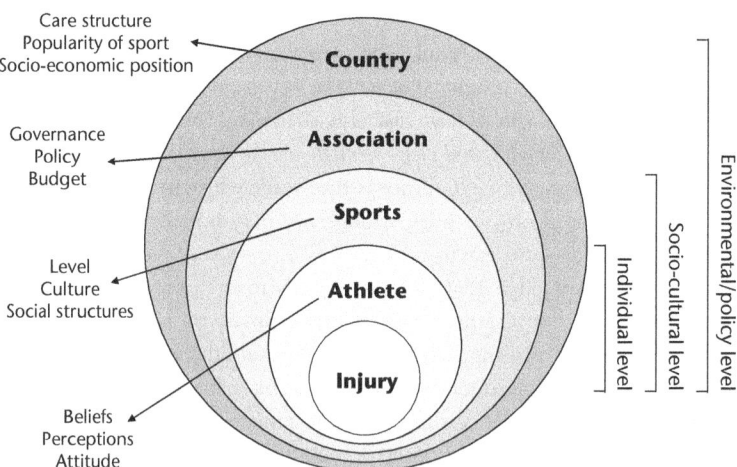

FIGURE 11.2 The socio-ecological model of sport injury, highlighting the athlete's position within a layered cultural context.[32]

relationships, and helping athletes cope with the challenges of their chosen professional path. This is easier said than done, of course. Healthcare providers are often employed by the athlete's club or organization and there's a tricky balance for them, acting in the athlete's best interest while having a responsibility to the success of the team. This means there's no standard approach that works for all contexts because of the diversity in daily practice for each individual.

For people working in sport, the only sensible practical recommendation is to learn more about the contexts of "your" athletes. Help them identify solutions to make the environment work in their favor instead of against them. To do this, we need to understand that all the factors we covered in this chapter (money, fame, glory, the Culture of Risk, commodification, the banalization of pain and injury, pursuit of excellence, sport culture) are embedded in a system where the athlete is just one piece. It's difficult to grasp the boundaries of that system when you're also part of it, and this applies to athletes as well as those who support them. If the goal is to be able to embrace this big picture and not only help athletes navigate it, but also improve the system from within, then continued critical assessment of professionalized sport is a good place to start.

Notes

i For those who are now singing this hook along with us, you're welcome. But for anyone who wasn't on top of the American rap music scene circa 1997, this might be a fringe reference. Do yourself a favor and check out The Notorious B.I.G.'s *Life After Death* album (if you're under 18, only the Clean Edition please).

ii Ok, this might be another obscure reference, but it's too perfect to pass up. *Logan's Run* is a 1967 sci-fi classic by William F Nolan and George Clayton Johnson. The story is set in an ageist future where the population is kept in a state of equilibrium by terminating everyone at age 21. It's a quick read (and an even quicker film) if you've got some time to spare and are comfortable with dystopian angst. And consider this recommendation your reward for getting 2/3 of the way through the book!

iii Although beyond the scope of this chapter, the construct of *hegemonic masculinity* has been a traditional foundation of professional sport (though alternative discourses are emerging). This is defined as any practice that legitimizes men's dominance in society and justifies the subordination of "common" men and women, and is often linked to structures that uphold the Culture of Risk. For a fascinating read on the intersection of hegemonic masculinity, injury, and media coverage, read Sanderson et al.'s comparison of two high-profile NFL quarterback injuries[28] or Miele's thesis on the portrayal of NHL injuries in the news.[29]

References

1 https://www.torrens.edu.au/blog/business/why-the-sports-industry-is-booming-in-2020-and-which-key-players-are-driving-growth. Accessed April 14, 2021.

2 Heitner D. Sports industry to reach $73.5 billion by 2019. Available at: https://www.forbes.com/sites/darrenheitner/2015/10/19/sports-industry-to-reach-73-5-billion-by-2019/#7278bab51b4b. Accessed April 14, 2021.

3 https://www.statista.com/statistics/1120190/broadcasting-rights-sports-by-source/. Accessed April 14, 2021.

4 Ryan D, Lewin C, Forsythe S, et al. Developing world-class soccer players: an example of the academy physical development program from an English Premier League team. *Strength and Conditioning Journal* 2018;40(3):2–11 doi:10.1519/SSC.0000000000000340.

5 https://www.businessinsider.com/michael-calvin-shocking-statistic-why-children-football-academies-will-never-succeed-soccer-sport-2017-6?r=US&IR=T. Accessed April 14, 2021.

6 Bergeron MF, Mountjoy M, Armstrong N, et al. International Olympic Committee consensus statement on youth athletic development. *Br J Sports Med* 2015;49(13):843–851; doi:10.1136/bjsports-2015-094962.

7 Gould D. The professionalization of youth sports: it's time to act! *Clin J Sport Med* 2009;19(2):81–82; doi:10.1097/JSM.0b013e31819edaff.

8 Myer GD, Jayanthi N, DiFiori JP. Sports specialization, Part II: alternative solutions to early sport specialization in youth athletes. *Sports Health* 2016;8(1):65–73; doi:10.1177/1941738115614811.

9 https://time.com/magazine/us/4913681/september-4th-2017-vol-190-no-9-u-s/. Accessed April 14, 2021.

10 Allen SV, Hopkins WG. Age of peak competitive performance of elite athletes: a systematic review. *Sports Med* 2015;45(10):1431–1441; doi:10.1007/s40279-015-0354-3.

11 Kalen A, Rey E, de Rellan-Guerra AS, et al. Are soccer players older now than before? Aging trends and market value in the last three decades of the UEFA Champions League. *Front Psychol* 2019;10:76; doi:10.3389/fpsyg.2019.00076.

12 Smith AL, Ntoumanis N, Duda JL, et al. Goal striving, coping, and well-being: a prospective investigation of the self-concordance model in sport. *J Sport Exerc Psychol* 2011;33:124–145; doi:10.1123/jsep.33.1.124.

13 Hays K, Thomas O, Maynard I, et al. The role of confidence in world-class sport performance. *J Sports Sci* 2009;11(27):1185–1199; doi:10.1080/02640410903089798.

14 Phillips KE, Hopkins WG. Determinants of cycling performance: a review of the dimensions and features regulating performance in elite cycling competitions. *Sports Med-Open* 2020;6:23; doi:10.1186/s40798-020-00252-z.

15 Bruner MW, Munroe-Chandler KJ, Spink KS. Entry into elite sport: a preliminary investigation into the transition experiences of rookie athletes. *J Appl Sport Psychol* 2008;20(2):236–252; doi:10.1080/10413200701867745.

16 Stambulova N, Franck A, Weibull F. Assessment of the transition from junior-to-senior sports in Swedish athletes. *Int J Sport Exerc Psychol* 2012;10(2):79–95; doi:10.1080/1612197X.2012.645136.

17 Finn J, McKenna J. Coping with Academy-to-first-team transitions in elite English male team sports: the coaches' perspective. *Int J Sports Sci Coach* 2010;5(2):257–279; doi:10.1260/1747-9541.5.2.257.

18 Nelson NW, Albright C. Injury reporting in collegiate soccer players and the impact of non-reporting. *Internet J Allied Health Sci Pract* 2020;18(4):19.

19 Whatman C, Walters S, Schluter P. Coach and player attitudes to injury in youth sport. *Phys Ther Sport* 2018;32:1–6; doi:10.1016/j.ptsp.2018.01.011.

20 Hawkins RD, Fuller CW. An examination of the frequency and severity of injuries and incidents at three levels of professional football. *Br J Sports Med* 1998;32(4):326–331; doi:10.1136/bjsm.32.4.326.

21 Drawer S, Fuller CW. Evaluating the level of injury in English professional football using a risk based assessment process. *Br J Sports Med* 2002;36(6):446–451; doi:10.1136/bjsm.36.6.446.

22 Boykoff J, Carrington B. Sporting dissent: Colin Kaepernick, NFL activism, and media framing contests. *Int Rev Sociol Sport* 2020;55(7):829–849; doi:10.1177/101269021 9861594.

23 Hughes R, Coakley J. Positive Deviance among Athletes: the Implications of Overconformity to the Sport Ethic. *Sociol Sport J* 1991;8:307–325; doi:10.1123/ ssj.8.4.307.

24 Nixon HL. Accepting the risks of pain and injury in sport: mediated cultural influences on playing hurt. *Sociol Sport* 1993 Jun 1;10(2):183–196; doi:10.1123/ssj.10.2.183.

25 Safai P. Healing the body in the "culture of risk": examining the negotiation of treatment between sport medicine clinicians and injured athletes in Canadian intercollegiate sport. *Sociol Sport J* 2003 Jun 1;20(2):127–146; doi:10.1123/ssj.20.2.127.

26 Weinberg R, Vernau D, Horn T. Playing through pain and injury: psychosocial considerations. *J Clin Sports Psychol* 2013;7(1):41–59; doi:10.1123/jcsp.7.1.41.

27 Jessiman-Perrault G, Godley J. Playing through the pain: a university-based study of sports injury. *Adv Phys Educ* 2016;6:178–194; doi:10.4236/ape.2016.63020.

28 Sanderson J, Weathers M, Grevious A, et al. A hero or a sissy? Exploring media framing of NFL quarterbacks injury decisions. *Commun Sport* 2016;4(1):3–22; doi:10.1177/ 2167479514536982.

29 Miele R. *Hegemonic masculinity and the ideal male hockey player: the constructions of NHL injuries in popular Canadian newspapers 2016-2017* [dissertation]. The University of Western Ontario 2020.

30 Pollock AM, White AJ, Kirkwood G. Evidence in support of the call to ban that tackle and harmful contact in school rugby: a response to World Rugby. *Br J Sports Med* 2017;51:1113–1117; doi:10.1136/bjsports-2016-096996.

31 Black AM, haggle BEE, Palacios-Derflingher L, et al. The risk of injury associated with body checking among Pee Wee ice hockey players: an evaluation of Hockey Canada's national body checking policy change. *Br J Sports Med* 2017;51:1767–1772; doi:10.1136/ bjsports-2016-097392.

32 Bolling, C, van Mechelen, W, Pasman, HR, et al. Context matters: revisiting the first step of the "sequence of prevention" of sports injuries. *Sports Med* 2018;48:2227–2234. doi: 10.1007/s40279-018-0953-x.

33 Hainline B, Turner JA, Caneiro JP, et al. Pain in elite athletes—neurophysiological, biomechanical and psychosocial considerations: a narrative review. *Br J Sports Med* 2017;51:1259–1264; doi:10.1136/bjsports-2017-097890.

34 Bolling C, Delfino Barboza S, van Mechelen W, Pasman HR. How elite athletes, coaches, and physiotherapists perceive a sports injury. *Transl Sports Med* 2019;2(1):17–23; doi:10.1002/tsm2.53.

35 Bolling C, van Rijn RM, Pasman HR, et al. In your shoes: a qualitative study on the perspectives of professional dancers and staff regarding dance injury and its prevention. *Transl Sports Med* 2021; doi:10.1102/tsm2.226.

36 Soligard T, Steffen K, Palmer D, et al. Sports injury and illness incidence in the Rio de Janeiro 2016 Olympic Summer Games: a prospective study of 11274 athletes from 207 countries. *Br J Sports Med* 2017;51:1265–1271; doi:10.1136/bjsports-2017-097956.

37 Soligard T, Palmer D, Steffen K, et al. Sports injury and illness incidence in the PyeongChang 2018 Olympic Winter Games: a prospective study of 2914 athletes from 92 countries. *Br J Sports Med* 2019;53:1085–1092; doi:10.1136/bjsports-2018-100236.

38 Lampe J, Groneeberg DA, Ohlendorf D, et al. Pain in female dancers and dance teachers: perception, assessment, and related behaviour. *Scand J Med Sci Sports* 2019;29(4):623–632; doi:10.1111/sms.13387.

39 McEwen K, Young K. Ballet and pain: reflections on a risk-dance culture. *Qualitative Research in Sport, exercise and health* 2011;3(2):152–173; doi:10.1080/2159676X.2011.572181.

40 Clark R, Stanfill AG. A systematic review of barriers and facilitators for concussion reporting behavior among student athletes. *J Trauma Nurs* 2019 1;26(6):297–311; doi: 10.1097/JTN.0000000000000468.

41 Reardon CL, Hainline B, Aron CM, et al. Mental health in elite athletes: International Olympic Committee consensus statement. *Br J Sports Med* 2019;53:667–699; doi:10.1136/bjsports-2019-100715.

42 Altfeld S, Schaffran P, Kleinert J, et al. Minimising the risk of coach burnout: from research to practice. *Int Sport Coach J* 208;5(1):71–78; doi:10.1123/iscj.2017-0033.

43 Hill DM, Matthews N, Senior R. The psychological characteristics of performance under pressure in professional rugby union referees. *Sport Psychol* 2016;30(4):376–387; doi:10.1123/tsp.2015-0109.

44 Vamplew W. The commodification of sport: exploring the nature of the sports product. *Int J Hist Sport* 2018;35:659–672; doi:10.1080/09523367.2018.1481832.

45 Horne J. *Sport in consumer culture*. Hampshire: Palgrave 2005.

46 Hylton K. *Race and sport: critical race theory*. New York: Routledge 2008.

47 Zanin AC. Structuring bodywork: control and agency in athlete injury discourse. *J Appl Commun Res* 2018;46(3):267–290; doi:10.1080/00909882.1465578.

48 Menke DJ, Germany ML. Reconstructing athletic identity: college athletes and sport retirement. *J Loss Trauma* 2019 24(1):17–30; doi:10.1080/15325024.2018.1522475.

49 Samuel RD, Tenenbaum G. The role of change in athletes' careers: a scheme of change for sport psychology practice. *Sport Psychol* 2011;25:233–252; doi:10.1123/tsp.25.2.233.

50 Wallace DF. *This is water: some thoughts, delivered on a significant occasion about living a compassionate life*. New York: Little, Brown 2009.

51 Sharma S, Ferreira-Valente, de C, Williams AC, et al. Group differences between countries and between languages in pain-related beliefs, coping, and catastrophizing in chronic pain: a systematic review. *Pain Med* 2020;21(9):1847–1862; doi:10.1093/pm/pnz373.

52 Ekstrand J, Lundqvist D, Davison M, et al. Communication quality between the medical team and the head coach/manager is associated with injury burden and player availability in elite football clubs. *Br J Sports Med* 2019;53:304–308; doi:10.1136/bjsports-2018-099411.

53 Bekker S, Clark AM. Bringing complexity to sports injury prevention research: from simplification to explanation. *Br J Sports Med* 2016;50:1489–1490; doi:10.1136/bjsports-2016-096457.

12

WHEN INJURIES LEAD TO RETIREMENT: CALLING IT A DAY

Carly McKay and Stephen Mellalieu

When the Game Ends and the Race Is Run

In 2018 the UK-based Professional Players Federation (PPF) published a com-missioned survey in partnership with the Rugby Players Association, the Professional Cricketers Association and the Professional Footballers Association.[1] The research covered 800 former professional players ranging from 17 to 79 years old and indicated that a significant number of them struggled both financially and mentally in the first few years after retiring from professional sport. Alarmingly, over 70% of those surveyed indicated they were unable to choose when they stopped playing professional sport, citing reasons like injuries, general wear and tear or being unable to obtain a new contract. Such an unceremonious end to one's career can present all kinds of challenges, some of which are entirely relatable to non-athletes and others that are unique to this group.

As inevitable as death and taxes is the occasion when we must walk away from an activity or sport that we love, something that may have been a lifelong passion pursued from childhood through to early adulthood or into middle age. For most of us normal 'Joes' for whom sport is a pastime rather than a profession, that decision will have been an active one, brought on by increasing study, family or work commitments reducing the amount of time we can dedicate to training or engaging in that activity. Sure, we may miss playing soccer on a Sunday morning with our former college mates or getting up before sunrise to catch perfect waves in the ocean, but we can console ourselves with the pleasure we derive from achievements in other parts of our lives, such as seeing our young family grow up or nailing the big contract in work and securing a promotion. We can be com-fortable in the knowledge that a trip to the gym on the way home from work or a run through the neighbourhood will keep our wellbeing balance maintained. But, for one group of this planet's population – professional athletes – the decision to

DOI: 10.4324/9781003088936-12

stop engaging in sport can often prove more difficult, as it's usually their sole means of earning a living and the singular feature that defines them. For these individuals, it's often not as simple as trading off priorities and finding fulfilment from other pursuits.

Ideally, an elite athlete will call it a day when they feel the time is right. This may be because they no longer have the desire to make the significant sacrifices associated with the high demands of their sport, or they've accomplished all they wanted to. Or, the reality is that while the mind may still be willing, often the body is not. Time catches up with us all and elite athletes are no exception. The lucky ones acknowledge they're not able to physically perform to the level required to allow them to compete at the professional end of the game, and so make the call to get out. Leaving sport on one's own terms like that usually brings with it a sense of closure, but the decision can often be expedited by the selection choices of the head coach or manager of the team, deciding not to renew an athlete's contract due to their age and performance level. That can be hard to take, but the most difficult of exits for elite athletes to acknowledge comes from injury-forced retirement. Whereas age, loss in motivation, and deselection all offer the athlete a degree of autonomy in their decision to retire, career-ending injury offers no such affordance. A career ending injury means no opportunity for the athlete to go out on top, no final standing ovation from the crowd, teammates or global TV audience at the final whistle, no lap of honour. No chance to properly celebrate a lifetime of commitment and investment into a passion, a profession that is now gone for the rest of their living days.

Poring over the back pages of most newspapers on a daily basis you'll be greeted with announcements of athletes who are unable to compete and have therefore been forced to retire on medical grounds. This doesn't just include those who have been told by Doctors not to continue, either. Elite athletes are increasingly making the decision to retire themselves, fearing permanent damage to their health. In the UK, Sam Warburton, one of Wales' and the British Lions' most successful professional rugby union captains, decided to call time on his career at 29 years of age, a time when most rugby players are at the peak of their playing and earning potential. After attempting to rehabilitate from the latest of what was a long list of injuries suffered in his professional career, Warburton noted he had made the decision to retire with his health and wellbeing as a priority.[2] That kind of Sophie's Choice[i] isn't reserved for contact sport athletes. Graham Onions, former fast bowler with England cricket, retired at 37 years old after suffering a back injury, also citing the need to protect his health and wellbeing in future years.[3] This scenario is also apparent in younger athletes who retire because of the fear of injury, or the concern about the long-term consequences of participating at the elite level. One such high profile case is Chris Borland who, in 2014 following a successful rookie season as a line-backer with the San Francisco 49ers, decided to quite the game to preserve his mental health due to anxieties over the prospective consequences of brain injuries, particularly chronic traumatic encephalopathy.[4] We can debate whether such choices made on medical grounds are indeed voluntary or whether athletes' hands have been forced by the circumstances, but either way the results are largely the same.

In contrast with the typical retirement age for most occupations in the western world (i.e., beyond 60 years of age), forced retirement from professional sport often occurs in the early to mid-thirties, or even younger. This can have meaningful psychological, social, financial, and health consequences across a significant portion of the lifespan. So, although we must not forget that amateur athletes can also experience some degree of challenge to their mental health and wellbeing if they're forced to cease participation, the situation former professionals find themselves in creates some very particular issues. We can begin to unpack these by exploring how sport shapes the way athletes define themselves, and what happens when retirement challenges that self-concept.

Hero to Zero

It's often said that a sports star will die twice, the first time at retirement. The "death" of a sportsperson through career termination can lead to dramatic changes in their personal, social and occupational lives which, in turn, can have a significant mental, emotional and behavioral impact. The social and professional changes induced by retirement from sport can cause distressful reactions leading athletes to experience feelings of emptiness in their lives. Much of this distress can be put down to the loss of the athlete's identity - what defines them, and what gives them a sense of purpose and confidence to function in life. An individual's identity may contain numerous dimensions. For example, a functioning adult may see their identity as comprising part spouse or partner, part parent, part friend, part office worker, and part exerciser/athlete. However, it's possible for one specific identity to become the preferred or dominant one, which then becomes a lens through which the other aspects of one's identities are viewed. This is often the case for elite athletes. The concept of *athletic identity* is viewed as the extent to which an individual identifies with their role as an athlete and looks to others for acknowledgement of that role.[5] The neglect of other roles as a consequence of this singular focus can result in subsequent identity issues. When a loss of a preferred or dominant identity occurs, such as through forced retirement from sport, the individual's self-concept becomes threatened. Our self-concept is essentially our overarching view of how we think about, evaluate, or perceive ourselves. When that's in jeopardy, we can experience an identity crisis (questioning who we are and how we think about ourselves). Those sportspeople with a strong athletic identity at the time of forced retirement are therefore more likely to experience a higher degree of emotional adjustment difficulties.[6] Indeed, many athletes who have struggled to come to terms with their retirement experience a profound sense of loss in their lives when they become an "ex-athlete", a label which inwardly and outwardly can be tough to take.

Sport-related identity loss is often a one-two punch, as well. *Social identity* is a person's self-concept based on their membership of social groups and cultures.[7]

Feeling part of, or being able to identify with a group, team or organization, helps to reinforce one's social identity. When an athlete is forced to retire, they can abruptly lose the ability to identify with their team or sport. The feeling of being part of something, the daily routine of interacting with fellow athletes, is quickly lost and can further contribute to the crisis of *Who Am I?* and the journey from hero (athlete) to zero (ex-athlete). Threats to social identity are also accompanied by changes in social networks, and therefore the social support mechanisms, athletes will be used to drawing upon to maintain their sense of worth. While competing, elite athletes typically have access to a strong network to support them (teammates, training partners, coaches, doctors, training staff, psychologists, analysts, nutritionists, agents, press office, player development/performance lifestyle managers... the list is endless). All of these individuals not only provide *instrumental support* (tangible assistance) during the athlete's professional career, but also offer *emotional support* (care and concern) to assist with the various challenges faced on the journey.[7] Upon retirement, a large portion of these networks become inaccessible. Some athletes have professional player associations or unions that provide aftercare and a degree of support during retirement, but athletes who have strong athletic identities and fractured social networks outside of their profession often experience further distress coming to terms with life after sport.

The Hidden Side of Injury

The 2018 PPF survey of former UK pro athletes suggested that 54% of past players had, at some time since retiring, experienced concerns about their mental and emotional wellbeing.[1] Concerningly, only 4 in 10 of them had sought help. Career termination induces significant changes in an athletes' personal, social and occupational lives, which can potentially affect how an individual thinks, feels and behaves. Among these reactions, clinical depression is front and centre as a common consequence. Multiple Olympic swimming champion Ian Thorpe, former Northern Ireland international soccer player and Celtic Football Club Manager Neil Lennon, and double Olympic champion Dame Kelly Holmes are just a few of the high-profile athletes who have made their depression public after their retirement from elite sport.[8] Research has shown that symptoms of depression, anxiety, distress, and sleep disturbance affect an estimated 15–25% of athletes in the first few years after their retirement.[9–11] Importantly, forced retirement appears to double the risk of these problems[10] and those retiring specifically due to injury may be up to three times more likely to have clinically relevant depression scores.[12] Ongoing pain and stronger athletic identity also appear to increase the likelihood of depressive symptoms post-retirement, though reliance on small samples with a high risk of selection bias[ii] and measurement tools with unknown validity in sporting populations mean that there's uncertainty around all of these estimates.[9] Regardless, numerous accounts of suicidal ideations and attempts (and some tragic events)[13,14] reinforce the evidence that the mental health challenges faced by retired athletes warrant significantly greater attention in both research and public domains.

Unfortunately, the mental health challenges of forced retirement are often accompanied by dysfunctional or destructive attempts to cope with distressful feelings. One behavioral manifestation of the impact of coping with symptoms such as depression and loss is alcohol and substance (ab)use. Alcohol and substance use is common in many professional sports, typically associated with social activities related to victory celebrations or drowning sorrows after defeat. Alcohol consumption can also be an ingrained feature of a sport culture. Studies in the Americas, Europe, Africa, and Australia have shown that between 20–70% of professional athletes engage in adverse alcohol use like binge drinking.[15] These behaviors often begin to emerge during adolescence for both boys and girls,[16] and are generally more prevalent in team sports compared to individual sports.[17] During an athletic career, alcohol use can be regulated to some extent by demanding training and competition schedules, but once that routine or schedule is no longer present (e.g., during injury or retirement), alcohol can become a destructive coping mechanism. A study of 38 former South African cricketers (10 of whom retired due to injury) found that 22% reported alcohol misuse over a four-week study period,[18] whereas samples from other settings have shown alcohol is used as a coping mechanism by 1–32% of athletes in the 10 years after retirement.[11] Importantly, the 2018 PPF survey suggested 7% of past players had sought help for drug, alcohol or gambling problems following retirement from sport, suggesting drinking is not the only salient behavior during this time.[1]

Stories of professional athletes who've sought solace in recreational substances are not uncommon, and cases following retirement have been well documented.[19,20] For example, one prevalent form of substance abuse associated with former injured athletes is opioid addiction. In 2011 a research team commissioned by ESPN, with additional funding provided by the US National Institute on Drug Abuse, published a study of 644 retired National Football League (NFL) players regarding their use of prescription painkillers.[21] They found that 52% of players reported taking painkillers at some time in their career; 71% reported abusing these substances, and 15% continued to do so in retirement. The overall rate of misuse during NFL play was reported as 37%, a rate 2.9 times higher than the lifetime rate of non-medical use of opioids among the general population of a comparable age (12.7%). This is a much higher rate than in the general population and presents a serious vignette of athletes being susceptible to substance use disorders. There are, of course, various reasons why this might happen. For instance, painkillers enable athletes to keep playing through injuries and taking prescribed medications for extended periods of time can lead to physical dependency. Another proposed explanation is the release of the neurochemical dopamine. Exercise releases endorphins, such as dopamine, which control the pleasure and reward centres of the brain. After retiring, many athletes describe "withdrawal-like" experiences, sometimes using addiction metaphors to describe what it's like to no longer get the "high" of playing and competing.[13] When athletes no longer receive the same levels of endorphins that they're accustomed to, they sometimes turn to chemical replacements.[13] This alteration in brain functioning can trigger a vicious cycle, whereby substance abuse leads to the development of depression and anxiety, which subsequently drives addiction.

Of course, these behaviors can exacerbate some of the often-overlooked outcomes associated with forced retirement from sport. Emotional struggles can place great strain on family and marital relations as retired athletes come to terms with their change in circumstance and regain or develop of new sense of identity. Figuring out how that fits with those nearest and dearest to them can be difficult, and the lack of structure to the day, increased free time, and subsequent changes in social circles can mean athletes spend more time with their partners than both parties are accustomed to. Relationship strain is not uncommon, with reports of 1 in 4 athletes experiencing some form of marital breakdown after retirement.[1] Many former athletes also struggle financially. A study commissioned by the National Bureau of Economic Research (NBER) examined the financial status NFL players who had been drafted between 1996 and 2003.[22] The authors found that bankruptcy filings began relatively soon after retirement and continued all the way through the first dozen post-retirement years. 78% of players either filed for bankruptcy or struggled financially once they retired (1 in 6 declared bankruptcy during the first twelve years of retirement). Of course, while many retired athletes are employed, self-employed or retired from a second career, the majority will have had to accept a drop in salary once they stop playing. Managing this loss of income, alongside failed or misguided investments and perceived or actual pressure to maintain previous financial commitments, are all relevant stressors, particularly if retirement is sudden (e.g., without any time to prepare). As many as 1 in 5 athletes cite financial worries as the largest single factor impacting negatively on their mental health.[1] An athlete's social and financial world can therefore further heighten the psychological struggles of retirement, with forced retirement through injury likely to make these issues even worse.

Knees of a 70-Year-Old

Now, we'd be remiss if we focused on the mental health aspects of retirement in isolation. After all, mental and physical wellbeing are intertwined, perhaps even more so for people who made a career from being in peak condition. A review of the literature identified involuntary retirement, participation in collision/high contact sports, concussion history, increased body mass index (BMI), and osteoarthritis as contributing factors to worse mental and physical quality of life among former athletes.[23] Though retired elite sportspeople generally have lower overall morbidity and better self-reported health in later years compared with the general population, they also report ongoing pain and musculoskeletal dysfunction. To illustrate, a survey of 3357 retired Olympians from 131 countries identified that one-third of participants attributed current pain and functional limitations to injuries during their Olympic career.[24] Once athletes retire, they must adapt to physical changes and this can affect their psychological state. For many, their body (and their body image) plays a key role in the construction of their athletic and social identities.[25] They train for years to reach their best physical condition and when this starts to deteriorate, it can be incredibly impactful. Dealing with weight gain, loss of muscular mass and bodily pain is often not something they're prepared for.

No matter whether we talk about or women or men in sport, body image, low self-esteem and changed perception of one's own physical capabilities are things that can negatively affect healthy transitions during the retirement process. Dealing with ongoing injury-related physical complaints can compound this, especially after losing access to the medical resources that are typically provided during a sporting career. Learning to deal with one's own physical health can therefore be a further demand that challenges the former athlete's health and wellbeing.

Ignore, Express or Confront?

As humans, we can deploy several strategies when attempting to cope with stressful encounters in life.[26] The effectiveness of these strategies very much depends on the fit between the approach we choose and the demands of the situation. In this way, strategies can be seen as either adaptive and constructive or maladaptive and deconstructive. *Adaptive coping* generally involves confronting problems directly, forming reasonably realistic assessments of the issues, recognizing and changing unhealthy emotional reactions, and trying to prevent adverse effects on our bodies. In sport, those athletes who experience forced retirement through injury but engage in adaptive coping strategies will be the ones who choose to accept the impact of the injury on themselves as a person and an athlete, reflect positively on their career achievements, and actively set and pursue goals in their lives outside of sport.

Maladaptive coping strategies work by decreasing symptoms of distress for a short period of time, without directly affecting their cause. Once these strategies have ceased, the problem remains.[iii] For example, alcohol and substance use are common maladaptive coping strategies used by athletes to 'numb' the emotional or physical pain associated with forced retirement. Another common maladaptive strategy is what's termed *avoidance-focused coping*. This is when a person changes their behavior to avoid thinking about, feeling, or doing difficult things (i.e., burying your head in the sand). Procrastination, passive-aggressiveness, and rumination are examples of unhelpful coping mechanisms that athletes may consciously or unconsciously use to avoid coming to terms with no longer being able to play sport or facing uncomfortable thoughts like *who am I and what next?* Unhelpfully, these behaviors tend to focus attention on one's feelings of helplessness (caused by an inability to change what's happened or uncertainty about how to correct the situation in the future), which can make the athlete feel even more powerless and more stressed.

Healthy or Crisis Transition?

So, what does all of this mean for athletes navigating their exit from sport? Well, for a long time, athlete retirement was viewed similarly to retirement from other forms of employment; however, given the vast difference in chronological age and cognitive and physical ability between elite athletes and other retirees, this line of enquiry wasn't that productive. Instead, sport psychologists have sought to develop a context-specific understanding of the factors that lead to healthy vs crisis transition for athletes.[27] In the 1990s, Taylor and Ogilvie proposed a sport-specific model to explain adaptation to retirement.[28] The model considers how the quality of retirement adaptation after sport – whether athletes experience a healthy transition or a crisis – is determined by the causes of retirement itself (i.e., forced, of own volition), factors specific to the athlete, and resources available to deal with the adaptation experience. Some 25 years on, this model is still used and it encompasses several potential factors affecting athletes who are forced to retire due to injury.

According to the model, one of the most prominent contributors to a successful transition out of sport is the developmental or life experiences athletes have accumulated. The most fundamental of these is the degree to which athletes define their self-worth in terms of their participation and achievement in sports. As we've discussed, elite athletes often have a self-identity composed almost exclusively of their sports involvement. Following forced retirement, without the input from their sport, these athletes have little to support their sense of self-worth and few options to channel their energies or reinforce their ego in other activities to the same extent. This is frequently the context in which terms such as 'loss' and 'dying' are used by athletes when discussing their transition experiences.[29] Many athletes also define themselves in terms of their popularity or social status.[28] Though this recognition is typically short-lived for most, some athletes question their self-worth when out of the public eye and feel the need to regain lost esteem. Athletes whose socialization process occurred primarily in the sports environment are often described as 'role restricted' in that they have only learned to assume certain social roles specific to the sport setting and are only able to interact with others within the narrow context of sport. As a result, their ability to assume other roles following retirement is hampered. Individuals who have a broad-based social identity that includes non-sport family, friends, education, and occupational ambitions are therefore likely to experience a healthier adaptation to forced retirement because of a diffuse social identity and more robust self-worth.

In addition to intrapersonal factors, social, cultural and environmental variables can influence transition success as well. For starters, simply having extra leisure time without a fixed schedule can be overwhelming at first,[iv] and newly retired athletes sometimes feel at loose ends, particularly if they don't have a strong family or non-sport social circle to anchor them. Coming to terms with a sudden increase in personal freedoms and responsibilities is pivotal to transition success, but this can be affected by how much stability the athlete perceives in their social life and the resources available to them. For example, those who are financially dependent on sports participation and possess few skills to earn a living outside of sport, or have limited financial resources to fall back on, will likely see retirement as more threatening. This may be most significant when interacting with perceived or real limitations on post-sport career opportunities that can be shaped by socio-economic status, gender, and ethnic background. Pre-retirement planning can alleviate some of this distress, but that's not always possible when a career terminates unexpectedly (e.g., due to injury). Moreover, athlete health at the time of retirement will further contribute to adaptation quality. Individuals with lingering medical needs or chronic disabilities may, as a result of their injuries, have limited choices in their post-sport activities and careers. This has obvious implications for how smoothly the immediate transition period might go but in the long run, athletes need to negotiate the process of re-positioning themselves in their new world – essentially constructing who they are now and how they'll function for the rest of their lives. Fitting into a culture outside of sport (e.g., at home or in a new work role) takes time for some, and whether this becomes a period of personal growth or personal crisis can be largely attributed to how the athlete perceives the demands of their situation.

This is where the athlete's coping skills become so important. The quality of their retirement adaptation will depend largely on the manner in which they manage the changes in their environment. Having effective coping skills at one's disposal will facilitate this process and reduce the likelihood of difficulties. A related factor is access to social support. When actively playing, athletes often lean on others in their sport setting to get through challenging situations, but that isn't always possible when they leave. Combined with a loss in their popularity status and social identity, this may leave athletes isolated and lonely, which can trigger maladaptive behaviors. So, athletes who receive support from family and friends tend to experience an easier transition.[30] Access to formal pre-retirement counselling programs can also have a big impact by promoting coping strategies like continuing education, occupational and investment goal setting, and social networking. These all help to enhance perceptions of control over the situation and diversify social identity. A note of caution here, though. Despite all the evidence and advice available to professional athletes, it's common for them to resist planning for their lives after the end of their careers. This is often influenced by maturity and youthful perceptions that they have years before they have to worry about life after sport. Often there's been no planning until a serious injury occurs, at which point there's a reality check that motivates thoughts of the future. Such enthusiasm generally dissipates, however, once the athlete is back to fitness and competing again, as sport takes over the focus. This kind of avoidance coping (putting off the inevitable rather than confronting it) is seen in athletes across the career spectrum and sets many up for difficult transitions when that time eventually comes.

Time to Intervene

Right, what signs should one look for if an athlete is experiencing a crisis transition? Generally, it will manifest in experiences of worry, low mood, anger or temper outbursts, behavioral problems, physical complaints or headaches, difficulty concentrating or sleeping, and avoidance of situations, tasks or people. Occupational and financial problems, relationship issues, and psychopathological symptoms such as anxiety or depression can also be key indicators. Given the complex and multifaceted nature of these factors, treatment or support for an athlete in crisis can take many forms. For example, clinical intervention may be required for someone experiencing acute mental health difficulties, or they may need family/social counselling, financial advice, or occupational guidance. When identifying appropriate professional help, it's important to consider that there is no one person or magic bullet to resolve a crisis transition. Contemporary mental health care typically works toward a group or community-based approach with a range of individuals (personal and professional) offering a support structure for the athlete.

Support after injury-forced retirement can come in many forms - cognitive, emotional, behavioral, social, and organizational. In the first instance, research suggests that prevention is better than cure, and pre-retirement planning (cognitive and organizational support) offers one of the best chances for successful transition out of sport.[30] This usually revolves around exploration of some form of post-sport career development through formal vocational or educational training. In addition to providing tangible qualifications for alternative employment, such activities also help to reduce exclusive identification with an athlete's sporting role and expand their self-identity, thereby reducing the potential for crisis transition. However, in acknowledging that many athletes struggle with their careers ending (especially when this happens abruptly), options to remain engaged in their sport in some form (coaching, media, and management) can minimize disruption to wellbeing and life satisfaction. Some athletes will find lasting roles in these areas and others will use them as stepping stones to other opportunities. Either way, time spent in such positions affords the chance to identify and make use of key transferrable skills developed throughout an athlete's sporting career. Common transferable skills for elite athletes include the ability to perform under pressure, problem solving, organization skills, the ability to meet deadlines and challenges, setting and achieving goals, dedication, self-motivation, and team-related interpersonal skills. Many of these are attractive to employers outside of the sport sector and can be emphasized during career counselling sessions.

During the retirement process, athletes may also need help developing a range of adaptive coping strategies to manage acute psychological distress (emotional, behavioral and social support). Encouraging strong relationships with significant others who care about their personal growth is an important part of this. Stress management, sleep hygiene, exercise, action planning, and in some cases medication will minimize acute crisis transition experiences. Social support networks can promote and enable these strategies, but professional intervention may be particularly beneficial in both preventative and therapeutic capacities. Sport psychologists, lifestyle counsellors, and career advisors can help athletes develop coping skills to be relied upon during the career transition process and/or explore additional adaptation techniques during acute crisis.

In the longer term, once the immediate challenges have been managed, athletes also need to deal with the other elephant in the room: learning to love (and look after) their body and their physical health. This may be through an exercise program for the specific management of the injury which forced their retirement, or through a broader regime focused on maintaining a general level of health and fitness. This kind of training will likely be very different than the sport performance training they're used to, and may require them to establish a new relationship with fitness. Former athletes whose sense of self includes exercise identity alongside athletic identity are more likely to stay physically active in retirement but, for others, finding a personal motivation to exercise is key. This might involve seeking opportunities for alternative competition. For instance, many retired athletes take up activities which allow them to challenge themselves physically and mentally (e.g., Ironman, Triathlon). Similarly, diet and nutrition become salient concerns through retirement. During an athlete's sporting career they require highly specialized and programmed nutrition practices (e.g., quality and quantity of food, calories, nutrients and supplements) in order to meet the high physical demands of training and competition. Appropriate dietary choices and calorie consumption habits commensurate with their post-retirement needs have to be considered, and this is something that many athletes struggle with.[25] Research has indicated that eating disorders and other maladaptive dietary behaviors are prevalent after sport retirement,[13,15,24] so ongoing behavioral support around this aspect of personal care can be really valuable.

Epilogue: What Is the Price of Success ... and Who Pays for It?

So, what makes the difference between positive and negative transition experiences? By all accounts, the primary factor is the level of aftercare and preparation for life after sport that an athlete receives. Many professional sports have players' associations that offer some level of support, though their resources vary significantly. Some provide salary guarantees for those suffering career-ending injuries, or services to help players better transition into life after sport. Others don't, and while the medical insurance policies players take out when they become professionals provide a degree of security, they often don't cover the psychological or social support that newly retired athletes might need. This prompts some moral reflection. Although elite sport at the highest level enables a select few to share in a multi-billion dollar industry, do those who profit the most (sponsors, media companies) have an obligation to support athletes' transitions out of sport, particularly when their exit is driven by what is essentially a workplace injury? And away from professional sport, elite athletes who represent their country at Olympic level also provide an interesting dilemma. Sporting success on the global stage has traditionally been a way to demonstrate political power. Many nations' Olympic athletes are therefore state funded, and tax payers may reasonably hold expectations for success; however, along with that expectation there doesn't seem to be a corresponding duty of care at a national level to look after athletes once they retire or are forced to retire through injury. An argument might be made in parallel to existing policies in many countries that support armed forces personnel injured in the line of duty. Although there are obvious differences between the level of physical and psychological trauma military personnel experience compared to athletes, and we don't mean to equate their experiences, there's still a significant health risk associated with performing/competing for one's country which bears greater societal acknowledgement. When national team athletes feel like they're *"just a coat rack for the medal [with] no value as a person"*[31] or being left to fend for themselves once they've *"done their job"* for their country,[32] it's clear that the complexities of athlete experiences during forced retirement have not yet been fully addressed in research or in practice.

Notes

i *Sophie's Choice* is a 1979 novel by William Styron (and 1982 award-winning film of the same name) that details a heart-wrenching life and death choice made by the titular character. The term has been co-opted to mean any difficult choice where both outcomes are equally bad and in a forced-retirement situation, that's exactly what athletes are faced with.

ii When did you last fill out a customer satisfaction survey? Odds are, you probably did it if you had either a really good or a really bad experience (when we're somewhere in the middle, we don't often bother giving feedback). This is an example of *selection bias*. When people are more likely to take part in a study – say, because they've been having mental health challenges and want to tell someone about them – the dataset will over-represent those people, so it looks like there are more cases than there actually are across the whole population. It's also possible that those in severe distress wouldn't respond to a survey, so we might underestimate the prevalence of extreme cases. Together, this creates imprecision in our estimates.

iii Who hasn't put off washing the dishes only to be faced with a mountain of stuck-on food scraps that would've been easier to clean if you hadn't let them sit … maladaptive coping in its rawest form!

iv Though not a perfect analogy, some of us experienced this firsthand during enforced COVID-19 lockdowns. Whereas some people continued on as usual (or were scrambling to keep up with massive new workloads, but let's not get into THAT), others found themselves idle at home with time to spare. This caused all kinds of different reactions – for some it was a chance to focus on hobbies or new pursuits, but many others experienced significant isolation and mental distress.

References

1 The Professional Players Federation. *Initial career transition research findings (2018)*. Available at: https://www.ppf.org.uk/ppf-org-uk/_img/images/doc/PPF%20Past%20Player%20Research%202018.pdf Accessed May 9, 2021.

2   *Sam Warburton calls time on illustrious career (2018, July 18)*. Available at: https://www.cardiffblues.com/news/sam-warburton-calls-time-on-illustrious-career Accessed May 9, 2021.

3   *Graham Onions: Lancashire & ex-England bowler retires (2020, September 4)*. Available at: https://www.bbc.co.uk/sport/cricket/54026658 Accessed May 9, 2021.

4   Maske, M. *The 'most dangerous man in football' traded an NFL career for an internship*. The Washington Post 2016. Available at: https://www.washingtonpost.com/sports/the-most-dangerous-man-in-football-traded-an-nfl-career-for-an-internship/2016/06/07/8087971c-2c21-11e6-9b37-42985f6a265c_story.html Accessed May 9, 2021.

5   Brewer BW, Van Raalte JL, Linder DE. Athletic identity: Hercules' muscles or Achilles heel? *Int J Sport Psychol* 1993;24:237–254.

6   Lavallee D, Grove JR, Gordon S. The causes of career termination from sport and their relationship to post-retirement adjustment among elite-amateur athletes in Australia. *Aust Psychol* 1997;32:131–135; doi:10.1080/00050069708257366.

7   Brewer BW, Van Raalte JL, Petitpas A. Self-identity issues in sport career transitions. In: D Lavallee, P Wylleman (eds.). *Career transition in sport: international perspectives*. Morgantown, WV: Fitness Information Technology 2000.

8   Lovett S. *Your identity disintegrates: the mental strain of retirement and life after sport*. Independent 2019. Available at: https://www.independent.co.uk/sport/sporting-mind-series-mental-health-sport-ellie-simmonds-retirement-kelly-holmes-a8942516.html Accessed May 9, 2021.

9   Barth M, Güllich A, Forstinger CA, et al. Retirement of professional soccer players – a systematic review from social sciences perspectives. *J Sport Sci* 2021; 39:903–914; doi: 10.1080/02640414.2020.1851449.

10   Brown JC, Kerkhoffs G, Lambert MI, et al. Forced retirement from professional rugby union is associated with symptoms of distress. *Int J Sports Med* 2017;38:582–587; doi: 10.1055/s-0043-103959.

11   Gouttebarge V, Kerkhoffs GM. A prospective cohort study on symptoms of common mental disorders among current and retired professional ice hockey players. *Phys Sportmed* 2017;45:252–258; doi:10.1080/00913847.2017.1338497.

12   Sanders G, Stevinson C. Associations between retirement reasons, chronic pain, athletic identity, and depressive symptoms among former professional footballers. *Eur J Sport Sci* 2017;17:1311–1318; doi:10.1080/17461391.2017.1371795.

13   Cosh SM, McNeil DG, Tully PJ. Poor mental health outcomes in crisis transitions: an examination of retired athletes accounting of crisis transition experiences in a cultural context. *Qual Res Sport Exerc Health* 2020;1–20; doi:10.1080/2159676X.2020.1765852.

14   Smith A. Depression and suicide in professional sports work. In: M Atkinson (ed.). *Sport, mental illness, and sociology (research in the sociology of sport*, vol. 11). Bingley: Emerald Publishing Limited 2018.

15   Gouttebarge V, Hopley P, Kerkhoffs G, et al. A 12-month prospective cohort study of symptoms of common mental disorders among professional rugby players. *Eur J Sport Sci* 2018;18:1004–1012; doi:10.1080/17461391.2018.1466914.

16   Boyes R, O'Sullivan DE, Linden B, et al. Gender-specific associations between involvement in team sport culture and Canadian adolescents' substance-use behavior. *SSM Popul Health* 2017;3:663–673; doi:10.1016/j.ssmph.2017.08.006.

17   O'Farrell A, Kingsland M, Kenny S, et al. A multi-faceted intervention to reduce alcohol misuse and harm amongst sports people in Ireland: a controlled trial. *Drug Alcohol Rev* 2018;37:14–22; doi:10.1111/dar.12585.

18 Schuring N, Kerkhoffs G, Gray J, et al. The mental wellbeing of current and retired professional cricketers: an observational prospective cohort study. *Phys Sportmed* 2017;45:463–469: doi:10.1080/00913847.2017.1386069.

19 Palmer C. Drugs, alcohol, and addiction in sport. In: M Atkinson (ed.) *Sport, mental illness, and sociology (research in the sociology of sport*, vol. 11). Bingley: Emerald Publishing Limited 2018.

20 Wylleman P. A developmental and holistic perspective on transiting out of elite sport. In: MH Anshel, TA Petrie, JA Steinfeldt (eds.). *APA handbooks in psychology series. APA handbook of sport and exercise psychology, vol. 1. sport psychology.* Washington: American Psychological Association 2019.

21 Cottler LB, Abdallah AB, Cummings SM, et al. Injury, pain, and prescription opioid use among former National Football League (NFL) players. *Drug Alcohol Depend* 2011;116:188–194; doi:10.1016/j.drugalcdep.2010.12.003.

22 Carlson K, Kim J, Lusardi A, et al. Bankruptcy rates among NFL players with short-lived income spikes. *Am Econ Rev* 2015;105:381–384; doi:10.1257/aer.p20151038.

23 Filbay S, Pandya T, Thomas B, et al. Quality of life and life satisfaction in former athletes: a systematic review and meta-analysis. *Sports Med* 2019;49:1723–1738; doi:10. 1007/s40279-019-01163-0.

24 Palmer D, Cooper DJ, Emery C, et al. Self-reported sports injuries and later-life health status in 3357 retired Olympians from 131 countries: a cross-sectional survey among those competing in the games between London 1948 and PyeongChang 2018. *Br J Sports Med* 2020;55:46–53; doi:10.1136/bjsports-2019-101772.

25 Buckley GL, Hall LE, Lassemillante ACM, et al. Retired athletes and the intersection of food and body: a systematic literature review exploring compensatory behaviours and body change. *Nutrients* 2019;11:1395; doi:10.3390/nu11061395.

26 Lazarus, RS, Folkman S. *Stress, appraisal, and coping.* New York: Springer 1984.

27 Alfermann D, Stambulova N. Career transitions and career termination. In: G Tenenbaum, RC Eklund (eds.). *Handbook of sport psychology.* New Jersey: John Wiley & Sons Inc 2007.

28 Taylor J, Ogilvie BC. A conceptual model of adaptation to retirement among athletes. *J Appl Sport Psychol* 1994;6:1–20; doi:10.1080/10413209408406462.

29 Blinde EM, Stratta TM. The "sport career death" of college athletes: involuntary and unanticipated sport exits. *J Sport Behav* 1992;15:3–20.

30 Park S, Lavallee D, Tod D. Athletes' career transition out of sport: a systematic review. *Int Rev Sport Exerc Psychol* 2013;6:22–53; doi:10.1080/1750984X.2012.687053.

31 Cooper L. *Former elite athletes reveal mental health struggles after retirement.* Huffpost 2017. Available at: https://www.huffingtonpost.com.au/2017/04/11/former-elite-athletes-reveal-mental-health-struggles-after-retir_a_22035114/ Accessed May 9, 2021.

32 Coverdale D. *We are chewed up and spat out ... where's the duty of care?' Many of our retired Olympic medal winners are plagued by mental health issues and much of it stems from a lack of support.* Daily Mail 2020. Available at: https://www.dailymail.co.uk/sport/olympics-2020/article-8001263/Many-British-Olympic-medallists-plagued-mental-health-issues-stemmed-lack-aftercare.html Accessed May 9, 2021.

13

CAN WE CONVINCE PEOPLE THAT PREVENTION IS IMPORTANT?: "BUT BROCCOLI IS GOOD FOR YOU!"

Carly McKay

Humans are funny creatures. We like to think of ourselves as rational beings capable of great things, and in a lot of cases that's been true. We've developed complex social systems, cured diseases, and put people in space! But we're also the same group who decided that eating laundry detergent was a good idea,[i] so we're clearly not above making some questionable choices. Behavior is a complex phenomenon and the reasons why people do things, or don't do them for that matter, aren't always straightforward. How about all those times you knew you shouldn't do something but went ahead and did it anyway? It's one of the remarkable features of humanity that we often insist on acting in ways that seem to be contrary to our own best interests, and this is exactly the challenge with sport injury prevention. On the surface of it, you'd think that athletes would want to avoid getting hurt but, as we'll discover in this chapter, promoting self-protective behaviors isn't actually all that simple.

Our Own Worst Enemy

We know that injuries in sport cause a number of detrimental outcomes for individuals, teams, and organizations. At a personal level, they can lead to significant physical and mental health problems, lost benefits from social/school/employment engagement, setbacks in training and sport development, direct and indirect treatment costs, and possibly a lost place on a team or the end of an athletic career. We also know that teams that sustain more injuries in a season tend to be less successful.[1–4] Along with societal burdens in terms of costs and lost productivity,[5] one would have to argue that there are compelling reasons to prevent as many sport injuries as possible. The good news is that plenty of injury prevention strategies have been developed over the last few decades and there's overwhelming evidence that many of them work.[6–8] The bad news is, it's tough to convince

DOI: 10.4324/9781003088936-13

athletes and their coaches to use them. For example, the "11+" is a warm-up program that's been shown to reduce injury risk in soccer by 35–40% in experimental trials.[9] It includes a series of exercises that take about 20 minutes to complete, and teams that use it three times per week see the greatest benefits. This sounds amazing, right? Why wouldn't teams swap out their usual warmup for something a little more structured if it would eliminate a third (or more) of their injuries? Well, after promotional activities in over 80 countries, only 10% of national governing bodies endorsed the program[10] and studies have shown uptake amongst individual coaches is pretty low as well.[11] So, here we have a really good program but coaches, and consequently athletes, don't use it. It seems completely illogical, but these kinds of issues have been recognized as the single biggest limiting factor in sport injury prevention efforts, regardless of the nature or content of the intervention. In order to understand why this is the case, we need to consider some fundamentals about health behavior.

There's a common assumption that people who behave in an undesirable way simply "don't know any better" and there's historically been a belief that educating them will lead them to act differently (i.e., if they know better, they'll do better). It's an appealing solution and certainly has some merit, as we can't expect people to behave in specific ways if they don't understand the problem or know how to fix it. But how do we explain things like smoking, then? Massive public health campaigns have been launched worldwide to curb tobacco use, many of them incorporating explicit information on packaging and advertising about negative health consequences like respiratory diseases and cancer. Still, there are hundreds of millions of people around the world who continue to smoke, and it causes an estimated eight million deaths per year.[12] If behavior change was just a matter of education, surely those numbers would be lower or at least decreasing. This is an example of what we call the *knowledge-behavior gap*. Just because people have all the facts, it doesn't mean they'll behave any differently because turning information into action isn't a direct input-output process. There are a number of essential steps that have to happen in between and when interventions fail to account for that, they rarely have their intended impact on people's health outcomes.

One of the intermediates between knowledge and action is the process of intention formation. Obviously, people who have absolutely no intention of doing something probably won't, but when they want to achieve a certain outcome, they form a kind of instruction to themselves about doing so. This is a *goal intention* and it signals a commitment to act, though it can vary in strength (sometimes we half-heartedly decide to do something and sometimes we're really serious about it).[13] Producing a goal intention is a necessary part of the process and it's been shown to explain about a third of the variance in people's goal attainment;[13] however, research suggests that as many as 47% of people who intend to act don't end up doing it.[14] This is the *intention-behavior gap*, and it's an easy one to illustrate. Have you ever made a New Year's resolution, or know someone who has? Think about how long it lasted.[ii] If you're one of the few who managed to maintain your new behavior for the long term, try to keep the bragging to a minimum. The rest of us ran into problems like a lack of time and resource, competing demands, a change of interest, or any number of other things that got in the way, and we fell off the wagon early. As the well-known proverb goes, there are certain roads paved with good intentions and even when people genuinely set out to do something, they don't always see it through. So, even if athletes know about the risks of injury and how to prevent them, they might not end up taking proactive steps. That could be for all kinds of reasons, and we need to better understand these if we hope to improve intervention use in the community.

In the Eye of the Beholder

In the early days of sport medicine, research aimed to identify injury risk factors, create interventions that would modify those risk factors, then see if these interventions worked in some kind of randomized controlled trial (RCT) or cohort study. If successful, the interventions were packaged up and disseminated through academic papers, websites, and public presentations, under the assumption that if they were made available, people would want to use them. You can probably see the issue with this. Within a research study, conditions are tightly controlled and there's a lot of support to make sure that athletes use the interventions being investigated. Outside of a study, all bets are off and, when people have free choice about using an intervention or not, the knowledge/intention-behavior gaps become limiting factors. This means that interventions which seem really good in research might not have the same benefit in practice because they aren't being used as designed (or they aren't being used at all). Therefore, it soon became apparent to researchers that just putting successful interventions out there in the world was no guarantee that they'd be effective. So, in 2006, Caroline Finch developed the Translating Research into Injury Prevention Practice (TRIPP) model that introduced a new step into the research process.[16] Basically, it highlighted the necessity of understanding the *implementation context* of injury prevention strategies, or in other words, figuring out what unique factors might shape prevention behaviors within a particular environment. After all, you can design the best prevention program in the world but if it doesn't meet the needs of the people who are meant to use it, they won't, and what works for one group might not work for another. This spawned a huge number of studies in various sports to get a better grasp of the situational variables that might influence prevention strategy adoption. It's beyond us to detail all of their findings here, so instead let's focus on the evidence around two common sport settings: soccer and rugby.

As arguably the most popular sport on the planet, soccer comprises an incredible range of implementation contexts (e.g., different age groups, competitive levels, organizational structures, national policies, etc). It would be a colossal undertaking to investigate all of the situational permutations at once, so research has pragmatically focused on two settings where injury risk seems to be particularly high – adolescent girls' and professional men's leagues. Now, on the surface of it, these seem to be as far apart as you can get in terms of the factors that might influence behaviors. Yet, there are some surprising similarities in what shapes intentions in these two environments.

Let's start with the findings in adolescent girls' soccer. In a Canadian sample ($n_{coaches}$ = 29, $n_{players}$ = 258), it was determined that around 60% of coaches and 75% of players thought an inadequate warmup was a risk factor for injury, though they didn't think that a specific injury prevention warmup would necessarily be effective.[17] After being asked to use the 11+ for a season, it was determined that participant beliefs about injury risk didn't actually affect their adherence to the program all that much, but their years of playing experience did. Veteran coaches and players were less likely to use the 11+ than their less experienced counterparts.[17] All of the teams in the study had access to injury risk information and were given instructions on using the program (i.e., they had good knowledge), but their individual backgrounds were salient in the decision to use it. Maybe those who'd been around longer already had warm-ups that they thought worked for them and they didn't want to change, or perhaps they held some old school ideas that injuries were just "part of the game," and they had no intention of doing anything about them. Whatever the case, this goes to show that personal factors can affect injury prevention behaviors and that will become an important point in a moment.

Similar to the 11+, "Knee Control" is an exercise program developed in Sweden and it's demonstrated commensurate injury prevention benefits.[18] Three years after an RCT to investigate the program's effects, eight district football associations participated in a follow-up to see whether it was still being used. Around 82% of coaches from the original intervention group and 68% from the control group were in fact using it, and the adoption rate was 74% amongst other coaches in those districts who weren't part of the initial trial. Those are pretty decent numbers, but none of the football associations had formal policies regarding Knee Control implementation, and most of the coaches reported no formal club expectations for using it.[19] So, this suggests that situational variables are important, too. Coaches function within the rules and policies of their organizations, and when there aren't set guidelines for using an intervention, we see varying rates of uptake and people often start picking and choosing which parts they want to stick to. Low *fidelity* (i.e., not keeping to the recommended content and dosage) is common for interventions in practical settings where usage isn't enforced, and that's important point #2.

A qualitative study involving 20 coaches from Swedish female football teams investigated these situational factors further. The participants described a number of external *facilitators* and *barriers* that determined their ability to use Knee Control, such as available resources for training, social support from other coaches, and player buy-in.[20] They also reported that things like how well the program fit the needs of the team influenced whether or not they used it. Many coaches said they modified the exercises to make them more appealing to players, and although these changes could compromise the preventive effect, they made the program more feasible for their team.[20] The same thing happens in professional youth soccer teams, as well. A study of four boys' Academy teams found that over the course of 160 observed training sessions, 11+ exercises were performed in their original form only 12% of the time. They were modified in a further 28% of sessions and weren't used at all in most of the others.[21] Coaches changed the program to add more variation and individualization in order to align with specific training objectives or player needs. Together, these studies introduce the third important point: people might intend to prevent injuries, but their method of doing so needs to be tailored to their context.

Since we're on the topic of professional soccer, we can look at some research investigating that particular implementation context, too. Four professional men's soccer teams in four different countries took part in a study about their perceptions of injury prevention.[22] More than 90% of the participants believed that soccer carries a high risk of injuries and that players should perform evidence-based prevention exercises to minimize both individual and team-level consequences. However, perceptions varied regarding how and when these exercises should be performed. Around 47% thought the 11+ would need modification for use in their team and there was some disagreement about who holds the responsibility for injury prevention (e.g., coaches, players, medical staff, others).[22] It's interesting that these are some of the same themes that emerged in amateur soccer settings. At a personal level, having coach and player buy-in is essential no matter what the context, and to achieve that it seems that a degree of individualization is needed. It's also important that everyone thinks the exercises will work, but the more experience they have, the less convinced people seem to be about the benefit of pre-designed programs. At a structural level, a lack of policy from clubs has been repeatedly mentioned as a barrier, and this gets at the idea of whose responsibility it actually is to enact prevention strategies. Together, these issues speak to the complex interactions between personal and situational factors in the implementation context, and it turns out that similar patterns can be seen in other sports.

Two studies in youth rugby have demonstrated that despite good injury risk awareness and beliefs that warmup programs can prevent injuries, implementation of such programs is as challenging here as it is in soccer.[23,24] School rugby coaches in Canada (n = 48) and England (n = 106) reported that they thought some exercises in a pre-designed warmup program weren't as effective as others[23] and, when using "Activate" (a rugby equivalent to the 11+), they introduced modifications to better suit the needs and preferences of their team.[24] Common barriers to implementation, such as lack of time and player disinterest, were also highlighted.[24] A further comparison between English coaches (n = 106) and their players (n = 571) showed that the coaches had significantly greater risk perceptions and prevention program awareness and, amazingly, almost half of the players were unaware if they had used Activate.[24] This suggests that information about injury prevention wasn't passed along from coaches to athletes, even if it was being actively incorporated into their training. This raises another important point. We often think about injury prevention being targeted at athletes, but often their coaches are the *delivery agents* for injury prevention strategies (i.e., they're usually the ones who call the shots about training practices). That raises questions about who we should actually be targeting with injury prevention strategies.

So, what does all of this tell us about the implementation context for injury prevention interventions, at least in team sport? Well, first it says that individual-level behavioral processes are important. The evidence very clearly reinforces the idea that people's personal characteristics, such as their sport experience and perceptions, are crucial to intention formation. They need to believe that the intervention will work, and they need to feel as though they have the ability to use it (e.g., overcoming issues of player buy-in). This contributes to some of the variability in rates of intervention uptake and fidelity in the community. We also have to remember that in sport, performance is the top priority, so injury prevention often gets fit into the schedule around fitness and skill development activities. When teams only have so much time for training, they're unlikely to devote it to warmup exercises. Therefore, we also need to be aware that sport-related values are going to shape how much time and effort people are willing to devote to injury prevention compared to things they consider to be more important. And, even if they intend to engage in prevention behaviors, that doesn't necessarily prepare them for the effort needed to do that in a context with competing objectives like winning matches or having fun.[14] That makes the intention-behavior gap even harder to close.

Where Are the Sticking Points?

We've talked a bit about forming goal intentions and how that's the process of people committing to a desired behavior; however, considering all the barriers and other demands we encounter in life, it's probably not surprising that this isn't enough to ensure action on its own. It's a bit like having a destination in mind but not having a planned route to get there. Research has shown that people also need to form *implementation intentions*, which involves choosing effective goal-directed behaviors to help them make things happen. In practice, this means that coaches and athletes who intend to prevent injuries need to pick a method of doing so. This is an absolutely essential part of the process: a meta-analysis of 94 studies across a variety of behavioral domains found that forming an implementation intention has a medium to large effect ($d = 0.65$) on whether or not people achieve their goals.[14] Extending this to sport, prevention efforts might therefore fizzle out if coaches and athletes don't know how to go about it or if there isn't a fit for purpose intervention ready to go. It's also an issue when people report that they don't think programs like the 11+ and Activate will work, or that they're skeptical of pre-packaged routines in general.

As an interesting aside, coaches with stronger goal intentions might decide that if the perfect program doesn't exist, they'll create one of their own. This is where we start to see program modifications happening. Such changes are often seen by researchers and policymakers as a failure in rolling out an intervention because people aren't using it the way it was designed, and there's concern that the new combination of elements might not work as well as the original. It's probably time to challenge this viewpoint, though. Program modifications might actually indicate stronger implementation intentions and a narrower intention-behavior gap for those individuals. With any luck, this reflects a more robust behavior change process and a greater likelihood that they'll keep using the program over the longer term, though more research is needed to verify that.

And here we arrive at another big concept in injury prevention. It's one thing to start or *uptake* a new behavior, and another thing entirely to maintain it. If our New Year's resolution experiences have taught us anything, it's that giving something a try isn't nearly as hard as sticking with it. At the individual level, continual cost-benefit analyses around the value of the behavior, what motivates it, and whether or not barriers can be overcome on a day-to-day basis will determine how much effort goes into sustaining it. We must remember, though, that none of this happens without the influence of various contextual factors. In sport, there are little things that might make an injury prevention warmup harder to do, like having to share training space with another team or players turning up late. These create challenges on an immediate level, but there are bigger things with more systemic effects that we need to consider as well. For instance, coaches are clearly calling the shots around injury prevention in team sport, and although keeping players happy is important, what they do in training is generally a coach decision. But coaches also need to act in alignment with organizational policy (e.g., if the club has a standardized training program, they might not be allowed to adjust it). This highlights the issue of whose intentions are actually important when it comes to injury prevention. Yes, we're trying to help athletes, so it's ultimately their behavior that really matters, but they might actually have the least say over what goes on. Herein lies the complexity of the situation, and why implementing a really good prevention program isn't as straightforward as it seems.

Before we move on, let's take stock of where we've gotten to in this discussion. We know that (1) injury prevention isn't usually the top priority in sport; (2) even if it is a priority, intention often isn't enough to prompt action; (3) interventions aren't always applied as designed because people have different needs or encounter barriers in their environments; and (4) there are multiple layers of influence that shape athletes' injury prevention behaviors. It likely comes as no surprise then, that as research has acknowledged the ineffectiveness of passive dissemination strategies for injury prevention (e.g., putting content on a website and hoping people will use it), there has been a move toward developing implementation approaches that account for the contextual factors we've identified here. This process has involved a couple of key conceptual advancements that set the foundation for everything else we're going to talk about. First, just like with injury risk and recovery, athlete behavior is seen as a product of multiple levels of influence including interpersonal, institutional, cultural, and policy pressures.[25] Research has exposed a tension around who bears the responsibility for injury prevention in sport and in the absence of organizational policies or cultural norms putting safety above performance, coaches often bear the brunt of navigating these competing demands. This is why prevention strategies that target only one stakeholder group often don't work, and why more comprehensive approaches that address multiple levels of the hierarchy are needed.

This is related to the second big step forward, which is addressing the terminology we use to describe prevention program use. When we talk about people following rules or instructions given to them by someone in a position of authority, we're talking about *compliance*. This implies that people can either be compliant or not, in as much as they do as they're told, and it offers no grey area in between. To illustrate, policies like restriction on how much tackle training is allowed in American football practice or pitch count limits in youth baseball can be enforced on a compliance basis. The issue here is that compliance doesn't support people's autonomy – they aren't free to choose what works best for them, they're expected to conform to a one-size-fits-all intervention. This clearly has its place, particularly in zero tolerance situations like preventing catastrophic injuries or safeguarding young people, but it leads to behavior change because people are afraid of punishment rather than for its intrinsic value.[26] Think about running in physical education class in school. Most kids do it because they have to and the minute the teacher isn't looking, they stop or find ways to get out of it. That doesn't engender a love of running or appreciation of exercise, it makes for an unpleasant experience that deters a lot of people from sticking with it in the long term. It's the same thing with RCTs in injury prevention. People use the warmups because they have to in the study, but when the project is over a lot of them stop, even if it's been beneficial.[27]

Instead, striving for *adherence* to prevention strategies (i.e., acknowledging that the recommended intervention is one of many possible actions, and how much people use it can be dynamic and situation-specific) is a more flexible paradigm.[28] It permits program adaptations and accounts for the fact that people can use it less than, as much as, or more than recommended (i.e., there's an element of personal choice involved). Although aiming for adherence does mean that some people won't choose to engage in injury prevention behaviors at all, which isn't ideal, it embraces the idea that doing something is better than nothing and any degree of program use will be of benefit. It's a less restrictive stance that theoretically might be better for promoting sustained behavior change, though we'll need more research to know if that's the case.

Engineering Behavior

Armed with all this information, how do we translate what we know into actual injury prevention? Well, we have two basic methods: *top-down* approaches are based around setting policy to affect behavior through the structure of the sport environment, and *bottom-up* approaches are about supporting intention formation and individual behavior change. These can be complementary strategies and indeed, the most successful injury prevention campaigns typically include elements of both.[29] If we focus on top-down approaches to begin with, there's evidence that changing the rules of a sport can be very successful in reducing injury risk by removing dangerous elements of play, like changing scrum engagement laws in rugby union or increasing the age for body checking in ice hockey.[30,31] Of course, these are particularly aggressive forms of shaping behavior and they don't always sit well with people at first (messing with the tradition of a sport causes all kinds of cognitive and emotional distress amongst people in the community), but in the long run they can be really effective for athlete protection. As you might imagine, though, injury prevention is rarely at the top of the priority list for sport organizations where performance is the number one goal. So, relying on policy change as a go-to method of injury prevention isn't that efficient at the best of times, and the resource implications of coordinating and enforcing policy across an entire sport context is often beyond the means of sport governing bodies and clubs. Thankfully, there's an entire field of research and practice devoted to implementation science, which aims to address these broad-scale barriers to intervention scale up and sustainability. Though that work includes elements of organizational psychology and behavior change, it's a little outside the wheelhouse of this book so we won't get into all the detail here.[iii] From an injury psychology perspective, the really fascinating implementation work is happening at the bottom-up end of the spectrum, so we'll turn focus to that instead.

If we want to encourage injury prevention behaviors at the individual level, we have two choices. We can either change the content of existing interventions to make them easier/more enticing to use or we can deliver them in a way that supports people in forming intentions and applying them. If we go with the first option, it involves developing new interventions or adapting ones that already exist, both of which can be time consuming and costly processes. Delivering existing interventions in a different way has therefore been the focus so far, with promising results. Now, we know that there are a number of personal and situational factors that determine whether someone is likely to develop injury prevention intentions and convert those into behavior. A number of well-established behavior change theories describe this process, using a variety of terminology and perspectives on what motivates health-related actions. Most of these have been developed in other domains like exercise promotion, nutrition, and disease management, and they've all by and large helped to increase our understanding of why people behave in certain ways. You might recognize the names of some of them: The Theory of Reasoned Action, The Theory of Planned Behavior, and Protection Motivation Theory are some of the common ones.[32–34] It stands to reason, then, that we might use one of these theoretical models to help us shape injury prevention behavior. Historically, though, that hasn't been the case. In 2010, a review of 100 injury prevention studies found that behavioral theories were only used explicitly in 11 of them.[35] This has improved a little in recent years, but it's still an underdeveloped area of research.

That said, there have been some remarkable successes to report. Remember when, way back in chapter 2, we introduced the Health Action Process Approach

(HAPA) model and said that it would reappear later in the book? Well get excited, because here it is! As a quick refresher, HAPA is a theory of health behavior change that proposes two distinct phases: a motivational phase (forming an intention) followed by a volitional phase (performing the action).[36] Applied to injury prevention, it predicts that if a person thinks they're at risk of injury (risk perception), they're confident they can perform an injury prevention program (task self-efficacy), and that the program will work (outcome expectancy), then they're more likely to form an intention to use it. Risk perceptions are seen as the least influential predictor, whereas self-efficacy is likely the strongest. Action planning (figuring out how/when/where to use the program) and coping planning (how to deal with barriers) turn those goal intentions into implementation intentions, and confidence in their ability to stick with the program or start using it again after a setback or time off will help them maintain program use. And that's the key reason why injury prevention researchers have focused in on HAPA as a good model to use in this context – most other theories of behavior change aren't explicit about the processes that occur in the intention-behavior gap.[37] HAPA's specification of the role planning has in turning intention into action is really helpful for using the model to improve intervention delivery (Figure 13.1).

The first study to explore HAPA in an injury prevention context applied it in a study of intention to use the 11+ amongst 12 girls' soccer teams.[37] Results showed that task self-efficacy and outcome expectancies were positively associated with intention to use the 11+ during the season, but risk perceptions were not. Importantly, of the three determinants, self-efficacy was by far the strongest predictor. Not only did this support the tenets of the HAPA model, it reflected the knowledge-behavior gap (participants knew injury risk was high but that wasn't

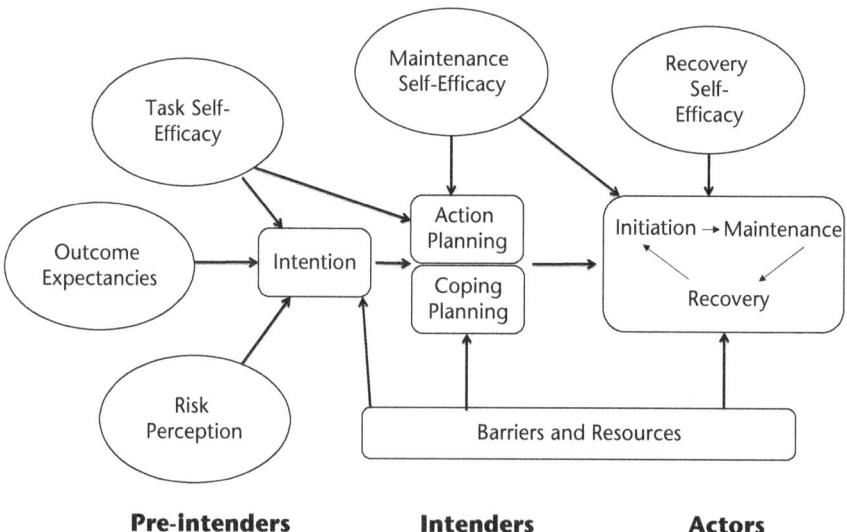

FIGURE 13.1   The Health Action Process Approach (HAPA) model.[36]

enough to kickstart preventive behavior) and highlighted the need to target task self-efficacy and outcome expectancies to promote intention formation.[37] Using this evidence, researchers have developed 11+ workshops to train coaches how to use the program with their teams. Built around HAPA constructs, the workshops include information sessions about injury risk in soccer and evidence for how effective the 11+ can be when used as designed (promoting accurate risk perceptions and outcome expectancies). There are also hands-on elements to teach coaches how to do the exercises properly and how to instruct their players. These field-based sessions draw on the four sources of self-efficacy postulated by Bandura in his original work on Self-Efficacy Theory: mastery experiences (practice coaching the exercises), vicarious experiences (learning from other coaches), verbal persuasion (testimonials from 11+ users), physiological states (what does correct exercise technique feel like?).[40] Early evidence suggests that these workshops successfully improve coaches' self-efficacy for using the program and for overcoming barriers in their environments.[41]

But do they lead to greater adherence? In rugby union, where similar coach workshops have been deployed to promote Activate use amongst youth teams, early evidence says that yes, they do. Coaches who attend workshops have significantly greater rates of Activate adoption and adherence through a season than coaches who don't, and this might be due to stronger intention formation driven by a focus on those HAPA predictors.[42] In a study of 54 coaches who attended an Activate workshop, those with stronger intentions were 49% more likely to maintain program use during the season and those with clear action plans were 33% more likely to stick with it.[43] These findings, although from small samples and with some limitations, imply that utilizing a health behavior change theory – and HAPA in particular – can be an effective way to design intervention delivery strategies to promote greater uptake. They also indicate that instead of focusing efforts on risk education, prevention self-efficacy is a far more helpful way forward.

Reverse Engineering Prevention

In one of the smartest pieces of environmental engineering you might ever see, campus planners at a Canadian university found themselves with an interesting opportunity. A new building had gone up and walkways needed to be laid to link it to neighbouring structures. When classes began in the spring term, however, the building was surrounded by grass and dirt. Through the whole summer, no concrete was laid, and people had to trudge across the landscaping to get to their classes. Just before the autumn term began, however, a series of paths miraculously appeared. The planners had waited to see where students wore tracks into the grass, knowing they'd choose the most efficient route between buildings, and they put the walkways down on top of them. The solution was elegant in its simplicity and illustrates the idea that we can study people's behavior to help us engineer more applicable interventions.

One example of this is the work of Matt Whalan and colleagues who have taken on board a number of the barriers that coaches have reported when using the 11+. In response to issues of limited training time and players being fatigued by some of the more difficult exercises, they've experimented with "rescheduling" part of the program. Instead of being done all at once as a warmup, the most demanding components have been shifted to a post-session activity. In a study of 25 semi-pro clubs, this approach maintained the injury preventive effect of the 11+ and the rescheduled group had 35% better compliance.[44] So, instead of dictating what injury prevention "should" look like, which has so far led to problems with implementation, maybe we can work backward to figure out what fits with the context and then design strategies around it. This is the principle behind passive interventions, like putting down rubber crumb in playgrounds instead of cement or creating breakaway stirrups for equestrians. There has also been some interest in integrating prevention exercises into physical education classes instead of making them sport-specific in order to confer benefit to all kids and take the pressure off coaches.[45] We're just starting to appreciate the benefits of these reverse engineered approaches for supporting behavior change, and there's likely going to be more work in this area over the coming years.

We need to proceed cautiously, though. There's a fine ethical line between making prevention accessible to those who would benefit from it and manipulating behavior based on what someone else thinks is in an athlete's (or coach's) best interest. Whether it be changing policy, engineering the environment, or even designing programs to be more persuasive, there's a constant debate about whether it's appropriate to force people to behave in particular ways instead of supporting their autonomy to choose what's right for them. We won't solve this issue today, but it's worth a small note in our chapter as an important issue to consider in future research and practice.

Forging New Territory

Prevention behavior is the newest addition to the sport injury psychology family and in its short history, a lot of progress has been made. From the early days of assuming dissemination would lead to behavior change, things have progressed to the application of theory and environmental engineering in the space of only 20 years. In research terms, that's the blink of an eye, and it's a really promising area of practical work. There's still a long way to go, though. With so much emphasis on intervention uptake, much less is known about the psychosocial factors that drive prevention behavior maintenance. Systematic longitudinal evaluation is therefore needed, along with much more robust methods for assessing the interacting contributions of different levels of influence in the sport context. With evolutions of the original TRIPP model now appearing in the literature[46] and increasing application of the principles of implementation science, there's scope for research and practice in this domain to take another big leap forward toward the goal of wide-scale injury prevention in sport.

Notes

i In 2018, the "Tide Pod Challenge" had people taking bites out of laundry detergent pods and posting video of it to their social media accounts. Ingesting toxic levels of ethanol and hydrogen peroxide is NEVER a good idea, and yet it still took a big public health campaign to put an end to it. If simple messages like "don't eat poison" aren't enough to affect behavior, it's no wonder more complex interventions struggle!

ii If it happened to be a fitness-related goal, it in all likelihood stalled out around January 19, which is the date digital fitness giant Strava™ has termed "Quitter's Day" based on trends in uploaded exercise activities.[15]

iii This is a really interesting area of sport injury research though, and if you're interested in some introductory reading, you might try Bauer et al.'s introduction to Implementation Science or Grimshaw et al.'s Knowledge Translation explainer.[38,39]

References

1 Hoffman DT, Dwyer DB, Bowe SJ, et al. Is injury associated with team performance in elite Australian football? 20 years of player injury and team performance data that include measures of individual player values. *Br J Sports Med* 2020;54:475–479; doi: 10.1136/bjsports-2018-100029.

2 Goggins L, Peirce N, Stokes K, et al. Negative association between injuries and team success in professional cricket: a 9-year prospective cohort analysis. *J Sci Med Sport* 2021;24(2):141–145; doi: 10.1016/j.jsams.2020.07.007.

3 West SW, Wiiliams S, Kemp SPT, et al. Training load, injury burden, and team success in professional rugby union: risk versus reward. *J Athl Train* 2020;55:960–966; doi: 10.4085/1062-6050-0387.19.

4 Williams S, Trewartha G, Kemp SPT, et al. Time loss injuries compromise team success in elite rugby union: a 7-year prospective study. *Br J Sports Med* 2016;50:651–656; doi: 10.1136/bjsports-2015-094798.

5 Ozturk S, Kilic D. What is the economic burden of sports injuries? *Eklem Hastalik Cerrahisi* 2013;24(2):108–111; doi: 10.5606/ehc.2013.24.

6 Barden C, Bekker S, Brown JC, et al. Evaluating the implementation of injury prevention strategies in rugby union and league: a systematic review using the re-aim framework. *Int J Sports Med* 2020;42:112–121; doi: 10.1055/a-1212-0649.

7 Steib S, Rahlf AL, Pfeifer K, et al. Dose-response relationship of neuromuscular training for injury prevention in youth athletes: a meta-analysis. *Front Physiol* 2017;8:920: doi: 10.3389/fphys.2017.00920.

8 Van Dyk N, Behan FP, Whiteley R. Including the Nordic hamstring exercise in injury prevention programmes halves the rate of hamstring injuries: a systematic review and meta-analysis of 8459 athletes. *Br J Sports Med* 2019;53(21):1362–1370; doi: 10.1136/bjsports-2018-100045.

9 Sadigursky D, Braid JA, De Lira DNL, et al. The FIFA 11+ injury prevention program for soccer players: a systematic review. *BMC Sports Sci Med Rehabil* 2017;9:18; doi: 10.1186/s13102-017-0083-z.

10 Bizzini M, Dvorak J. FIFA 11+: an effective programme to prevent football injuries in various player groups worldwide—a narrative review. *Br J Sports Med* 2015;49:577–579; doi: 10.1136/bjsports-2015-094765.

11 O'Brien J, Young W, Finch CF. The delivery of injury prevention exercise programmes in professional youth soccer: comparison to the FIFA 11+. *J Sci Med Sport* 2017;20(1):26–31; doi: 10.1016/j.jsams.2016.05.007.

12 World Health Organization. WHO launches year-long campaign to help 100 million people quit tobacco. Available at: https://www.who.int/news/item/08-12-2020-who-launches-year-long-campaign-to-help-100-million-people-quit-tobacco Accessed June 11, 2021.

13 Sheeran P. Intention-behavior relations: a conceptual and empirical review In: W Stroebe, M. Hewstone (eds.). *European review of social psychology* (vol. 12). New York: Wiley 2002.

14 Gollwitzer PM, Sheeran P. Implementation intentions and goal achievement: a meta-analysis of effects and processes. *Adv Exp Soc Psychol* 2006;38:69–119; doi:10.1016/S0065-2601(06)38002-1.

15 Barr S. What is quitter's day and when does it take place? Available at: https://www.independent.co.uk/life-style/quitters-day-new-years-resolutions-fitness-january-exercise-active-strava-a9288556.html Accessed June 11, 2021.

16 Finch C. A new framework for research leading to sports injury prevention. *J Sci Med Sport* 2006;9:3–9; doi:10.1016/j.jsams.2006.02.009.

17 McKay CD, Steffen K, Romiti M, et al. The effect of coach and player injury knowledge, attitudes and beliefs on adherence to the FIFA 11+ programme in female youth soccer. *Br J Sports Med* 2014;48:1281–1286; doi:10.1136/bjsports-2014-093543.

18 Waldén M, Atroshi I, Magnusson H, et al. Prevention of acute knee injuries in adolescent female football players: cluster randomised controlled trial. *BMJ* 2012;344:e3042; doi:10.1136/bmj.e3042.

19 Lindblom H, Waldén M, Carlfjord S, et al. Implementation of a neuromuscular training programme in female adolescent football: 3-year follow-up study after a randomised controlled trial. *Br J Sports Med* 2014;48:1425–1430; doi:10.1136/bjsports-2013-093298.

20 Lindblom, H, Carlfjord, S, Hägglund, M. Adoption and use of an injury prevention exercise program in female football: a qualitative study among coaches. *Scand J Med Sci Sports* 2018;28:1295–1303; doi:10.1111/sms.13012.

21 O'Brien J, Young W, Finch CF. The use and modification of injury prevention exercises by professional youth soccer teams. *Scand J Med Sci Sports* 2017;27:1337–1346; doi:10.1111/sms.12756.

22 O'Brien J, Finch CF. Injury prevention exercise programs for professional soccer: understanding the perceptions of the end-users. *Clin J Sport Med* 2017;27:1–9; doi:10.1097/JSM.0000000000000291.

23 Shill I, Raisanen A, Black AM, et al. Canadian high school rugby coaches' readiness for an injury prevention strategy implementation: evaluating a train-the-coach workshop. *Front Sport Act Living* 2021; doi:10.3389/fspo.2021.672603.

24 Barden C, Stokes KA, McKay CD. Implementation of the *Activate* injury prevention exercise programme in English schoolboy rugby union. *BMJ Open Sport Ex Med* 2021;7:e001018. doi:10.1136/bmjsem-2020-001018.

25 Wadey R, Day M, Cavallerio F, et al. Multilevel model of sport injury (MMSI): can coaches impact and be impacted by injury? In: R Thelwell, M Dicks (eds.). *Professional advances in sports coaching: research and practice.* London: Routledge 2018.

26 Deci EL, Ryan RM. Self-determination theory: a macrotheory of human motivation, development, and health. *Can Psychol* 2008;49:182–185; doi:10.1037/a0012801.

27 Myklebust G, Skjolberg A, Bahr R. ACL injury incidence in female handball 10 years after the Norwegian ACL prevention study: important lessons learned. *Br J Sports Med* 2013;47:476–479; doi:10.1136/bjsports-2012-091862.

28 McKay CD, Verhagen E. "Compliance" versus "adherence" in sport injury prevention: why definition matters. *Br J Sports Med* 2016;50:382–383; doi:10.1136/bjsports-2015-095192.

29 Viljoen W, Patricios J. BokSmart - implementing a national rugby safety programme. *Br J Sports Med* 2012;46:692–693; doi:10.1136/bjsports-2012-091278.

30 Reboursiere E, Bohu Y, Retière D, et al. Impact of the national prevention policy and scrum law changes on the incidence of rugby-related catastrophic cervical spine injuries in French Rugby Union. *Br J Sports Med* 2018;52:674–677; doi:10.1136/bjsports-2016-096122.

31 Black AM, Hagel BE, Palacios-Derflingher L, et al. The risk of injury associated with body checking among Pee Wee ice hockey players: an evaluation of Hockey Canada's national body checking policy change. *Br J Sports Med* 2017;5:1767–1772; doi:10.1136/bjsports-2016-097392.

32 Hale JL, Householder BJ, Greene KL. The theory of reasoned action. In: JP Dillard, L Shen (eds.). *The SAGE handbook of persuasion: developments in theory and practice.* London: Sage Publications 2002.

33 Ajzen I. From intentions to actions: a theory of planned behaviour. In: J Kuhl, J Beckman (eds.). *Action-control: from cognition to behaviour.* Heidelberg: Springer 1985.

34 Rogers RW, Prentice-Dunn S. Protection motivation theory. In: DS Gochman (ed.). *Handbook of health behaviour research 1: personal and social determinants.* New York: Plenum Press 1997.

35 McGlashan AJ, Finch CF. The extent to which behavioural and social sciences theories and models are used in sport injury prevention research. *Sport Med* 2010;40:841–858; doi:10.2165/11534960-000000000-00000.

36 Schwarzer R. The Health Action Process Approach (HAPA). Available at: http://www.hapa-model.de/ Accessed June 3, 2021.

37 McKay CD, Merrett CK, Emery CA. Predictors of FIFA 11+ implementation intention in female adolescent soccer: an application of the Health Action Process Approach (HAPA) model. *Int J Environ Res Public Health* 2016;13(7):657; doi:10.3390/ijerph13070657.

38 Bauer MS, Damschroder L, Hagedorn H, et al. An introduction to implementation science for the non-specialist. *BMC Psychol* 2015;3:32: doi:10.1186/s40359-015-0089-9.

39 Grimshaw J, Eccles MP, Lavis JN, et al. Knowledge translation of research findings. *Implement Sci* 2012;7:50; doi:10.1186/1748-5908-7-50.

40 Bandura A. Self-efficacy: toward a unifying theory of behavioral change. *Psychol Rev* 1977;84:191–215; doi:10.1037/0033-295X.84.2.191.

41 Owoeye O, McKay CD, Raisanen AM, et al. Psychosocial factors and the effects of a structured injury prevention workshop on coaches' self-efficacy to implement the 11+ exercise program. *J Exerc Sci* 2020;13:1459–1475.

42 Barden C, Stokes KA, McKay CD. Utilising a behaviour change model to improve implementation of the *Activate* injury prevention exercise programme in schoolboy rugby union. *Int J Environ Res Public Health* 2021;18:5681; doi:10.3390/ijerph18115681.

43 Hislop MD. *Injury risk factors and prevention strategies in schoolboy rugby union* [dissertation]. The University of Bath 2017.

44 Whalan, M, Lovell, R, Steele, et al. Rescheduling part 2 of the 11+ reduces injury burden and increases compliance in semi-professional football. *Scand J Med Sci Sports* 2019;29:1941–1951; doi:10.1111/sms.13532.

45 Emery CA, van den Berg C, Richmond SA, et al. Implementing a junior high school-based programme to reduce sports injuries through neuromuscular training (iSPRINT): a cluster randomised controlled trial (RCT). *Br J Sports Med* 2020;54:913–919; doi: 10.1136/bjsports-2019-101117.

46 O'Brien J, Finch CF, Pruna R, et al. A new model for injury prevention in team sports: the Team-sport Injury Prevention (TIP) cycle. *Sci Med Football* 2019;3:77–80; doi: 10.1080/24733938.2018.1512752.

14

LEARNING FROM MARKETING GIANTS TO SELL ATHLETE HEALTH: WHAT IF PREVENTION HAD A SLOGAN?

Carly McKay

Following a panel discussion at the 2016 conference of the World Rugby Science Network, an audience member posed an interesting question: *"what if a giant sports apparel/equipment brand sold injury prevention?"* The question got a few bemused looks and prompted some speculation at the time, though it was very much an off the cuff idea. Yet, over the intervening years, it's kept resurfacing periodically as a talking point. Given this staying power, you have to wonder if there might actually be something to it. So, let's take a step off the beaten path for a moment and explore this in earnest. What would happen if it wasn't researchers and practitioners pushing the prevention agenda?

Injury prevention has typically been promoted through conventional channels like presentations, awareness campaigns, and workshops. These are often academically led activities to share information, focused on convincing people that injuries can and should be avoided. This has only been passingly successful in most cases,[1] and there remains a diffusion of benefit as interventions move from research settings into the "real" world. This is likely because limited reach of prevention strategies into end-user communities, and poor adoption once they get there, results in *voltage drop* (i.e., the intervention loses potency moving from controlled to uncontrolled conditions) and *program drift* (i.e., deviation from protocol impacts its effectiveness).[1,2] This is considered a risk with any large-scale intervention, but maybe that's the biggest hurdle – researchers often view injury through a public health lens (e.g., supporting the greater good) that isn't compatible with the sport mentality (e.g., gaining a competitive advantage).

Herein lies the problem with standard intervention approaches. They rely on injury prevention being a priority for athletes, coaches, and the sport system in general. It requires considerable investment of time, energy, and resource from multiple stakeholders, and it regularly sits at odds with the reason people participate in the first place – to have fun, to win, and to achieve goals. Let's face it,

DOI: 10.4324/9781003088936-14

injury prevention isn't sexy. Winning trophies is, pulling off ridiculous moves is, ending up covered in mud and proud of one's accomplishments is. Warmups and protective padding are not, and that's one of the reasons why it's so difficult to engrain prevention into the collective sport psyche. It's the chore that nobody really wants to do, especially at recreational levels where total dedication to the game isn't driving people's behavior. They're there to train and compete. Obviously, maintaining athlete health is incredibly important from every perspective, but the actual nuts and bolts of doing so aren't exactly a feature when people sign up. In other words, prevention is a good product, but it doesn't sell.

Standing on the Shoulders of Giants

So, what if we came at this from a different angle and took a lesson from the best marketing teams of our times? After all, there are companies that can sell someone a new pair of running shoes, identical to the ones they bought only months ago, because now they come in a new color. They brand lifestyles and shape the way people experience media content, creating a dedicated customer base ready to model themselves after the latest spokesperson. Imagine if that power could be harnessed to "sell" prevention. Clearly, without a means of turning a profit, that's unlikely to be a successful venture and that's not what we're proposing. But maybe we can borrow some of their tricks to improve the way we design and deliver our "product".

We'll need to take a few conceptual liberties when applying some of these ideas to a prevention context, but one of the first things to consider is whether we should adopt a transactional or relationship marketing paradigm. The goal of *transactional marketing* is to make a sale and move on to find new customers, whereas *relationship marketing* aims to foster and retain a client base.[3] We could argue that specific scenarios might call for the former (e.g., one-and-done travel vaccinations before competing abroad), but the necessity of maintaining most prevention behaviors over time fits with the latter. Of course, these needn't be mutually exclusive; for instance, getting people to purchase safety equipment and then continue using it might need elements of both. From there, we can apply a classic *marketing mix* using the "4 Ps": product, price, place, and promotion. These are viewed as the traditional cornerstones of sales and although they've been expanded into countless derivatives, from an injury prevention standpoint the originals will serve just fine.[3,4]

Starting with the *product*, it's all about what the customer wants. We have to think about the needs our interventions will satisfy and whether they include attractive features or unnecessary extras. Despite the clear health benefits, this is the point to upsell what else prevention has to offer, like potential performance benefits that come along with it.[5] It's also important to incorporate feedback about components that people don't seem to like (e.g., specific exercises)[6] to make the product as attractive as possible. We also need to factor in the experience of using these interventions. Are they easy to apply without too many negative side effects?

Just as a customer would stop using a product that was more hassle than it was worth, so too will prevention program users. This is related to the *price* (i.e., what is the value of the product or service to the customer?) If we consider the cost of prevention in terms of not only financial implications but also its drain on resources like time, space, and attention span, then in sport we're working with customers who are particularly price sensitive. The value for investment therefore needs to be high, and interventions must compete with lower "priced" alternatives (like doing nothing at all, where injury risk may seem like a fair gamble).

This leaves us with *place* (where do people find our product?) and *promotion* (how do messages reach our audience?). Getting the distribution channels right is the key to successful marketing, and this is where prevention has struggled in the past. It's not just about raising awareness and getting information to the right people at the right time – the way it's delivered really matters. Messages can be *targeted* (directed at a particular group, like coaches) or *tailored* (fit to individual characteristics, like personality), to increase their persuasiveness[7] and in a sweeping review, Teeny et al.[8] identified four key factors in this process: characteristics of the recipient, message content, message source, and the setting in which the message is received. Within this framework, there are dozens of factors that we can use to match messages to the audience, such as a person's mood state, their goals and attitudes, or even their demographics and culture. For example, research has shown that matching the content of a message to the recipient's *approach/avoidance orientation* (e.g., promotion-focused people look for gains whereas prevention-focused people want to avoid losses) increases persuasion.[8] Moreover, abstract messages are better for alerting promotion-focused people about multiple options for attaining their goals and concrete messages engender more self-efficacy in prevention-focused people. This suggests that traditional intervention delivery, which tends to provide concrete information framed around avoiding injuries (e.g., losses) will appeal to health-conscious athletes and coaches, but if we're working with a group more interested in performance then we might need to use a different tactic. Because there are endless combinations of factors that influence how persuasive messages are, there's no single best way to encourage prevention behaviors. Instead, we may need to develop a suite of marketing resources to connect with a variety of users, much the same way companies advertise the same product differently from one setting to another (e.g., the same car can have different names from country to country).

There's also evidence that we're more receptive to messages that uphold the values of our social groups, particularly when these come from people who look or sound like us (i.e., members of our in-group).[8] This is why establishing authority is an important early step. Athletes and coaches might not buy into researchers' or practitioners' advice due to perceptions that "outsiders" don't understand the sport context. This is an example of the *in-group bias*, which is a tendency for people to favor others within their group over people without.[9] Businesses use this to build brand loyalty, and in injury prevention it's the idea behind training coaches to deliver programs to other coaches.[10] People trust information coming from relatable ("in-group") sources, and they also tend to trust "experts". How many television ads have you seen where a doctor or dentist endorses a product? *Authority bias* describes our inclination to attribute greater accuracy to the opinions of authority figures, suggesting that prevention messages coming from prominent sport figures or reputable scientists may hold sway in some settings, like grassroot sport with novice coaches. Of course, there's evidence that as athletes and coaches gain experience, they're less likely to change their behavior (e.g., they become the experts),[11] so this will probably only get us so far.

Word-of-mouth promotion can be useful to some extent within sport communities, but we might be inclined to take a page straight from the sport business playbook and consider endorsements. Many big sport companies have brand ambassadors and professional athlete spokespeople, trading on authority biases, wider market reach (e.g., through celebrity social media accounts), and *social comparison biases* (showing someone with desirable qualities that people aspire to) to increase their persuasiveness.[12] To illustrate, why did helmets suddenly become "cool" in snowboarding? Well, as "extreme" sports started to infiltrate mainstream media coverage and transition into the Olympics, the equipment and clothing worn by the athletes was associated with a particular alternative lifestyle. Modeling themselves after their idols, young riders began emulating their style and helmets became fashion, not safety equipment. It wasn't long before companies began branding them to sell an image.[13] Peer influence has been key in this as well, as the community has developed norms around wearing gear, supported by the big names in the sport who act as role models. In conjunction with industry-wide efforts to mandate helmet use at ski hills, this has resulted in general acceptance across the sector with far less resistance compared to what we've seen in other settings (e.g., cycling).[14]

In some sports, a role model has been instrumental in shaping prevention behavior, like helmet pioneers Tony Hawk in skateboarding or Olav Hagen in rollerskiing.[15] In other instances, high-profile incidents have been a flashpoint for increased uptake in safety equipment and prevention behaviors, such as Natasha Richardson's death while skiing or Sidney Crosby's concussion struggles in ice hockey. In both cases, public attention was captured by a story which simultaneously increased risk awareness and triggered emotional responses that prompted change across a wide cross-section of sport participants. These examples highlight how impactful narratives can be,[16] and they form a big part of contemporary marketing strategy for exactly that reason. As a sales tool, stories (a.k.a. *content marketing*) engage with customers in a relatable way, moving away from pitches in favor of vignettes that highlight the credibility and authenticity of the brand.[17] Perhaps the most well-known example from an athlete health perspective is the nearly legendary tale of how Gatorade was developed to prevent heat illness but ended up changing the fortunes of a lacklustre Florida Gators college football team, turning them into champions.[18] When people form an emotional connection with stories like that, they remember the key messages and that translates into substantial increases in sales volumes.[19] So, why not leverage this in injury prevention? Storytelling is emerging as a helpful element in injury rehabilitation[20] and increased presence of the athlete voice in intervention delivery might be equally effective.

Points for Creativity

Though integrating psychological principles from business marketing might be an uncomfortable step toward behavior manipulation, there are some prevention campaigns that have leaned into that world and been really successful. Though not an injury prevention program per se, the Centres for Disease Control and Prevention (CDC) in the United States capitalized on the incredible popularity of television shows like *The Walking Dead* to introduce "zombie preparedness" resources aimed at public emergency planning.[21] It turns out that the things you'd do to prepare for an undead apocalypse (stocking up on food and medication, mapping an escape route) mirror the recommendations for extreme weather events and pandemics. What began as a tongue-in-cheek way of encouraging people to be ready for worst-case scenarios has been remarkably well received and has even expanded into education packs for schools.[21] This is a prime example of how targeted messaging that taps into a group's shared identity (a particular fandom in this case) can "sell" an intervention in a fun and interesting way.

Another emerging marketing technique is *behavioral nudging*, which is exactly what it sounds like: encouraging people to make specific choices by altering the environment to facilitate automatic cognitive processes.[22] When people are under time pressure or decisions are complex, they often revert to heuristic judgments that are prone to environmental influence. The *availability heuristic* is one of these, which is a cognitive shortcut that makes it easier for us to recall some memories than others. Things that get a lot of media coverage, or times when we've had strong emotional reactions are easier for us to remember and have greater influence over our decisions than they would if we logically considered things. This is why people are worried about shark attacks and plane crashes even though getting in a car is far riskier. Nudging also takes advantage of the *social proof heuristic* (i.e., we look to what others are doing to guide our own behavior)[23] and the fact that people more often than not go with the default option when presented with a choice.[24,25] So, what does this have to do with marketing? Well, stores actually use nudges like putting more expensive things on shelves at eye level, displaying certain items near the cash registers, or planting "shoppers" in the aisles to draw attention to particular products. It seems really sneaky, but a Dutch company called iNudgeyou has shown that it can be used for injury prevention, too. They carried out a project to improve safety behaviors on staircases in a big office building, because even though we consider them relatively non-threatening, stairway falls actually lead to a surprisingly high number of severe injuries.[26] They traced silhouettes at the bottom of the stairs (like you'd see at a crime scene) with speech bubbles saying, "should have grabbed the handrail". Based on observational data, these nudges improved handrail use by approximately 10%.[27] Although that doesn't seem like much of an increase, it goes to show how behavior can be shaped through simple psychological techniques.

Of course, if subtlety isn't the goal, *guerilla marketing* (using unconventional strategies to attract interest) holds promise as well. The Community Against Preventable Injury is a Canadian organization dedicated to safety promotion and they're known for their attention-grabbing approaches.[27] Some of their more daring campaigns have involved staging an overturned boat along a lakeshore – complete with paddles floating nearby – with a message about the importance of wearing life vests etched on its bottom. They also had snowboarders go out to the slopes for a day with a sarcastic "you probably won't need a helmet today" on the backs of their jackets to challenge beliefs about head injury risk.[27,28] As the opposite of nudging, these are bold, in-your-face techniques for confronting unsafe behavior and opening a dialogue about how to improve it. Sometimes, jarring people out of their usual thought patterns can make them think more critically about what they're doing and why, and they're unlikely to forget the key message if it's something they don't see every day.

Testing the Market

If we asked a big sport company to market injury prevention, it's probably safe to say that it would look a lot different than it does now. Based on extensive market research, they would hone their advertising to hit just the right balance of images versus words and emotional versus informational content. They'd identify the precise colors, word choices, and catchphrases that would appeal to different end-user groups and we'd end up with slick campaigns using state of the art media, working toward brand saturation. But, that kind of expertise doesn't come cheaply and when you're working from a public health perspective, you can't monetize your product or service. So, until we can convince these companies to invest in athlete health to the same extent as performance, it's up to researchers and practitioners to learn what we can from business and apply it to what we do.

Though injury prevention isn't easy to glamourize, we can borrow some of the ideas that marketing firms use to highlight the value of what's on offer. We can shape the environment to make prevention an easier choice than the alternative, and we can better frame our messages to improve audience appeal. We can make prevention the "default setting" by enacting policies and improving access to safety equipment. We can also go with the tried-and-true approach of repeated exposure, which we know builds more positive attitudes toward products over time.[29] The psychology of consumer marketing is a largely untapped resource from an injury prevention point of view and presents an interesting opportunity to advance the field. While we're waiting for that research to develop, some pioneering injury prevention groups are already heading in that direction, and it will be really exciting to see what they come up with next.

References

1 Verhagen E, van Nassau F. Implementation science to reduce the prevalence and burden of MSK disorders following sport and exercise-related injury. *Best Prac Res Clin Rheumatol* 2019;33:188–201; doi: 10.1016/j.berh.2019.02.011.

2 Chambers DA, Glasgow RE, Stange KC. The dynamic sustainability framework: addressing the paradox of sustainment amid ongoing change. *Implement Sci* 2013;8:117; doi: 10.1186/1748-5908-8-117.

3 Zineldin M, Philipson S. Kotler and Borden are not dead: myth of relationship marketing and truth of the 4Ps. *J Consum Mark* 2007;24:229–241; doi: 10.1108/07363760710756011.

4 McCarthy J. *Basic marketing – a managerial approach.* Homewood, IL: Richard D. Irwin, Inc 1960.

5 Drew MK, Raysmith BP, Charlton PC. Injuries impair the chance of successful performance by sportspeople: a systematic review. *Br J Sports Med* 2017;51:1209–1214; doi: 10.1136/bjsports-2016-096731.

6 Donaldson A, Callaghan A, Bizzini M, et al. A concept mapping approach to identifying the barriers to implementing an evidence-based sports injury prevention programme. *Inj Prev* 2019;25:244–251; doi: 10.1136/injuryprev-2017-042639.

7 Schmid KL, Rivers SE, Latimer AE, et al. Targeting or tailoring? Maximizing resources to create effective health communications. *Mark Health Serv* 2008;28:32–37.

8 Teeny JD, Siev JJ, Briñol P, et al. A review and conceptual framework for understanding personalized matching effects in persuasion. *J Consum Psychol* 2021;31:382–414; doi: 10.1002/jcpy.1198.

9 Tajfel H. Social psychology of intergroup relations. *Annu Rev Pscyhol* 1982;33:1–39.

10 Barden C, Stokes KA, McKay CD. Implementation of the *activate* injury prevention exercise programme in English schoolboy rugby union. *BMJ Open Sport Ex Med* 2021;7:e001018; doi: 10.1136/bmjsem-2020-001018.

11 McKay CD, Steffen K, Romiti M, et al. The effect of coach and player injury knowledge, attitudes and beliefs on adherence to the FIFA 11+ programme in female youth soccer. *Br J Sports Med* 2014;48:1281–1286; doi: 10.1136/bjsports-2014-093543.

12 Knoll J, Matthes J. The effectiveness of celebrity endorsements: a meta-analysis. *J Acad Mark Sci* 2017;45:55–75; doi:10.1007/s11747-016-0503-8.

13 Critchell S. Helmets become the fashion in snow sports, including for Olympians. Available at: https://www.seattletimes.com/life/outdoors/helmets-become-the-fashion-in-snow-sports-including-for-olympians/ Accessed June 16, 2021.

14 Ledesma RD, Shinar D, Valero-Mora MP, et al. Psychosocial factors associated with helmet use by adult cyclists. *Transp Res Part F Traffic Psychol Behav* 2019;65:376–388; doi:10.1016/j.trf.2019.08.003.

15 Role of individual in history or how one man made wearing helmets cool. Available at: https://www.dailyskier.com/2018/08/28/role-of-individual-in-history-or-how-one-man-made-wearing-helmets-to-be-cool-visto-por-daily-skier-a-las-2343/ Accessed June 16, 2021.

16 Wadey R, Day M, Cavallerio F, et al. Multilevel model of sport injury (MMSI): can coaches impact and be impacted by injury? In: R Thelwell, M Dicks (eds.). *Professional advances in sports coaching: research and practice.* London: Routledge 2018.

17 Pulizzi J. The rise of storytelling as the new marketing. *Publishing Res Q* 2012;28:116–123; doi:10.1007/s12109-012-9264-5.

18 Gatorade heritage. Available at: http://www.gatorade.com.mx/company/heritage Accessed June 16, 2021.

19 We're ruled by our emotions, and so are the ads we watch. Available at: https://www.nielsen.com/us/en/insights/article/2016/were-ruled-by-our-emotions-and-so-are-the-ads-we-watch/ Accessed June 16, 2021.

20 Arrvinen-Barrow M, Clement D, Hemmings B. "This is the final jump," I respond. Why, why do I utter those words? Using storytelling in sport injury rehabilitation. In: R Wadey (ed.). *Sport injury psychology: cultural, relational, methodological, and applied considerations*. New York: Routledge 2020.

21 CDC. Zombie preparedness. Available at: https://www.cdc.gov/cpr/zombie/index.htm Accessed June 16, 2021.

22 Simon C, Tagliabue M. Feeding the behavioral revolution: contributions of behavior analysis to nudging and vice versa. *J Behav Economics Policy* 2018;1:91–97.

23 Cheung T, Kroese F, Fennis B, et al. The hunger games: using hunger to promote healthy choices in self-control conflicts. *Appetite* 2017;116:401–409; doi:10.1016/j.appet.2017.05.020.

24 Campbell-Arvai V, Arvai J, Kalof L. Motivating sustainable food choices: the role of nudges, value orientation, and information provision. *Environ Behav* 2014;46:453–475; doi:10.1177/0013916512469099.

25 Pichert D, Katsikopoulos KV. Green defaults: information presentation and pro-environmental behavior. *J Environ Psychol* 2008;28:63–73; doi: 10.1016-j.jenvp.2 007.09.004.

26 Jacobs JV. A review of stairway falls and stair negotiation: lessons learned and future needs to reduce injury. *Gait Posture* 2016;49:159–167; doi:10.1016/j.gaitpost.2016. 06.030.

27 Applying behavioural science to ensure stairway safety – a closer look at fall precention and occupational stairway behaviour. Available at: https://inudgeyou.com/en/applying-behavioural-science-to-ensure-stairway-safety/ Accessed June 16, 2021.

28 The Community Against Preventable Injuries. Available at: https://www.preventable.ca Accessed June 16, 2021.

29 Hamilton K, Johnson BT. Attitudes and persuasive communication interventions. In: MS Hagger, LD Cameron, K Hamilton, N Hankonen, T Lintunen (eds.). *The handbook of behavior change*. Cambridge, UK: Cambridge University Press 2020.

15

INJURY PSYCHOLOGY AND YOUNG ATHLETES: CHOOSING FROM THE KIDS' MENU

Carly McKay and Ulrika Tranaeus

"I thought it was pretty cool when I injured myself playing football and the ambulance came to take me to hospital. All my friends watched, and I was hero for a while. Now I know better. If someone is fetched by an ambulance, it's a serious injury. That means the person is in pain, have a lot of boring rehabilitation waiting, and a long journey back to sport. Sometimes even never get back to sport."

Sport psychology client, 16 years old

For many, sport or another kind of active play constituted some of the most formative events of our childhood years. Whether it be at home, at school, or simply around the neighborhood where we grew up, the intrinsic value of chasing around a ball – or each other – was cemented either by personal experience or the idealized versions of childhood portrayed on television. For those with firsthand knowledge, the perils of such pursuits included skinned knees and bruises, and it seemed everyone knew someone who had to be taken to the hospital for a broken bone. Of course, this nostalgic view doesn't represent the reality for all children, but it introduces some of the innate challenges and opportunities when working with young, active groups.

There are clear benefits of physical activity for children and adolescents. Active play and sports participation improve aerobic capacity, muscular development, and bone health.[1] Research also highlights the positive role of physical activity in promoting mental wellbeing, cognitive function, quality of life, and academic engagement.[2] All in all, to stave off the negative consequences of an inactive lifestyle, youth sport is an attractive option and enrolment around the world reflects this. For example, in the United States, there are roughly 60 million athletes between the ages of six and 18 participating in some form of organized sport.[3]

This is where some of the challenges arise. With physical activity comes the risk of injury, and national-level data indicate that sport and recreation injury burden is

DOI: 10.4324/9781003088936-15

highest in youth populations.[4,5] For instance, there's an annual incidence of 1.3 million hospital-treated sport injuries for those under 15 years of age across the European Union.[6] Beyond the immediate and future health consequences of these injuries, there are notable knock-on effects for physical activity in the longer term. Sport participation declines with age under the best of circumstances, particularly for girls, for several reasons including competing demands and interests, lack of access to affordable opportunities, and conformity to traditional gender norms.[7] Indeed, as many as 80% of youth drop out of sport by the time they're 15 years old.[8,9] Injury is also a major contributor to this. For instance, 20% of Canadian adolescent athletes reported injury as their reason for leaving sport in one study, and similar results have been seen in samples from a variety of sports and countries.[10,11] So, while we're trying to promote sport participation for its health benefits, in a way we're also setting kids up for all kinds of potential problems.[12]

Well, that paints a bleak picture, doesn't it? What about those lovely images of children chasing each other around the playground and having wholesome, character-building fun? Fear not, those ideals are still achievable, but in order to identify and maximize the opportunities for realizing them, we need to overcome some of these big challenges.

The Injury Landscape

Injuries occur in different contexts, such as at school, in recreational activities, and in organized sport. In many cases, there is considerable overlap between these settings, and it can be difficult to work out a denominator for youth sport exposure. Sure, we can figure out how many hours kids spend in physical education class, but how do we quantify the time they spend playing basketball in the front yard or running with the family dog? That makes comparing injury rates across different kinds of participation rather difficult but, such issues aside, injury surveillance in organized sport has shown us that (1) sport participation peaks during childhood and adolescence, and (2) injury rates are high in a lot of these activities.[11] To put this into perspective, a study of 8406 schoolchildren aged 11 to 15 years reported that 47% had sustained at least one injury related to physical activity in the previous 12 months.[13] Notably, injury prevalence was higher in organized sport (46%) compared to leisure time physical activities (30%) or school-based physical activities (18%). We also know that contact sports like American football tend to have the highest injury incidence (e.g., 2.0–17.8 injuries/1000 athlete exposures).[14] Non-contact sports like volleyball can be risky too (e.g., 1.7–10.7 injuries/1000 player hours),[15] though the mechanism and types of injuries may differ substantially from sport to sport.[16]

There are some reliable injury patterns that emerge in the youth context. For instance, overuse injury prevalence ranges from 37–68% across sports, and we start to see sex-specific increases emerge for some injury types through adolescence (e.g., threefold increased risk of anterior cruciate ligament [ACL] injury for girls compared to boys after puberty).[17] These distinct epidemiological features are largely attributed to factors associated with growth and maturation.[12] Carefully considering how and why these injuries happen can help us reduce risk and appropriately support athletes through rehabilitation.

Some Risk Factors Are Unique

As with adults, young athletes are susceptible to injury for all kinds of reasons. These include physical stressors, cognitive or emotional difficulties, improper training, or poor coaching. Whatever the cause, we need to evaluate risk with constant acknowledgement of the environment in which we're working. Youth sport is characterized by its many layers. The athletes are not autonomous; they participate within spheres of influence that include their coaches, parents, sport organizations, and competing demands of academics, social pressures, personal development, and myriad internal and external expectations.[12] So, when we think about the psychological elements of the injury experience, we must always account for their expression within the athlete's immediate context.

One of the primary contextual factors to consider is sport specialization. Defined as intense, year-round training in a single sport to the exclusion of others,[18] this practice is becoming more commonplace among younger athletes. As we discussed in chapter 11, professionalized systems have given rise to talent identification and increasing pressure for young athletes to enter developmental pathways. Although this can provide access to better coaching and other resources, it also significantly increases the risks of overuse injury, burnout, and other negative outcomes.[12] Multi-sport participation is common in younger cohorts as well, bringing its own unique challenges such as balancing competing demands and injury risks across different sport settings. Therefore, as we discuss injury risk factors and how best to work with young athletes toward injury prevention or recovery, we need to remember that one single approach isn't going to work for everyone.

Growth, Maturation, and Injury Risk

Right, let's get the obvious out of the way. Between childhood and adulthood, people undergo many physical changes, peaking during those angsty adolescent years. A number of comprehensive reviews have gone through this in detail,[19,20] but the summary notes are that *growth, maturation,* and *development* are related but independent processes that play central roles during this time period. *Growth* specifically refers to changes in body size, shape, and composition, whereas *maturation* is the act of progression toward the adult state and can be measured in multiple biological systems (e.g., skeletal, hormonal).[19] *Development* encompasses biological, motor, psychological, cognitive, emotional, and social changes in function that happen on the way to adulthood.[19] The flagship moment in each of these processes is the pubertal growth spurt, which usually occurs between 11–12 years old for girls and 13–14 years old for boys.[19] This is characterized by rapid gains in height and body mass. Altogether, the timing and tempo of these processes may increase or decrease young athletes' injury risk depending on their exposure to external factors such as larger/more mature competitors or heavy training loads.[12] To illustrate, let's consider an early maturing rugby player who is the same age, but substantially taller and heavier than the other kids in their league. In a tackle, they may be less likely to be injured (though their opponents could be at greater risk). Similarly, training volume and intensity typically increase with age, so a late-maturing gymnast may undergo their pubertal growth spurt during a time of high training load, thereby increasing injury risk.

The way individual athletes respond to these changes can vary widely. Self-perceptions and the reactions of others (e.g., peers, parents, coaches, teachers) can range from either positive evaluation, such as embracing the physical advantages provided by extra height or weight, to negative critique when comparing one athlete's sudden size or awkwardness to the appearance and performance of same-aged peers. Unfortunately, this can be a vehicle for team selection, as research has demonstrated the clear existence of maturation biases in elite sport pathways.[21] Larger, more mature kids are over-represented in team sports where size and strength provide competitive advantages, whereas smaller, less mature kids are preferentially selected in dance and gymnastics. *Self-presentation anxiety* (i.e., anxiety about how one's physique is evaluated by others) can become increasingly salient in these situations, leading to disengagement from training, sport drop-out, or malingering after injury to avoid social comparison.[22] Importantly, athletes sometimes engage in risky behaviors when faced with these pressures. Things like weight controlling (e.g., dieting, excessive exercise) and repetitive practice, undertaken in an effort to minimize noticeable changes in size or coordination, can actually increase the likelihood of injury and propagate negative body image.[23] It's therefore important to making sure that all athletes are supported to build realistic expectations around their abilities during periods of growth, no matter their maturity status.

Some of the injury types that maturing athletes experience are a direct result of biological changes occurring during adolescence. Things like physeal plate injuries, apophyseal injuries (e.g., Osgood-Schlatter and Sever's diseases), and stress fractures[i] are characteristic of those who are actively growing.[3,24] The difficulty with these injuries is that they have a gradual onset related to repetitive loading without sufficient rest, meaning that prevention efforts necessarily require athletes to take time off. Convincing young people to take a break from the activities they enjoy when they're healthy (e.g., to prevent injury) is no easy task. Plus, these injuries are typically managed with rest and exercises, but sometimes they require surgery. Addressing the psychological and social issues that arise during protracted rehabilitation can be difficult and is something coaches, parents, and practitioners should be prepared for.

Other Developmental Milestones

As we hinted a few paragraphs ago, maturation isn't just about physical changes. There are lots cognitive and social functions that also emerge through this process.

Did you know that our brains are not fully developed until we're in our early 20s?[25] That probably explains some of our cringeworthy personal choices[ii] in late adolescence and has terrifying implications for the responsibilities we inherit when we come of legal age, but those are topics of discussion for another book. From an injury perspective, the key point is that one of the last cognitive skills to develop is decision-making capacity, which is good to keep in mind when working with young athletes.

In early adolescence, analytic and problem-solving skills begin to emerge; however, emotional and impulse control are not yet fully established, which is why risk-taking behaviors are not uncommon in this age group.[26] Indeed, research has shown that adolescents engage in risky actions not because they don't appreciate the danger, but because their decisions are heavily swayed by emotion instead of rationality.[26] This means that the immediate outcomes of specific actions may be apparent, but young athletes might not understand the consequences for themselves or others in the longer term.[27] For example, tackling an opponent from behind might seem like a good defensive play, but the tackler might not consider the possibility of causing a life-altering injury in the process. It also means that future implications, such as the likelihood of osteoarthritis after a serious knee injury, may be incomprehensible. There's some evidence that adolescent athletes tend to incorrectly perceive injury risk and are unconcerned about potential long-term consequences, and that these factors increase injury risk.[28] Very little research has been done in this area, however, and it remains a topic of debate in the literature.

With increasing age, kids assume greater independence and are increasingly able to set realistic goals and prioritize events. So, this means that they should become more safety-conscious and be better equipped to make responsible choices about their behavior, right? Well, as anyone who has spent time being, parenting, or coaching an adolescent knows, that's not quite how this works. As adolescents begin to make choices for themselves, they are often heavily influenced by their peer group.[27] Whereas in early adolescence, family members tend to be a primary source of support, through the teenage years this wanes in favor of friends and teammates. In fact, much of the adolescent period is defined by comparing oneself to others and peer acceptance becomes vitally important. Many young people go to considerable lengths to achieve this, including spontaneous engagement in high-risk behaviors. For example, a cross-sectional study of 735 youth skiers and snowboarders found that kids were significantly more likely to engage in risky behaviors on the slopes when participating with peers.[29] They were more likely to use terrain parks with their friends than when alone (OR: 3.96; 95%CI: 1.71,9.20), or if they thought terrain parks were "cool" (OR: 5.84; 95%CI: 2.85,11.96). They were also more likely to video record sessions with friends (OR: 3.65, 95% CI: 1.45,9.18). In fact, peer norming was so influential that they were less likely to video record if their friends chose not to (OR: 0.36; 95% CI: 0.16,0.80).[29] Moreover, peer pressure and attempting skills beyond one's capability have been directly implicated in skiing and snowboarding injuries.[30]

Let's dig a bit deeper into these social pressures. Norms around acceptable/ unacceptable behaviors, appearances, and even vocabulary can be very pronounced in young social circles, and cliques often form around these characteristics. Attempting to fit in with a group that has such established features can prompt risk-taking behaviors (either to match what others are doing, or to impress them and gain acceptance). Here we need to consider the phenomenon of *groupthink*. This is defined as the practice of making decisions as a group, which often leads to poorly challenged and low-quality choices.[31] A simple example can be seen in any average horror movie – a group of people are being chased by a villain and decide to split up, which is a terrible plan because they'll all be more vulnerable alone, but nobody questions it, and we know how that story ends.[iii]

How does this relate to youth sport? Well, it's understandably tempting to consider risk taking as a product of individual characteristics (e.g., impulsivity) or peer pressure, but emerging research suggests that this doesn't capture the entire picture. Although not focused on the sport context specifically, a series of eight studies conducted across a variety of health, disease, and physical risk scenarios in university and general population settings (n = 4708) provides evidence that groupthink can change the way we perceive risk.[32] They demonstrated that people feel safest within their usual social groups and, because we trust the judgement of those we're closest to, we're more likely to perceive a behavior undertaken by the group as less risky than it is. As the authors state, *"ironically, this means the people we trust the most may sometimes post the greatest risk."*[32] So, if risk taking is at least partially driven by how closely young athletes relate to their peer groups, then we also need to consider how they come to self-categorize as part of those peer groups. In other words, how do they develop a *social identity*?

As it happens, identity formation is another developmental process occurring during adolescence. Now, we all establish social identities for ourselves. These might include particular roles like *caregiver, pet owner,* or *coach,* or they might exist along broader lines like belonging to religious or cultural communities. No matter how we define these, identity refers to the extent to which we see ourselves as members of a particular group, and we generally have greater affinity for others whom we see as belonging to the same groups as we do. We also tend to behave in ways that are congruent with our identities – if I see myself as a charitable person, I'll donate time or money to charity. So, *athletic identity* describes how much being an athlete dominates one's self-perception and social roles, and this often develops for youth who spend much of their time engaged in sports.[33] Having a strong athletic identity can facilitate continued sport engagement and healthy goal pursuit, but it can also cause people to push through pain, fatigue, and injury because they see themselves as an athlete. Uh-oh. We've seen this before, in chapter 11 where we talked about how professional athletes hold themselves to idealized versions of toughness and perseverance. Well, kids sometimes tie their self-worth into their sport achievements, and if you see yourself as an athlete, you're going to act the way you think athletes should. Estimation of one's own abilities is positively associated with risk taking, which could lead to greater injury risk for those who rate themselves highly because greater confidence may prompt them to undertake more challenging skills.[28] Although there isn't much research to rely on in this area, it certainly makes intuitive sense and bears further investigation as a potential injury risk factor.

Another challenge on the rise in youth populations is perfectionism. Between 1989 and 2016, many western nations have seen linear increases in *self-oriented perfectionism* (attaching irrational importance to being perfect, holding unrealistic expectations and being punitively self-critical), *socially prescribed perfectionism* (perceiving one's social context to be excessively demanding and believing others exert harsh judgment), and *other-oriented perfectionism* (imposing unrealistic standards on others).[34] Though some perfectionistic tendencies can be facilitative in sport – striving for excellence is inherent to competition, after all – there is accumulating evidence that that some dimensions of perfectionism leave athletes vulnerable to mental and physical harm.[35] In the last phase of adolescence, athletes are more prepared to cope with success and failure, and have greater ability to withstand pressure from others, but there is a risk of falling short of their own or what are perceived to be others', expectations. Coping mechanisms are not always fully established when this happens, particularly if this is the first major setback the young athlete has had, and resulting emotional difficulties (e.g., burnout and depression) are common.[36] The same can happen with injuries during this time, where they can seem like personal failures and insurmountable barriers to achievement.

In the first study of its kind, Madigan and colleagues[37] investigated the relationship between perfectionism and injury incidence among 80 junior athletes from a variety of sports (age range 16–19) over 10 months of training. They found that perfectionistic concerns significantly and positively predicted medical attention and time loss injury.[37] There's also emerging evidence from adult samples that these concerns are associated with treatment over-adherence and pain normalization during injury rehabilitation.[38] We don't yet know if this applies to young athletes, but clinical research has shown that child and parent perfectionism is associated with pain duration, catastrophizing, and functional disability in chronic pain populations.[39] Parents, coaches and practitioners therefore need to be vigilant when monitoring training and rehabilitation practices. Right then. How are we supposed to do that? Well, let's consider some different ways of supporting young athletes through the injury process.

Re-defining "Risk"

Okay, we've just spent a good chunk of this chapter talking about the challenges of youth sport. What about the opportunities we promised? We've established that expecting young athletes to appreciate the risks of their sport and always behave in ways to protect their own health is completely unrealistic. So, the first thing we need to figure out is how to recalibrate our interpretation of "risk".

Step one is determining who is responsible for risk management in youth sport. In a way, there's an easy answer: when you're under the legal age of majority, your parent or a caregiver is in charge. But the situation is more complex than simply delegating responsibility to a single group of stakeholders. Providing a tidy synopsis of the current youth sport climate, Watchman and Spencer-Cavaliere[40] point out that while parents value the life skills (e.g., sportsmanship, teamwork) and social bonds their children build through sport, they also express concerns about safety. There's a modern trend toward making sport as risk-free as possible (i.e., the so-called "bubble-wrapped" children phenomenon),[41] and parents need to negotiate social expectations to keep children safe while simultaneously allowing them to develop some independence.[42] This is a complex task, made trickier by the additional influence of coaches, teachers, family, friends, community norms, sport organizations, cultural and parenting ideologies, and public policies. Is it any wonder, through all these layers of structure and regulation, that young athletes' wellbeing has become a shared responsibility? And in doing so, it has compounded the number of perspectives involved in implementing safety measures to the point that there's often confusion about what is best for kids and their health.[42,43]

Of course, "zero risk" is not an attainable goal, but we can't treat young athletes like miniature adults and leave them to their own devices, either. Therefore, step two involves thinking about how children assess risk and understand consequences. Children generally learn in a variety of ways that involve trial-and-error progression and the response they receive when they attempt something new. By distinguishing between *hazards* (potentially harmful elements with little chance of positive outcome) and *risks* (potentially beneficial elements where possible negative outcomes are mild in severity) in the youth sport environment, we can begin to facilitate experiences that allow young children to explore their thresholds for fear vs excitement.[42] For instance, if a six-year-old wanted to try surfing we probably wouldn't let them loose in the ocean unsupervised, but letting them test out the shallows with a parent nearby would help them develop judgement, risk assessment, and physical capacity while having fun.[42] As kids get older and their understanding of causality and consequence matures, less oversight is necessary, and they can assume greater autonomy in making risk-reward decisions. Importantly, overprotection has been shown to have negative effects on young adults' internalized levels of self-efficacy,[44] so ensuring they foster a sense of self-reliance and competence is an important consideration. This may be accomplished by having age-appropriate discussions about risk to support the formation of analytic skills, setting social norms about what levels of risk are acceptable in the sport context, or teaching self-regulation through positive adult role modeling.[45,46]

A quick note on modeling. Learning by copying others is common in sport and is a good way of developing technical skills. In fact, there's an entire generation of YouTube-savvy kids who are proficient in techniques that their predecessors could only dream of, based entirely on a watch-and-try approach. This can work in our favor. We know that young athletes develop at different rates, and this applies to risk assessment as well – not all members of a team will have the same risk thresholds and they aren't all going to recognize the demands/dangers of various situations.

Exposing young athletes to role models whom they aspire to be like, or peer models who are relatable (e.g., people who look and sound like them), can be a method for shaping their interpretation of risk and reward. It can encourage them to take positive risks, like trying a new skill even if they're afraid of being evaluated by others,[45] and discourage them from taking negative risks by reinforcing their own situational assessments. Establishing models from within a team can help to set norms, which is great for supporting those who are a bit slower to develop, but it also has its drawbacks. If as coaches (or parents and practitioners) we don't practice what we preach, how can we expect young athletes to behave any differently? So, make sure you warm up before training and don't try to one-up somebody on the ski slope, because you never know who's watching!

Right, back to the main story. Step three in re-defining risk is making sure that all stakeholders are on the same page.[47,48] Kids are experts at pointing out inconsistencies and contradictions, and teenagers generally enjoy proving adults wrong, so making sure that everyone is promoting the same behaviors is critical. If coaches are telling young athletes one thing and their parents another, they'll pick and choose which side they're going to take and that can cause stress and confusion for everyone. Knowing who should deliver important messages is equally important (e.g., younger children listen mostly to their parents, whereas adolescents may actively avoid doing so). Matching communication channels to athletes' stages of development is a small but helpful way of transmitting information for maximum uptake.

Aside from consistently supporting injury prevention strategies and adherence to rehabilitation, there are other ways of sharing responsibility. Young athletes don't always recognize the risks of playing sport while injured or in pain, often listening to coaches' instructions rather than to their own bodies.[49,50] This is a particular problem for those competing at high level or who have been selected to a team they aspired to.[23,51] What young athlete is going to say they want to stop while trying to make a positive impression on their coach and teammates, competing for a position, or simply having fun? Being on the lookout for signs they need a break and adjusting expectations/demands to the athlete's development is something all stakeholders can help with.[52] Sometimes, adults also unintentionally push young athletes beyond their physical and cognitive limits. For instance, if a sport is paid for, parents might insist their child participate in every session even though they're tired from other activities. The language we use also has an effect – asking "did you win?" emphasizes the importance of results, whereas "did you have fun?" fosters more open and honest communication, enabling young athletes to build self-confidence and be less afraid of voicing their concerns.

Exciting Opportunities

Anybody who has tried to feed a picky child knows that it's nigh impossible to convince them that certain "adult" foods are, in fact, tasty. No matter how many times we try to feed them onions or cabbage or [insert delicious item here], their palates simply do not respond the same way, and it's a doomed exercise from the start. That's why restaurants have "Kid's Menus". Well, when it comes to psychosocial interventions for sport injury, it helps to take the same view − what works for grown-ups won't always work for younger groups, so we need to adapt our approaches.

We've established that childhood and adolescence are characterized by periods of increased stress associated with growth and maturation, and some struggles are unique to these age groups, such as balancing the demands of both school and sport. Unrealistic expectations from coaches and parents,[53,54] major life events, and daily hassles[55] are also prevalent through adolescence, exacerbated by underdeveloped coping skills.[56] Although theoretical models suggest that ineffective stress responses may be a factor in injury risk,[57,58] none of these have focused specifically on youth. Yet, hypotheses that the accumulation of stressors can increase injury risk for kids as they do for adults[55,56,59] have been partially supported. Research has shown that trait anxious youths who have experienced several stressful events during the previous 12 months (e.g., moving, family illness, divorce) and do not have effective coping strategies are at increased risk for injuries.[56] Subjective low well-being has also been related to increased injury risk and may have a relationship with injury severity.[60] So, interventions that help with stress management and coping are likely to be impactful and this is borne out in the research literature.

Meta-analytic evidence suggests that psychosocial interventions can reduce sport injury risk.[61] In studies of younger groups, successful strategies have included *acceptance-commitment therapy* (ACT),[62] *mindfulness-acceptance-commitment (MAC)*,[63] and *psychological skills training (PST)*.[64–67] As a modern take on the ever-popular cognitive behavioral therapy,[iv] ACT aims to provide athletes with psychological flexibility by increasing their willingness to accept negative thoughts and emotions rather than fighting them.[68] For adolescent athletes this may consist of dealing with sources of stress through normalizing feelings, accepting the situation, and focusing on personal goals and values.[62] Taking it one step further, a MAC intervention could include elements of mindfulness, using exercises to enhance the feeling of 'being present' and noting where the athlete is directing their attention, reflecting on which behaviors do/don't lead toward their goals.[69,70] Though more research is needed with younger athletes, these approaches also show promise during injury rehabilitation,[71] but the key is in using metaphors suitable for younger athletes and explaining concepts in age-appropriate terms.

More traditional PST interventions have their place in youth sport as well. Common components such as goal setting, concentration development, and arousal regulation can help with stress management and promote adaptive coping behaviors much like ACT and MAC do.[66,67] Goal setting can be particularly helpful during injury rehabilitation for maintaining motivation and enhancing self-efficacy, especially when a series of short-term goals (e.g., increasing range of motion) is coupled with a longer-term goal (e.g., clearance for return to play). With younger athletes, however, it's important that goals are realistic. When injury information and prognosis may not be easily understood or involve some uncertainty, involving parents, coaches, and/or medical practitioners in moderating goals can be a good idea. It's also important to review and revise them on a regular basis, as recovery setbacks can be emotionally difficult for younger athletes and it's important to reframe these as normal parts of the process rather than failures.

Working on attentional control can also be useful. You may be familiar with the Buddhist metaphor of the *monkey mind*, which describes how our thoughts can be unruly and jump from one object to another. It addresses how our inner voices can sometimes be critical and sow doubt, too. This "chatter" can manifest behaviorally in young athletes, so developing concentration ability can help reduce injury risk and improve rehabilitation outcomes by limiting distraction and improving self-confidence. Getting ahead of negative self-talk by identifying problematic messages and replacing them with instructional or motivational self-talk is one approach.[72–74] A combination of assigned and self-determined self-talk can provide a good balance for kids who are learning to self-regulate and using the monkey metaphor is a good way of explaining, even to young children, how all this works. Most kids can imagine "training the mischievous monkey" that lives in their heads, so regular practice with focusing on single tasks and speaking kindly to themselves can be a simple way to introduce these ideas.

Alongside attentional control, arousal regulation can help minimize the effects of life stress on injury risk and recovery. In other words, we can try to incorporate "rest and relaxation" into young athlete's routines. Not getting enough sleep is often reported in specialized sport settings and stress clearly affects sleep quality, but how much rest young athletes need is often underestimated. Teenagers need to sleep 8.5–9.5 hours per night for hormone production and the development of neurological systems during puberty.[23] Moreover, fatigue is a known risk factor for injury, and may independently influence mental health and the risk of burnout.[59] Setting norms around sleep hygiene and facilitating periods of rest are therefore some of the best ways to support health and wellbeing. And, while kids are awake, managing fluctuations in stress is equally important. We know that relaxation can be muscular (contraction of one muscle group at a time and relax), cognitive (thinking of one body part and feel a heaviness/warmth cover it up), or centering (using breathing to induce calm), and all three are effective arousal regulators. Tailoring relaxation exercise descriptions to match kids' vocabulary (e.g., "make a fist and squeeze" vs "contract your forearm") can be helpful here, and they might need to close their eyes to stop them from giggling, but otherwise young athletes can benefit greatly from these techniques.

Another big opportunity to overcome the challenges of the youth sport environment is leveraging the power of peer influence. We can see how effective this can be when looking at safety equipment uptake across sport settings. Getting kids to wear bicycle helmets can be a battle, yet most young skiers and snowboarders wear helmets and other protective gear even when mandatory use policies aren't in place. Promoting equipment within young circles through modeling (e.g., Olympic athletes wear it) and marketing (e.g., "must have" pieces of fashion) relies on social acceptance and norming, which become strong behavioral drivers through adolescence. In fact, research has shown that youth are more likely to wear safety gear if their peers are, or if they are in an environment where it is socially acceptable to do so.[75] Dealing with perceptions of invulnerability when wearing equipment can be trickier,[28] but injury risk can be reduced when prevention efforts work with, rather than against, the desire to fit in. Other positive behaviors can be socially enhanced as well. For example, during injury rehabilitation it is useful to identify others who have had a similar injury and successful recovery. This might be someone rehabilitating at the same training facilities or a sport hero who has spoken openly about their injuries.[73] Building motivation and self-efficacy through vicarious experience is a compelling way to help young athletes set goals, overcome setbacks, and normalize the healing process. Some of this comes down to "if they can do it, so can I", but modeling can also foster an element of social support. Turning to others for help can buffer negative injury responses by providing practical solutions to problems, distraction from emotional issues, and setting realistic expectations.[74]

Whatever approach we use, working with young athletes requires some unique considerations.[76] As with adults, interventions should be chosen based on individual needs, but kids aren't always able to articulate what those needs are. Building a trustful communication climate and giving sound explanations of what is going to happen and why can help them express their thoughts and preferences. It's vital to respect children's autonomy and let them decide when issues discussed privately can be shared with others (and who those others should be). This can help to alleviate pressure and facilitate informed decision-making, even in age groups where these abilities are still developing.[77–80]

Putting It into Practice

It's evident that youth sport injury psychology is under-researched.[81] The features of this environment create challenges, and although there are opportunities to adapt techniques that we already use with adults, we need to tailor them for younger groups. This means that for parents, coaches, and practitioners, there's a fine line to tread between being supportive but not adding pressure, focussing on achievements but not results, being protective but encouraging independence. To maximize the benefits of youth sport and uphold those valuable ideals of fun and play, we must therefore take a multi-level approach that accounts for athlete development and maturity status. After all, kids' aren't just little adults, and best practice needs to take that into account.

Notes

i Some of these terms might not be familiar. Physeal plates are also known as "growth plates" and are translucent, cartilage-like discs at the end of our long bones that allow them to lengthen during growth spurts. Apophyseal injuries happen because bones grow faster than muscles and tendons, and this can cause inflammation or fractures around the spots where those structures connect to each other. Osgood Schlatter occurs when this happens at the top of the tibia (shin) where the patellar ligament attaches. Sever's happens where the Achilles' tendon attaches to the calcaneus (heel).

ii There is nothing quite as humbling as revisiting your own teenaged photographs and remembering how cool you thought you were at the time. Many haircuts are prime illustrations of decision-making capacity that isn't yet fully formed.

iii Well, if you're a horror film aficionado, you do. If that genre really isn't your thing, let us explain: [SPOILER ALERT] they all get caught. They do not make it to the final scene.

iv Cognitive behavioral therapy (CBT) focuses on changing unhelpful patterns of thinking and acting. It's based on collaboration between an individual and a practitioner to develop better coping strategies through, e.g., role play, problem-solving, facing fears, and relaxation techniques.

References

1 Harrison CB, Gill ND, Kinugasa T, et al. Development of aerobic fitness in young team sport athletes. *Sports Med* 2015;45:969e83; doi:10.1007/s40279-015-0330-y.

2 Jewett R, Sabiston C, Brunet J, et al. School sport participation during adolescence and mental health in early adulthood. *J Adolesc Health* 2014;55:640e4; doi:10.1016/j/jadohealth.2014.04.018.

3 DiFiori JP, Benjamin HJ, Brenner JS, et al. Overuse injuries and burnout in youth sports: a position statement from the American Medical Society for Sports Medicine. *Br J Sports Med* 2014;48(4):287–288; doi:10.1136/bjsports-2013-093299.

4 Koester MC. Youth sports: a pediatrician's perspective on coaching and injury prevention. *J Athl Train* 2000;35(4):466–470; PMID:16558664.

5 Conn JM, Annest JL, Gilchrist J. Sport and recreation related injury episodes in the US population, 1997-99. *Inj Prev* 2003;9:117e23; doi:10.1136/ip.9.2.117.

6 Kisser R, Bauer R. The burden of sport injuries in the European Union. Research report D2h of the project "Safety in Sports." Vienna: Austrian Road Safety Board (Kuratorium für Verkehrssicherheit) 2012.

7 Crane J, Temple V. A systematic review of dropout from organized sport among children and youth. *Eur Phys Educat Rev* 2014;21:114e31; doi:10.1177/1356336X14555294.

8 Normand JM, Wolfe A, Peak K. A review of early sport specialization in relation to the development of a young athlete. *Int J Kinesiol Sport Sci* 2017;5(2):37e42; doi:10.7575/aiac.ijkss.v.5n.2p.37.

9 Brenner JS. Sports specialization and intensive training in young athletes. *Pediatrics* 2016;138(3):e20162148; doi:10.1542/peds.2016-2148.

10 Butcher J, Lindner KJ, Johns DP. Withdrawal from competitive youth sport: a retrospective ten-year study. *J Sport Behav* 2002;25(2):145e63.

11 Crane J, Temple V. A systematic review of dropout from organized sport among children and youth. *Eur Phys Educat Rev* 2014;21:114e31; doi:10.1177/1356336X14555294.

12 McKay CD, Cumming SP, Blake T. Youth sport: friend or foe? *Best Prac Res Clin Rheumatol* 2019;33(1):141–157; doi:10.1016/j.berh.2019.01.017.

13 Räisänen AM, Kokko S, Pasanen K, et al. Prevalence of adolescent physical activity-related injuries in sports, leisure time, and school: the National Physical Activity Behaviour Study for children and Adolescents. *BMC Musculoskelet Disord* 2018;*19*(1):58; doi:10.1186/s12891-018-1969-y.

14 Peterson AR, Kruse AJ, Meester SM, et al. Youth football injuries: a prospective co-hort. *Orthop J Sports Med* 2017;5(2):1–7; doi:10.1177/2325967116686784.

15 Kilic O, Maas M, Verhagen E, et al. Incidence, aetiology and prevention of muscu-loskeletal injuries in volleyball: a systematic review of the literature. *Eur J Sport Sci* 2017;6:765–793; doi:10.1080/17461391.2017.1306114.

16 Patel D, Yamasaki A, Brown K. Epidemiology of sports-related musculoskeletal injuries in young athletes in United States. *Transl Pediatr* 2017;6(3):160–166; doi:10.21037/tp.2 017.04.08.

17 Voskanian N. ACL injury prevention in female athletes: review of the literature and practical considerations in implementing an ACL prevention program. *Curr Rev Musculoskelet Med* 2013;6:158e63; doi:10.1007/s12178-013-9158-y.

18 Jayanthi N, Pinkham C, Dugas L, et al. Sport specialization in young athletes: evidence-based recommendations. *Sports Health* 2013;5(3):251e7; doi:10.1177/1941738112464 626.

19 Malina RM, Bouchard C, Bar-Or O. Growth, maturation, and physical activity. second ed. Champaign, Ill: Human Kinetics 2004.

20 Blakemore SJ. Brain development in adolescence. *J Neurol Neurosurg Psychiatry* 2014;85:e3; doi: 10.1136/jnnp-2014-308883.3.

21 Beunen G, Malina RM. Growth and biologic maturation: relevance to athletic per-formance. In: *The young athlete.* New Jersey: Blackwell Publishing Ltd 2007.

22 Podlog L, Dimmock J, Miller J. (2011). A review of return to sport concerns following injury rehabilitation: practitioner strategies for enhancing recovery outcomes. *Phys Ther Sport* 2011;12(1):36–42; doi: 10.1016/j.ptsp.2010.07.005.

23 Bergeron MF, Mountjoy M, Armstrong N, et al. International Olympic Committee consensus statement on youth athletic development. *Br J Sports Med* 2015;49(13):843–851; doi:10.1136/bjsports-2015-094962.

24 Read PJ, Oliver JL, De Ste Croix MBA, et al. The scientific foundations and associated injury risks of early soccer specialization. *J Sports Sci* 2016;34(24):2295e302; doi:10.1 080/02640414.2016.1173221.

25 Brown, KA, Patel, DR, Darmawan, D. Participation in sports in relation to adolescent growth and development. *Translation Pediatri* 2017;6(3):150–159; doi:10.21037/tp.201 7.04.03.

26 Steinberg L. Cognitive and affective development in adolescence. *Trends Cogn Sci* 2005;9(2):69–74; doi:10.1016/j.tics.2004.12.005.

27 McInerney DM. A discussion of future time perspective. *Educ Psychol Rev* 2004;16:141–151; doi:10.1023/B:EDPR.0000026610.18125.a3.

28 Kontos AP. Perceived risk, risk taking, estimation of ability and injury among adoles-cent sport participants. *J Pediatr Psychol* 2004;29(6):447e55; doi:10.1093/jpepsy/jsh048.

29 Russell K, Arthur S, Goulet C, et al. Understanding youth's attitudes and practices regarding listening to music, video recording and terrain park use while skiing and snowboarding. *BMC Pediatrics* 2020;20:389; doi:10.1186/s12887-020-02292-6.

30 Paquette L, Dumais M, Bergeron J, et al. The effect of personality traits and beliefs on the relationship between injury severity and subsequent sport risk-taking among ado-lescents. *Pediatr Res Int J* 2016;405500; doi:10.5171/2016.405500.

31 McCauley C. (1989). The nature of social influence in groupthink: compliance and in-ternalization. *J Pers Soc Psychol* 1989;57(2):250–260; doi:10.1037/0022-3514.57.2.250.

32 Cruwys T, Greenaway KH, Ferris LJ, et al. When trust goes wrong: a social identity model of risk taking. *J Pers Soc Psychol* 2021;120(1):57–83; doi:10.1037/pspi0000243.

33 Brewer BW, Van Raalte JL, Linder DE. Athletic identity: Hercules' muscles or Achilles heel? *Int J Sport Psychol* 1993;24:237e54.

34 Curran T, Hill AP. Perfectionism is increasing over time: a meta-analysis of birth cohort differences from 1989-2016. *Psychol Bull* 2019;145(4):410–429; doi:10.1037/bul0000138.

35 Hill AP, Mallinson-Howard SH, Madigan DJ, et al. Perfectionism in sport, dance and exercise: an extended review and reanalysis. In: G Tenenbaum, RC Eklund (eds.). *Handbook of Sport Psychology* (4th ed.). New Jersey: John Wiley & Sons, Inc 2020.

36 Smith EP, Hill AP, Hall HK. Perfectionism, burnout, and depression in youth soccer players: a longitudinal study. *J Clin Sport Psychol* 2018;12(2):179–200; doi:10.1123/jcsp.2017-0015.

37 Madigan DJ, Stoeber J, Forsdyke D, et al. Perfectionism predicts injury in junior athletes preliminary evidence from a prospective study. *J Sports Sci* 2018;36(5):545–550; doi:10.1080/02640414.2017.1322709.

38 MacWilliam, KR, Gotwals JK, Sanzo P, et al. Perfectionism and rehabilitation over-adherence among injured athletes. *J Exerc Movement Sport* 2018;50(1):146.

39 Randall ET, Smith KR, Kronman CA, et al. Feeling the pressure to be perfect: effect on pain-related distress and dysfunction in youth with chronic pain. *J Pain* 2018;19(4):418–429; doi: 10.1016/j.jpain.2017.11.012.

40 Watchman T, Spencer NLI. Times have changed: parent perspectives on children's free play and sport. *Psychol Sport Exerc* 2017;32:102–112; doi: 10.1016/j.psychsport.2017.06.008.

41 Malone K. The bubble-wrap generation: children growing up in walled gardens. *Environ Educ Res* 2007;13(4):513e527; doi: 10.1080/13504620701581612.

42 Harper N. Outdoor risky play and healthy child development in the shadow of the "risk society": a forest and nature school perspective. *Child Youth Serv* 2017;38(4):318–334; doi:10.1080/0145935X.2017.1412825.

43 Watchman T, Spencer NLI. "What are you doing for your kids?" Exploring messages and Canadian Parents' decisions and perspectives in children's sport and free play. *Leisure* 2019;39(3):341–354; doi: 10.1080/02614367.2019.1703140.

44 Van Petegem S, Antonietti JP, Nunes CE, et al. The relationship between maternal overprotection, adolescent internalizing and externalizing problems, and psychological need frustration: a multi-informant study using response surface analysis. *J Youth Adolesc* 2020;49:162–177; doi:10.1007/s10964-019-01126-8.

45 Duell N, Steinberg L. Positive risk taking in adolescence. *Child Dev Perspect* 2019;13(1):48–52; doi:10.1111/cdep.12310.

46 Geldhof GJ, Fenn ML, Finders JK. A self-determination perspective on self-regulation across the life span. In: M Wehmeyer, K Shogren, T Little, S Lopez (eds.). *Development of self-determination through the life-course.* Dordrecht: Springer 2017.

47 Ageberg E, Bunke S, Nilsen P, et al. Planning injury prevention training for youth handball players: application of the generalisable six-step intervention development process. *Inj Prev* 2020;26(2):164–169; doi:10.1136/injuryprev-2019-043468.

48 Finch C. A new framework for research leading to sports injury prevention. *J Sci Med Sport* 2006;9(1-2):3–9; doi:10.1016/j.jsmas.2006.02.009.

49 Stambulova N, Wylleman P. Athletes' career development and transitions. In: *Routledge companion to sport and exercise psychology: global perspectives and fundamental concepts.* New York, NY: Routledge/Taylor & Francis Group 2014.

50 Wylleman P. Sport psychologists assisting young talented athletes faced with career transitions. In: CJ Knight, CG Harwood, D Gould (eds.). *Sport psychology for young athletes.* London: Routledge 2017.

51 Capranica L, Millard-Stafford ML. Youth sport specialization: how to manage competition and training? *Int J Sports Physiol Perform* 2011;6(4):572–579; doi:10.1123/ijspp.6.4.572.

52 DiFiori JP, Guellich A, Brenner JS, et al. The NBA and youth basketball: recommendations for promoting a healthy and positive experience. *Sports Med* 2018;48(9):2053–2065; doi:10.1007/s40279-018-0950-0.

53 Burgess NS, Knight CJ, Mellalieu SD. Parental stress and coping in elite youth gymnastics: an interpretative phenomenological analysis. *Qual Res Sport Exerc Health* 2016;8(3);237–256; doi:10.1080/2159676x.2015.1134633.

54 Jayanthi NA, Post EG, Laury TC, et al. Health consequences of youth sport specialization. *J Athl Train* 2019;54(10):1040–1049; doi:10.4085/1062-6050-380-18.

55 Ivarsson A, Johnson U, Lindwall M, et al. Psychosocial stress as a predictor of injury in elite junior soccer: a latent growth curve analysis. *J Sci Med Sport* 2014;17(4):366–370; doi:10.1016/j.jsams.2013.10.242.

56 Johnson U, Ivarsson A. Psychological predictors of sport injuries among junior soccer players. *Scand J Med Sci Sports* 2011;21(1):129–136; doi:10.1111/j.1600-0838.2009.01057.x.

57 Appaneal R, Perna F. (2014). Biopsychosocial model of injury. In: R Eklund, G Tenenbaum (eds.). *Encyclopedia of sport and exercise psychology*. Thousand Oaks: SAGE Publications, Inc 2014.

58 Williams JM, Andersen MB. Psychosocial antecedents of sport injury: review and critique of the stress and injury model. *J Appl Sport Psychol* 1998;10(1):5–25; doi: 10.1080/10413209808406375.

59 Brenner JS, LaBotz M, Sugimoto D, et al. The psychosocial implications of sport specialization in pediatric athletes. *J Athl Train* 2019;54(10):1021–1029; doi:10.4085/1062-6050-394-18.

60 von Rosen P, Heijne A. Subjective well-being is associated with injury risk in adolescent elite athletes. *Physiother Theory Pract* 2019;July18:1–7; doi:10.1080/09593985.2019.1641869.

61 Ivarsson A, Johnson U, Andersen MB, et al. Psychosocial factors and sport injuries: meta-analyses for prediction and prevention. *Sports Med* 2017;47(2):353–365; doi:10.1007/s40279-016-0578-x.

62 Kiens K, Larsen CH. A case study with a young basketball player. In: K Henriksen, J Hansen, C Hvid Larsen (eds.). *Mindfulness and acceptance in sport: how to help athletes perform and thrive under pressure*. New York: Routledge 2019.

63 Ivarsson A, Johnson U, Andersen MB, et al. It pays to pay attention: a mindfulness-based program for injury prevention with soccer players. *J Appl Sport Psychol* 2015;27(3):319–334; doi:10.1080/10413200.2015.1008072.

64 Edvardsson A, Ivarsson A, Johnson U. Is a cognitive-behavioural biofeedback intervention useful to reduce injury risk in junior football players? *J Sports Sci Med* 2012;11(2):331–338; PMID:24149207.

65 Noh YE, Morris T, Andersen MB. Psychological intervention programs for reduction of injury in ballet dancers. *Res Sports Med* 2007;15(1):13–32; doi: 10.1080/15438620600987064.

66 Tranaeus U, Ivarsson A, Johnson U. Evaluation of the effects of psychological prevention interventions on sport injuries: a meta-analysis. *Sci Sports* 2015;30(6):305–313; doi:10.1016/j.scispo.2015.04.009.

67 Tranaeus U, Johnson U, Engstrom B, et al. A psychological injury prevention group intervention in Swedish floorball. *Knee Surg Sports traumatol Arthrosc* 2015;23(11):3414–3420; doi:10.1007/s00167-014-3133-z.

68 Henriksen K, Hansen J, Larsen CH. *Mindfulness and acceptance in sport: how to help athletes perform and thrive under pressure.* New York: Routledge 2019.

69 Moore ZE. Theoretical and empirical developments of the Mindfulness-Acceptance-Commitment (MAC) approach to performance enhancement. *J Clin Sport Psychol* 2009;3(4):291–302; doi:10.1123/jcsp.3.4.291.

70 Schwanhausser L. Application of the mindfulness-acceptance-commitment (MAC) protocol with an adolescent springboard diver. *J Clin Sport Psychol* 2009;3(4):377–395; doi: 10.1123/jcsp.3.4.377.

71 Baranoff J, Appaneal RN. Helping the injured athlete to accept and refocus. In: K Henriksen, J Hansen, C Hvid Larsen (eds.). *Mindfulness and acceptance in sport: how to help athletes perform and thrive under pressure.* New York: Routledge 2019.

72 Arvinen-Barrow M, Walker N. *The psychology of sport injury and rehabilitation.* New York, NY: Routledge 2013.

73 Hall C, Duncan L, McKay C. *Psychological interventions in sport, exercise, and injury rehabilitation.* Dubuque, IA: Kendall Hunt 2014.

74 Nippert AH, Smith AM. Psychologic stress related to injury and impact on sport performance. *Phys Med Rehabil Clin N Am* 2008;19(2):399; doi:10.1016/j.pmr.2007.12.003.

75 Peterson AR, Brooks MA. Pilot study of adolescent attitudes regarding ski or snowboard helmet use. *WMJ Official Publication of the State Medical Society of Wisconsin* 2010;109(1):28–30.

76 Chase MA. Children. In: SJ Hanrahan, MB Andersen (eds.). *Routledge handbook of applied sport psychology.* Oxon: Routledge 2013.

77 Hallquist C, Fitzgerald UT, Alricsson M. Responsibility for child and adolescent's psychosocial support associated with severe sports injuries. *J Exerc Rehabil* 2016;12(6):589–597; doi:10.12965/jer.1632814.407.

78 Hamstra KL, Cherubini JM, Swanik CB. Athletic injury and parental pressure in youth sports. *Athl Ther Today* 2002;7(6):36–41; doi:10.1123/att.7.6.36.

79 Oosterhoff JHF, Bexkens R, Vranceanu AM, et al. Do injured adolescent athletes and their parents agree on the athletes' level of psychologic and physical functioning? *Clin Orthop Relat Res* 2018;476(4):767–775; doi:10.1007/s11999.0000000000000071.

80 Shrier I, Safai P, Charland L. Return to play following injury: whose decision should it be? *Br J Sports Med* 2014:48(5):8; doi:10.1136/bjsports-2013-092492.

81 Steffen K, Engebretsen L. More data needed on injury risk among young elite athletes. *Br J Sports Med* 2010;44(7):485–489; doi:10.1136/bjsm.2010.073833.

16
INJURY PSYCHOLOGY AND PARA ATHLETES: SAME SAME, BUT DIFFERENT

Carly McKay, Lisa Callaghan, Marelise Badenhorst, Phoebe Runciman, and Wayne Derman

Let's start out with a bit of trivia. Do you know what the "Para" in Paralympic means? It's a word that many of us take for granted, but a general ignorance of its etymology is actually symbolic of the Para sport experience more broadly. The Olympic Movement has been in existence since ancient Greece and sport for able-bodied individuals is significantly more developed than for those with impairment. Indeed, it was only after World War II that the Paralympic Movement really started to gain traction, with the first official Paralympic Games held in Rome in 1960. In the short time since then, Para sport has become internationally recognized, commercially funded, and popular, with more than 4,300 athletes competing at the Rio 2016 Paralympic Games. But back to the original question, the "Para" prefix formally indicates the parallel nature of the Games, with the Olympics and Paralympics being held in the same city over the same period. So, even by nature of its title, Para sport is automatically seen as "other" or secondary to the traditional able-bodied Games that occupy centre stage over the same time and space.

This highlights the conflict within the Paralympic Movement regarding who makes the decisions and on whose behalf. Indeed, the presence of ableism (celebrating athletes who are closest to "normal") in elite Para sport is pervasive and difficult to change. Para athletes and experts have raised this as a problem, and there's been a steady improvement in awareness and representation; however, in the world of sports injury research, investigations with Para athletes are still novel. In practice, this means that medical practitioners and coaches are still forced to transfer methods demonstrated in able-bodied athletes to Para athletes in their care via trial and error. When it comes to understanding injury and illness experiences, the same can be said. Only in the past few years has impairment-specific information started filtering into standard practice for injury surveillance, for example. The International Olympic Committee (IOC) and International Paralympic Committee (IPC) have committed

DOI: 10.4324/9781003088936-16

to protecting the health of all athletes, both Para and able-bodied.[1,2] In order to do that, we need to better understand how the history of Para sport has shaped the lived experiences of its athletes, recognizing that the physical, psychological, and social contexts of injury and illness are inherently different in this setting. This requires a critical look at the emergence of Para sport through the 20th century.

Where It All Began

The Stoke Mandeville Games[i] and subsequent large-scale competitions for in-dividuals with impairment have their roots in post-war England, where a physician named Ludwig Guttmann used wheelchair archery as a form of rehabilitation for veterans returning from World War II with spinal cord injuries. Through the 1940s and 1950s, sport was used as an end-phase rehabilitation tool to promote individuals' return to society. Then, at the height of the global human rights movement in the mid-1960s, people started to take notice that Para athletes were representing individuals with impairment at the highest levels. This contrasted starkly with the general state of human rights for individuals with impairment, where support structures and protective legislation were lacking. Consequently, the Para sport Movement developed from a rehabilitation-specific intervention into a platform for visibility, equality, and inclusion for the entire community.

It took a while to get organized, though. At first, rehabilitation events operated as separate entities to able-bodied sport, but between 1960 (the first official Paralympic Summer Games) and 1976 (the first Paralympic Winter Games), the IOC began to bring the two halves into closer alignment. Over this time there was significant growth in available sports and participating athletes, so by the mid-1980s, there was a need to co-ordinate various Para sport governing bodies. Initially, this saw the co-operation of the International Stoke Mandeville Games Federation (ISMGF), International Sport Organisation for the Disabled (ISOD), International Blind Sports Federation (IBSA), and Cerebral Palsy International Sports and Recreation Association (CPISRA). The International Sports Federations for Persons with an Intellectual Disability (INAS-FID) and International Committee of Sport for the Deaf (CISS) soon joined the group but maintained their own agendas. In 1989, the IPC was founded and has been focusing on elite participation and performance since then. From all this, there has been exponential growth with regard to sporting op-portunities for individuals with impairment. Initiatives like the Warrior Games in the USA and Invictus Games in the UK have founding dates as recent as 2014, indicating that Para sport is still growing and we're likely to see even greater developments over the coming years.

A Unique Challenge

Classification is one of the cornerstones of Para sport. Although not a new concept – fighters and rowers have weight classes, for example – classification in Para sport holds different implications. Each Para athlete's impairment is assessed and classified with the aim of grouping athletes with similar impairments together, to even the playing field.[3,4] Not all sports cater for all impairment categories, though. For example, 5-a-side football is only for athletes with visual impairment, so classifications must be sport-specific. This can be done by medical (e.g., visual impairment, for which an ophthalmologic exam is required), categorical (Para athletics, where the categories of impairment are presented in order, such as T/F 31–34 for non-ambulant individuals with cerebral palsy and T/F 35–38 for ambulant individuals), or functional criteria (Para swimming, where different impairments are grouped together but exhibit similar functional deficits).[3] However, impairment presentation differs from person to person, the tests are not always sensitive, and the classifiers are only given short time periods in which to do their assessments. This results in a somewhat subjective process. Unfortunately, as classification determines the field against which an athlete must compete, to be incorrectly classified can have catastrophic results for an athlete's ranking. Furthermore, changes in impairment-related function can result in a change in classification scoring. In reality, the complex nature of impairment cannot be covered by a single system, and consequently, some athletes are excluded from competition based on minimum eligibility requirements. It's not unheard of for a severely affected individual to be classified as non-eligible, merely because they don't present with "typical" impairment-related limitations and fit neatly into the pre-determined categories. New classification rules are passed regularly as well, and athletes who have been competing and succeeding for many years can be suddenly re-classified as non-eligible, putting an end to their sporting careers.

Imagine the anxiety inherent in this process! For able-bodied athletes who compete in sports with weight classifications, they can plan and train and prepare themselves to ensure that they end up exactly where they want to be. Para athletes don't have the same advantage. Some have a condition that isn't static (e.g., cerebral palsy) and they're training to compete to their best abilities but there's a chance their classification might change at the last minute. Others who have non-changing impairments (e.g., amputation) may not experience the same kind of constant uncertainty, but they still encounter events where classifications are combined so the competitive landscape is different than expected. Anecdotally, these athletes report feeling as though they're at the mercy of a subjective system that they can't anticipate or manage well, and that has implications for their pre-competition stress responses. As a known injury risk factor, this has the potential to cause problems before the event even takes place.

Similarities and Differences

Of course, not all injury risks in Para sport can be attributed to psychological stress, but there are some striking patterns in the medical surveillance data. The first investigations into injuries in the Para athlete population were conducted at the Salt Lake City 2002, Torino 2006, and Vancouver 2010 Paralympic Winter Games.[5,6] From the London 2012 Paralympic Games onward, a larger epidemiological study of injury and illness has been conducted by the IPC medical commission.[7–10] This work has identified a significantly higher injury rate in Para athletes compared with able-bodied athletes. For instance, the injury rate at the Sochi 2014 Paralympic Games was three times higher than the corresponding Olympic Games[6] Evidence also shows that the injury rate in the Winter Games is twice that of the Summer Games.[7–10] So, straight away it's clear that the context of injury in Para sport is unique and needs to be considered if we hope to support athletes appropriately.

In earlier chapters we've established that sports injuries are complex phenomena, resulting from the interaction of various determinants within a specific context.[11,12] This complexity is evident even when we try to define what an injury actually is.[13,14] From a medical point of view, it's understood that Para sport includes a diverse population of athletes with different impairments and, by definition, competitors have an altered baseline state of health.[15] This means that a sport-related health problem is defined as a change to a "less healthy" state relative to the athlete's starting point.[15] We know that for able-bodied athletes, injury definitions are fluid and not necessarily based on symptoms, but on the consequences for sports performance.[16] Part of this is an acknowledgement that contextual factors, such as differences in sports demands or the athlete's baseline health status, may mean that what's performance-limiting for one person may not be for another.[16] We therefore need to rely on athletes' perspectives and experiences to build our understanding of what injuries mean to them in terms of health and other sports outcomes (e.g., the benefits of an insider's vs an outsider's view).[17,18] However, research exploring the injury experiences of Para athletes is severely limited, so we have a generally poor idea of how they define injury and, consequently, what the effects of those injuries might be.

It's helpful at this point to overlay some of our theoretical understanding of injury risk and rehabilitation. If you recall back to Chapter 2 (go ahead and flip back to remind yourself, it's been a while), we can conceptualize the role of psychological factors using a number of different models. For our purposes, let's focus on the Integrated Model of Response to Sport Injury which postulates that cognitive appraisals, emotional responses, and behaviours are shaped by the athlete's personal and situational factors.[19] These will be unique to each athlete, so whether it's applied in an able-bodied or Para sport setting, the model should be applicable. Of course, this only describes injury responses at an intraindividual level. The Multilevel Model of Sport Injury (MMSI) highlights that the athlete sits at the centre of a layered context consisting of interpersonal, institutional, cultural, and policy influences.[20] In Para sport, this includes athletes' immediate social networks, their physical environment and available support services, broader cultural effects of the media and prevailing narratives, and standards for duty of care and societal responsibility. In the absence of sufficient research evidence around Para athletes' experiences, we can use these models as a starting point to understand the information that we do have and to direct future research toward important areas of enquiry. Why don't we start by seeing how they fit with the evidence that we do have?

What little research has been conducted in Para sport has revealed both similarities and differences to the able-bodied literature. In a qualitative study exploring Paralympic athletes' (n = 18) experiences of sport-related injuries, Fagher and colleagues'[21] participants believed injuries can occur due to overuse or risk behaviours related to training intensity and technique. This is much the same as for able-bodied athletes, yet they also saw injuries as a secondary effect of their impairments. They expressed concerns that their bodies were more vulnerable, with a reduced capacity for recovery, which would represent an inherent risk factor unique to this population. Importantly, all of the athletes had experienced pain while training and/or competing and regarded that pain as a fundamental part of Paralympic sport. The athletes had difficulties admitting to themselves that they were injured, and the authors postulated that Para athletes may have a different perception of pain (or the level of threat associated with it) because of repeated exposure to pain in their daily lives.[21] This clearly has implications for injury reporting and speaks to the cognitive appraisals (e.g., attributions) that Para athletes may form in response to an injury event.

In terms of emotional responses, many of the descriptions offered by the Para athletes in Fagher et al.'s study were similar to those we hear from able-bodied athletes.[21] These included concentration difficulties, sadness, depression, anxiety, and decreased motivation. Many athletes also experienced guilt for having an injury or had feelings of failure.[21] So, it appears there are some stable patterns in the way that athletes react to injury, regardless of the setting; however, the magnitude and source of these cognitive and emotional responses might differ. Paralympians reported that injury was a psychological stressor, often leading to feelings of concern, fear, and insecurity about what could happen to their bodies. Though able-bodied athletes experience similar things, the implications are not the same. For Para athletes, the consequences of a sports injury may include severe functional limitations that would restrict their ability to perform activities of daily life. For example, an athlete with a spinal cord injury who uses a wheelchair for mobility is at heightened risk of a shoulder injury which would severely impact daily needs like transfers and other necessary activities for which assistance may then be required. Regardless of their impairment type, Para athletes have reported that tasks in daily life also consume more energy when they're injured and that transportation, household work, and life, in general, becomes much more difficult.[21] As one athlete said, *"I'm often thinking, what will happen if I get an injury to my non-disabled side, I wouldn't be able to manage my daily life. That's what I am afraid of."*[8] Stemming from this is a tension around the value of elite Para sport in general. Athletes have perceptions that it's dangerous and harmful, yet they often state that their choice to compete is worth it despite the risks.[21] Exploring how these apparently conflicting views shape post-injury responses is an important next step in understanding what injury means to Para athletes and how they affect rehabilitation outcomes.

We also need to bear in mind that injury in Para sport happens within a context where coaches sometimes don't have enough knowledge of impairments and the effects that training might have on them. From the theoretical perspective of the MMSI, interactions at this interpersonal level can clearly influence injury risk and recovery, but little is known about the psychological climate of the coach-athlete relationship in this setting. Preliminary evidence suggests that there's an important social function in this dynamic, where coaches can offer necessary emotional and tangible support for athletes before and after injury.[22] This fits with what we know about the importance of social support as a buffer against negative stress responses. But coaches are also seen as a source of stress – many Para athletes find that coaches don't appreciate that sport is just one of the challenges they face every day.[22] Though many say that they want to be treated as an athlete first, there's a need for coaches to empathize and consider adaptations to their approach to accommodate the athlete's needs.[22] Otherwise, there's significant potential for negative physical and psychological outcomes to emerge, whether that be in the form of a primary sports injury, exacerbation of an existing condition, or a longer-term health problem.

Expanding our contextual view as per the MMSI, we can consider the potential influence of factors at institutional, cultural, and policy levels. Para sport injury is set against the backdrop of a health care system that often doesn't provide adequate support for those with disabilities and Para athletes themselves have reported having insufficient access to medical care outside of competition.[21,23,24] Moreover, there's a pervasive cultural narrative that Para sport is not "elite", which exacerbates inequalities in resource allocation between Para and able-bodied athletes. We can use a case study to illustrate how this often plays out.

Lisa Callaghan represented Ireland in athletics at three Paralympic Summer Games. From her perspective:

> *"Now Para athletes are getting the same experiences and treatments as able-bodied people. This wasn't always the case. When I first started, you were lucky if you had a Physiotherapist going with you to an event [and there was] no such thing as high performance."*

In 1999, Para sport was funded by Sport Ireland off the back of international medal achievements and increased promotion, and at home, Lisa finds that *"people are more familiar [with Para sport] and Para athletes are recognized as world class athletes."* Even in this environment, though, she recalls the challenges she faced around injury during her career. As a competitor in discus and javelin events, Lisa experienced regular ligament strains in her lower body. She has mild cerebral palsy that affects the left side of her body and suggests that:

> *"This may have occurred because I wasn't positioned correctly when throwing. As a result of poor balance and coordination, one has to find a technique that suits them best. I also had a tendency to put pressure on my good side rather than my weak side (for fear of falling.)"*

This is consistent with the early research in this area, showing that injury attributions can be centred around an athlete's impairment, and it raises some interesting questions. Evidence from able-bodied athlete samples suggests that those who make stable internal attributions for injuries experience less mood disturbance than those who attribute injuries to external or unstable causes.[25] It's unclear whether this is also the case in Para sport, or if these cognitions may be shaped by the environment, but finding out could help in the development of psychological interventions down the road.

For Lisa, her injury experience was also affected by her access to medical services. She saw a specialized therapist for her ligament injuries and remembers *"the reason I got this treatment was because my Mam was a nurse and got me the appointment within the hospital setting."* So even for a Paralympian within a funded sport system, resource allocation affected her rehabilitation process. For Para athletes in other circumstances, such obstacles may pose greater risks to their recovery, or indeed be insurmountable. Along with ableism and other structural biases that disadvantage those with impairments, these contextual factors can determine rehabilitation behaviours by limiting access to care or by contributing to negative cognitive appraisals and emotional responses. For instance, a common theme in Para sport discourse is that Para athletes are not always the ones making decisions on their own behalf and are instead at the mercy of the system around them. This lack of autonomy can be damaging to motivation and result in feelings of helplessness or apathy, leading to negative physical and mental health outcomes.[26]

Lisa's story perfectly illustrates how institutional (e.g., rehabilitation services), cultural (e.g., public support), and policy (e.g., national-level funding) levels of influence can interact to produce a unique injury context. Their effects may be positive or negative, or a combination of both, but they undoubtedly determine an athlete's pathway through the injury process. What we don't fully understand is what the psychological effects of all this might be. Much more research is clearly needed, but in the meantime, we can take some cues from the narratives that are emerging from within the Para sport community.

Taking Control of the Story

Let's stick with the medical side of things to begin with. Obviously, athletes themselves tend to be the focus in sport injury situations, but we can learn from the experiences of the clinicians who support them as well. Professor Wayne Derman has served on the IPC Medical Commission and fulfilled the positions of Chief Medical Officer for the South African Team to the Sydney 2000, Athens 2004 Olympic Games, and Chief Medical Officer for the South African Paralympic Team to Beijing 2008 and London 2012. Reflecting on his experiences, he's noted a number of key similarities between Olympic and Paralympic athletes. In his words, both groups are *"the ultimate achievers,"* typifying elite sport at its highest level and sacrificing everything to win. But as a group, Para athletes seem to display particularly adaptive coping strategies when faced with challenges:

"Perhaps the most lasting impressions I have taken away from my work with Paralympians is an overwhelming sense of gratitude displayed by the Paralympic athletes. In my time travelling with them, I did not hear one complaint from a single athlete, not a word expressing difficulty. On reflection, I think that the ability to deal with adversity is learnt through adopting a mindset, which is the gift of perspective. When one has to face the most challenging circumstances that life may have to offer (often the cause of the disability) and have accepted and integrated that into one's being... If I am allowed to generalize, I would say that Paralympic athletes clearly have the gift of being able to see the bigger picture and somehow do not seem to get caught up in complaining about the minutia. Another striking observation is that of profound resilience in the characters of these athletes, as well as an excellent sense of humor. If one is able to laugh at oneself, the ego is removed or suppressed, and when the ego has been reduced, this allows one to be fully present and fully engaged with the task at hand."

We've talked about coping and resilience before (Chapter 7 has all the details), and this vignette is (quite literally) a textbook example. Positive adaptation to circumstantial difficulties and seeing adversity as a challenge instead of a threat are characteristic responses associated with elite-level athletes in general.[27,28] They're also hallmark features of positive injury outcomes, usually indicating that athletes have robust coping strategies that allow them to find meaning in their situation and actively engage in the recovery process. Whilst many able-bodied athletes need to develop these skills, Para athletes may be much better equipped by virtue of their life experience. Having to regularly overcome challenges can help to build a coping reserve, which in turn buffers against emotional distress and its knock-on effects on physical and psychological health.[29] Although research in this area is really limited at present, understanding how resilience shapes the meaning of injury for Para athletes will be key to better supporting them.

As an interesting evolution of resiliency, which we think of as a psychological construct, there's also some very early evidence that Para athletes may have a physical capacity to withstand challenges as well. A case study of two Paralympians with acute grade I-II hamstring injuries described how they were able to return to competition in under a week, setting personal bests in sprinting and jumping events.[30] This is remarkable, considering the usual recovery period for such injuries is around 27 days, and return to sport wouldn't typically occur before the two-week mark.[30] Para athletes generally report more sport-related muscle pain than able-bodied athletes and it may be that adaptation to training with pain allows modulation of its effects.[31,32] The ability to "transcend" injury may therefore reflect a biopsychosocial process of pain interpretation and an increased sensitivity to the meaning (and limits) associated with bodily sensations as a result of continually managing the effects of impairment. This ties into some of the concepts we discussed in Chapter 6 and, as an extension of our standard interpretation of resiliency, represents a really fascinating area of exploration in Para sport injury psychology.

But we've digressed slightly. Another of Professor Derman's observations focuses on the bigger narrative surrounding Para sport and how that might shape the meaning of injury as well:

> *"It seems that when the athletes who are victorious at the Paralympic Games make it to the podium, the medal represents a victory not only in the race or event, but a victory of that athlete over their impairment and the various hurdles that come along with it. Without a doubt, the Paralympics are as competitive an event as the Olympic Games, however with an additional mission to raise awareness and provide a global perspective on the unique and remarkable capabilities of individuals with an impairment. Athletes with disabilities are just as dedicated, train and compete equally as hard as their able-bodied counterparts. Yet, the Paralympians manage to see the bigger picture. As disappointing as losing a medal might be, many of these athletes have at some stage lost something much bigger in their life."*

The key statement here is the idea of the Paralympics serving a dual purpose of sport and social activism (i.e., advocating for individuals with impairments). This is important for gaining some perspective on the context in which injuries occur. Specifically, in this setting injuries don't just impact a single athlete or their team, they also affect the public image of Para athletes more broadly. Research has established that injuries can pose a meaningful threat to an athlete's personal identity and self-presentational concerns often emerge when this happens, resulting in anxiety and a number of maladaptive behaviours (e.g., risk-taking, avoidance).[33] What happens when it isn't just your personal identity at stake, but also the identity of your community? In Para sport, some unique narratives have been structured around this issue to reflect both the sport and social activism elements that athletes perceive as being central to their context. One of these revolves around the "Supercrip" concept and the other is about establishing individual value and reward through sport participation.

Hold on, wait a second! "Supercrip" is a term that makes a lot of people uncomfortable, so as a disclaimer upfront, it's not a word we've come up with. Its origins aren't particularly clear, but it seems to have emerged within the disability rights community sometime in the 1970s.[ii] In contemporary use, it implies "overcoming" a perceived deficit associated with impairment. Given widespread biases – and maltreatment – against people with disabilities in society at large, the Supercrip term implies a kind of social reverence toward those who achieve "in spite of" their challenges, and it supports the "inspirational" commentary that accompanies Para sport. Now, given all the horrible stereotypes about disability, the Supercrip phenomenon seems okay on the surface – there's absolutely nothing wrong with being inspired by Para athletes' achievements, after all. But, as you might have guessed by our liberal use of quotation marks, this discourse has some problematic undercurrents that need to be acknowledged.[35]

For starters, implicit in the idea of the Supercrip is the notion that people with impairments aren't expected to achieve in the first place, so those who do must be exceptional.[34,35] This reflects society's ableist perspective on what life is (or should be) for people with disabilities. Herein emerges a contradiction within the narrative. On the one hand, it reinforces a disempowering presentation of people with disabilities who are seen as being extraordinary for doing ordinary things (e.g., playing on a sports team); on the other, it venerates people with disabilities for doing something rare (e.g., competing at a Paralympic Games).[36,37] So already, we can see how injuries in recreational Para sport may occur in a very different social context to those in elite settings. We can imagine, for example, an injury reinforcing disability stereotypes within community sport but being seen as heroic at the Paralympic level. This leads into a second problem, whereby many Para athletes don't encounter the same barriers as other people with disabilities. The role of privilege in their achievements is often overlooked and as such, white and/ or wealthy individuals have both a greater likelihood of sports achievement and of being glorified in the Supercrip narrative.[34,35] Not only can this set unreasonable expectations about what people with disabilities can or "should" be able to do, but it also has the potential to feed into racial and/or classist stereotypes that can affect Para athletes' sport and health outcomes disproportionately depending on their personal characteristics and level of competition.

From an injury psychology point of view, the most salient issue within the Supercrip phenomenon is the fact that the discourse has become ingrained within the Para sport community itself. Don't get us wrong, there's empowerment in athletes taking control of their own narratives (particularly in a setting where agency and autonomy have been limited); however, some athletes internalize it to an extreme. Whether it's entangled with or supersedes, athletic identity hasn't been determined,[22] but some Para athletes believe that their sport achievements are what signal their equality with others.[35] When an athlete thinks that to be respected as a person they must perform at the highest level, it generates incredible pressure and will likely lead to physical and mental health consequences (e.g., overtraining, injury, burnout). By claiming personhood based on their Supercrip identity, there's also a significant risk that injury may cause devastating effects on self-perceptions and trigger a cascade of negative emotional and behavioural outcomes.[35] There's an added layer of complexity to think about in Para sport, too. In other chapters, we've considered how identity shapes and is shaped by injury experiences, but a Para athlete's relationship with their own impairment, and whether they see it as intrinsic to who they are, will be part of this dynamic.[38] Though we can't speculate about how that might affect responses to injury, investigating the nature of that relationship and whether it differs for those with congenital or acquired impairments will be an important area of research moving forward.[iii]

Of course, not all Para athletes accept the Supercrip narrative as a reflection of their experiences.[35] For instance, a qualitative study involving five Paralympic swimmers[38] found that none of the participants viewed themselves as disabled, nor as Supercrips. Instead, their social environments (including family and non-sport networks) reinforced a holistic vision of themselves, and swimming facilitated self-

and social acceptance that was central to their identity development. They suggested that they saw themselves as athletes, not athletes with disabilities, and sport success had given them increased visibility as such in the public eye. So, we must be careful not to superimpose the Supercrip narrative (or any others) onto Para sport injury research or practice, because as with any other contextual factor, its effects are likely to be individual to each athlete.

Considerations for Mental Health

As a final topic for consideration, we'd be remiss not to broach the issue of mental health. We know that sport, regardless of who participates in it, generally has physical and mental health benefits.[42] That said, from the limited available evidence, we don't know if that's always the case for Para athletes. Some of that uncertainty is due to conflicting evidence in the few studies that have been conducted. To illustrate, a study of Brazilian Paralympians (n=40) found that athletes presented with positive mood states, good sleep quality, and average levels of anxiety prior to competition.[43] In contrast, a high prevalence of psychological distress was identified in South African Para athletes (n=125) at provincial, national, and international levels when compared to the general South African population.[44] Of concern was the high rate of sub-clinal symptoms identified in this group – 76% had high symptom ratings but didn't meet the criteria for diagnosis of a specific disorder. It's reasonable to suggest that some psychological stressors may be unique, or magnified, for Para athletes.[35,45] Things like costs (e.g., expensive specialist equipment with no/limited funding), lack of sufficient adaptive sports facilities, being misclassified for competition, experiencing chronic pain, and managing complex medical situations are all likely sources of difficulty.[35,46] It must also be considered that a substantial proportion of Para athletes have acquired disabilities, and that trauma may manifest in physical or psychological symptoms.[35] Anxiety and low mood, or other signs of distress, have been implicated in injury risk,[47] and clearly impact post-injury cognitions and behaviours.[19] It's therefore really important that we get a more complete picture of mental health in Para sport, both as a health outcome in its own right and for its contribution to injury experiences.

Looking Ahead

We've addressed a number of important topics in this chapter and perhaps we can best summarize the discussion with a few observations. Foremost, Para athletes view themselves as committed and serious sportspeople, but there are still pervasive views that question their legitimacy as such.[48,49] This forms a salient part of their sport experience, with potential effects on support and health care accessibility (which is a fundamental disability issue) as well as all of the other complexities of Para sport. When we think about the psychological factors that contribute to injury risk and rehabilitation, we can't lose sight of this. If athletes do indeed define their injuries by their consequences more so than their symptoms,[50] Para athletes are likely to experience significantly greater burden than their able-bodied counterparts and as researchers and practitioners, we have a responsibility to do something about that.

The biggest thing we can do is listen to athletes and learn from their experiences and expertise. This will facilitate research in which academics, athletes, clinicians, coaches, and the wider Para sport community work together to create meaningful change based on their needs. Part of this is increasing the diversity of the voices we hear. The lived experiences of Para athletes are specific to their environment, and our current narratives are largely structured around the perspectives of those from well-resourced nations. Para athletes from developing countries are sorely underrepresented in the literature, leaving a significant gap in our understanding and service provision. Similarly, there's been a lot of focus on Paralympic athletes with very little attention at amateur or recreational levels. The Paralympic Movement evolved to promote a more equitable society through sport. A step toward achieving these ideals of fairness and inclusivity is providing high quality medical and psychological care to everyone who participates, across the full range of Para sport participation. This is an important goal, and one that needs much more deliberate action if we hope to make progress.[51]

Notes

i On the day of the Opening Ceremony of the London 1948 Olympic Games (July 29, to be exact), Dr. Guttmann organized the first competition for 16 wheelchair archers, which he named the Stoke Mandeville Games. Thus, a legacy was born.

ii It seems "Supercrip" was a pejorative term for people with disabilities who were seen as "overachievers", though its obvious origin in the Superman story has been long acknowledged by scholars in the field.[34]

iii There's also a really interesting conversation emerging around sport technologies and the process of cyborgification (integrating mechanical/electronic and human functions), and the kind of hybrid identities that athletes develop as a result. It's still early days in this line of research, but Sparkes and colleagues have conducted an insightful study on the topic as a starting point if you're interested.[36,37,39–41]

References

1 International Olympic Committee Executive Board. Olympic movement medical code 2016. Available at: https://olympics.com/ioc/medical-research. Accessed June 8, 2021.

2 International Paralympic Committee General Assembly. International Paralympic Committee medical code 2011. Available at: https://www.paralympic.org/medical. Accessed June 8, 2021.

3 International Paralympic Committee. IPC athlete classification code 2015. Available at: https://www.paralympic.org/classification-code. Accessed June 8, 2021.

4 Webborn N, Willick S, Reeser JC. Injuries among disabled athletes during the 2002 Winter Paralympic Games. *Med Sci Sports Exerc* 2006;38:811–815; doi: 10.1249/01 .mss.0000218120.05244.da.

5 Webborn N, Willick S, Emery CA. The injury experience at the 2010 Winter Paralympic Games. *Clin J Sport Med* 2012;22:3–9; doi: 10.1097/JSM.0b013e31 8243309f.

6 Derman W, Schwellnus MP, Jordaan E, et al. High incidence of injury at the Sochi 2014 Winter Paralympic Games: a prospective cohort study of 6564 athlete days. *Br J Sports Med* 2016;50:1069–1074; doi: 10.1136/bjsports-2016-096214.

7 Derman W, Runciman P, Jordaan E, et al. High incidence of injuries at the Pyeongchang 2018 Paralympic Winter Games: a prospective cohort study of 6804 athlete days. *Br J Sports Med* 2020;54:38–43; doi: 10.1136/bjsports-2018-100170.

8 Willick SE, Webborn N, Emery C, et al. The epidemiology of injuries at the London 2012 Paralympic Games. *Br J Sports Med* 2013;47:426–432; doi: 10.1136/bjsports-2013-092374.

9 Derman W, Schwellnus M, Jordaan E, et al. Illness and injury in athletes during the competition period at the London 2012 Paralympic Games: development and implementation of a web-based surveillance system (WEB-IISS) for team medical staff. *Br J Sports Med* 2013;47:420–425; doi: 10.1136/bjsports-2013-092375.

10 Derman W, Runciman P, Schwellnus M, et al. High precompetition injury rate dominates the injury profile at the Rio 2016 Summer Paralympic Games: a prospective cohort study of 51 198 athlete days. *Br J Sports Med* 2018;52:24–31; doi: 10.1136/bjsports-2017-098039.

11 Bittencourt NFN, Meeuwisse WH, Mendonça LD, et al. Complex systems approach for sports injuries: moving from risk factor identification to injury pattern recognition - narrative review and new concept. *Br J Sports Med* 2016;50:1309–1314; doi: 10.1136/bjsports-2015-095850.

12 Bolling C, van Mechelen W, Pasman HR, et al. Context Matters: revisiting the first step of the "sequence of prevention" of sports injuries. *Sport Med* 2018;48:2227–2234; doi: 10.1007/s40279-018-0953-x.

13 Timpka T, Jacobsson J, Bickenbach J, et al. What is a sports injury? *Sports Med* 2014;44:423–428; doi: 10.1007/s40279-014-0143-4

14 Fuller CW, Ekstrand J, Junge A, et al. Consensus statement on injury definitions and data collection procedures in studies of football (soccer) injuries. *Clin J Sport Med* 2006;16:97–106. doi: 10.1097/00042752-200603000-00003.

15 Derman W, Badenhorst M, Blauwet C, et al. Para sport translation of the IOC consensus on recording and reporting of data for injury and illness in sport. *Br J Sports Med* 2021;bjsports-2020-103464; doi: 10.1136/bjsports-2020-103464.

16 Bolling C, Delfino Barboza S, van Mechelen W, et al. How elite athletes, coaches, and physiotherapists perceive a sports injury. *Transl Sport Med* 2019;2:17–23; doi: 10.1002/tsm2.53.

17 Bolling C. "Who me? I thought you would never ask!" Applying qualitative methods in sports injury prevention research. *Br J Sports Med* 2021;55:125–126; doi: 10.1136/bjsports-2020-102984.

18 Bekker S, Bolling C, H Ahmed O, et al. Athlete health protection: why qualitative research matters. *J Sci Med Sport* 2020;23:898–901; doi: 10.1016/j.jsams.2020.06.020.

19 Wiese-Bjornstal DM, Smith AM, Shaffer SM, et al. An integrated model of response to sport injury: psychological and sociological dynamics. *J Appl Sport Psychol* 1998;10(1):46–69; doi: 10.1080/10413209808406377.

20 Wadey R, Day M, Cavallerio F, et al. Multilevel model of sport injury (MMSI): can coaches impact and be impacted by injury? In: R Thelwell, M Dicks (eds.). *Professional advances in sports coaching: research and practice.* London: Routledge 2018.

21 Fagher K, Forsberg A, Jacobsson J, et al. Paralympic athletes' perceptions of their experiences of sports-related injuries, risk factors and preventive possibilities. *Eur J Sport Sci* 2016;16:1240–1249; doi:10.1080/17461391.2016.1192689.

22 Culver DM, Werthner P. Voices: para athletes speak. *Qual Res Sport Exerc Heal* 2018;10:167–175; doi:10.1080/2159676X.2017.1393004.

23 Badenhorst M, Verhagen E, Lambert M, et al. Accessing healthcare as a person with a rugby-related spinal cord injury in South Africa: the injured player's perspective. *Physiother Theory Pract* Published Online First: 2021. doi:10.1080/09593985.2021.1872753.

24 Eide AH, Mannan H, Khogali M, et al. Perceived barriers for accessing health services among individuals with disability in four African countries. *PLoS One* 2015;10:e0125915; doi:10.1371/journal.pone.0125915.

25 Brewer BW. Injury Prevention and Rehabilitation. In: BW Brewer (ed.). *Sport Psychology*. Chichester, UK: Wiley-Blackwell 2009.

26 Deci EL, Ryan RM. Self-determination theory: a macrotheory of human motivation, development, and health. *Can Psychol* 2008;49:182–185; doi: 10.1037/a0012801.

27 Luthar SS. Resilience in development: a synthesis of research across five decades. In: D Cicchetti, DJ Cohen (eds.). *Developmental psychopathology: risk, disorder, and adaptation (Vol. 3, 2nd ed.)*. New York, NY: Wiley 2006.

28 Fletcher D, Sarkar M. A grounded theory of psychological resilience in Olympic champions. *Psychol Sport Exerc* 2012;13:669–678; doi:10.1016/j.psychsport.2012.04.007.

29 Meichenbaum D. Stress inoculation training. In: D Meichenbaum. *The Evolution of Cognitive Behavior Therapy: A Personal and Professional Journey with Don Meichenbaum*. New York: Routledge 2017.

30 Derman W, Ferreira S, Subban K, et al. Transcendence of musculoskeletal injury in athletes with disability during major competition. *South African J Sports Med* 2011;23:95–97.

31 Hainline B, Turner JA, Caneiro JP, et al. Pain in elite athletes—neurophysiological, biomechanical and psychosocial considerations: a narrative review. *Br J Sports Med* 2017;51:1259–1264; doi:10.1136/bjsports-2017-097890.

32 Tesarz J, Schuster AK, Hartmann M, et al. Pain perception in Athletes compared to normally active controls: a systematic review with meta-analysis. *Pain* 2012;153:1253–1262; doi: 10.1016/j.pain.2012.03.005.

33 Brewer B. Self-identity and specific vulnerability to depressed mood. *J Pers* 1993;61:343–364; doi: 10.1111/j.1467-6494.1993.tb00284.x.

34 Schalk S. Re-evaluating the supercrip. *J Literary & Cult Disabil Stud* 2016;10:71–87.

35 Swartz L, Hunt X, Bantjes J, et al. Mental health symptoms and disorders in Paralympic athletes: A narrative review. *Br J Sports Med* 2019;53:737–740; doi:10.1136/bjsports-2019-100731.

36 Silva CF, Howe PD. The (in)validity of supercrip representation of paralympian athletes. *J Sport Soc Issues* 2012;36:174–194; doi:10.1177/0193723511433865.

37 Howe PD. From inside the newsroom: Paralympic media and the "production" of elite disability. *Int Rev Sociol Sport* 2008;43:135–150; doi:10.1177/1012690208095376.

38 Pack S, Kelly S, Arvinen-Barrow M. "I think I became a swimmer rather than just someone with a disability swimming up and down:" paralympic athletes perceptions of self and identity development. *Disabil Rehabil* 2017;39:2063–2070; doi:10.1080/09638288.2016.1217074.

39 Sparkes AC, Brighton J, Inckle K. "It's a part of me": an ethnographic exploration of becoming a disabled sporting cyborg following spinal cord injury. *Qual Res Sport Exerc Heal* 2018;10:151–166; doi:10.1080/2159676X.2017.1389768.

40 Sparkes AC, Brighton J, Inckle K. "I am proud of my back": an ethnographic study of the motivations and meanings of body modification as identity work among athletes with spinal cord injury. *Qual Res Sport Exerc Heal* Published Online First: 2020. doi:10.1080/2159676X.2020.1756393.

41 Berger RJ. Disability and the dedicated wheelchair athlete: beyond the "supercrip" critique. *J Contemp Ethnogr* 2008;37:647–678; doi:10.1177/0891241607309892.

42 Vita G, La Foresta S, Russo M, et al. Sport activity in Charcot–Marie–Tooth disease: a case study of a Paralympic swimmer. *Neuromuscul Disord* 2016;26:614–618; doi:10.1016/j.nmd.2016.06.002.

43 Rodrigues DF, Silva A, Rosa JPP, et al. Sleep quality and psychobiological aspects of Brazilian Paralympic athletes in the London 2012 pre-Paralympics period. *Motriz Rev Educ Fis* 2015;21:168–176; doi:10.1590/S1980-65742015000200007.

44 Badenhorst M, Runciman P, Brown JC, et al. Promotion of Para athlete well-being in South Africa (the PROPEL studies): profiles and prevalence of psychological distress. *J Sci Med Sport* Published Online First: 2021; doi:10.1016/j.jsams.2020.12.013.

45 Reardon CL, Hainline B, Aron CM, et al. Mental health in elite athletes: International Olympic Committee consensus statement (2019). *Br J Sports Med* 2019;53:667–699; doi:10.1136/bjsports-2019-100715.

46 Campbell E, Jones G. Sources of stress experienced by elite male wheelchair basketball players. *Adapt Phys Act Q* 2002;19:82–99; doi:10.1123/apaq.19.1.82.

47 Andersen MB, Williams JM. A model of stress and athletic injury: prediction and prevention. *J Sport Exerc Psychol* 1988;10:294–306 doi: 10.1123/jsep.10.3.294.

48 Webborn N, Van De Vliet P. Paralympic medicine. *Lancet* 2012;380:65–71; doi:10.1016/S0140-6736(12)60831-9.

49 Van De Vliet P. Paralympic athlete's health. *Br J Sports Med* 2012;46:458–459; doi: 10.1136/bjsports-2012-091192.

50 Bolling C, Delfino Barboza S, van Mechelen W, et al. How elite athletes, coaches, and physiotherapists perceive a sports injury. *Transl Sports Med* 2019;2(1):17–23; doi: 10.1002/tsm2.53.

51 Swartz L, Bantjes J, Rall D, et al. "A more equitable society": the politics of global fairness in Paralympic sport. *PLOS One* 2016;10.1371/journal.pone.0167481.

17

CONCLUSIONS: WHERE DO WE GO FROM HERE?

Carly McKay

Right, well, you've made it to the end! Thanks for sticking with it - hopefully it's been an interesting and worthwhile read. We've covered a lot of ground through this book and it's probably worth summarizing the big points, at least as I see them. You might have picked up on some other interesting nuggets along the way, but from my perspective, there are a few major issues that bear reinforcement if we hope to learn and develop the practice of sport injury psychology further.

Point #1

If you take away only one idea from all of this, I hope it's the concept that injury risk and rehabilitation are complex processes. They aren't simply cause-and-effect situations where factors affect each other in a linear fashion, but instead, they're driven by a web of interconnected features that interact in different (and sometimes surprising) ways. If we really want to understand how personal and environmental factors increase injury susceptibility, or why some athletes fare well through recovery while others don't, we need to embrace this. That means changing the research paradigm that's served us so well up to this point, which is going to require some significant buy-in. It'll involve bringing together different disciplines (physiology, biomechanics, sociology, data science) and seeking patterns in the data rather than just looking for simple associations between variables. The upshot will be a more holistic appreciation for the context in which athletes experience injuries and more precise information about which factors should be targeted by interventions. It's a big step, though, and is probably going to be a gradual transition rather than an immediate about-face. That will allow some time for non-psychologist stakeholders to get in on the action (insert shameless advertisement for community involvement here).

DOI: 10.4324/9781003088936-17

Point #2

The second big idea that we've discussed is that no, injuries aren't really a good thing, but they don't always lead to negative outcomes either. Sport injury-related growth is a real phenomenon and we're just scratching the surface of why it happens, what it means, and how we can promote it. After a few decades of focusing primarily on the detrimental effects, this represents a really exciting step forward in exploring the entire spectrum of athlete responses to injury. Categorizing people into groups is cognitively efficient and helps to simplify otherwise complicated situations; however, thinking that athletes either suffer or excel misses out on all of the nuances in between those extremes. Acknowledging that there are as many different journeys through injury as there are athletes who go through them might free us up to approach things more creatively. The need for individualized intervention has always been implicit in the sport injury psychology literature, but perhaps it's time to be very upfront about it. Instead of seeking a single "best" way to manage injury, tailored approaches are probably more effective, taking into account the athlete's personal and situational environment. This is an unbelievable amount of work, though, and there will always be an element of trial and error in that process. It also seems to negate the need for research – why bother if we're saying that it all depends on the person, and we'll have to sort things out on the fly anyway? Well, going back to the first big point, taking a complex systems approach can help us figure out some stable patterns in the way that variables interact with each other. This can help us narrow in on which intervention options are most likely to succeed, much like a doctor's differential diagnosis helps them whittle down the list of available treatments. Not every medication will work for every patient, but with a little tinkering, they can usually get the type and dosage right. Looking at it that way could be helpful when trying to fit psychology into a traditional medical model.

Point #3

We've devoted a couple of chapters to athlete monitoring and the digital revolution in sport, and that speaks to where the current momentum is taking us. Technology is here to stay, and it brings with it a host of benefits and potential drawbacks that deserve some more attention than they've received up to this point. Part of this is due to the relentless speed of the industry. Equipment is upgraded on incredibly rapid timescales, which are wholly incompatible with the pace of academic research. This creates a "wild west" frontier in terms of how technology is deployed in practice. Even if we carried out rigorous studies to inform the process, they would be obsolete by the time they were published. So, what are we to do? All I can advise is, let's try to avoid opening a Pandora's Box by thinking critically about how and why these tools are being used in the first place. Their primary function is performance and they've been reasonably useful in that regard, so there's no need to launch an anti-tech campaign. Instead, it's imperative that we're careful about the potential for surveillance to create unintended consequences for athletes' mental health and wellbeing. Making sure that we're only using these tools for discrete and transparent purposes is a good place to start and minimizing their intrusiveness in future versioning will be important, too. There's no telling just how advanced things might become, so setting some ground rules for acceptable use[i] might be a low-hanging objective to focus on in the meantime.

Point #4

Focusing on injury prevention for a second, which happens to be my personal area of interest, we can clearly see traditional methods of implementing interventions are not working as well as we'd hoped. Some of that can be chalked up to the relative naivety of early research in this area. Just because people know better, it doesn't mean they'll do better, and human beings don't always act in their own best interest. Or, more accurately, we cannot impose a value system on people that determines what their best interests should be. Sport is an environment where this becomes very apparent, particularly in the tension between promoting performance whilst trying to protect health at the same time. This is why old school assumptions that awareness campaigns would lead to change are doomed to mediocre results at best. Sure, some folks are really logical and will behave in self-protective ways, but that's not everyone's top priority. Letting go of this idea has been a rocky road in the sport medicine community, but the tide has turned and there's now much greater support for integrating the principles of behaviour change and implementation science into intervention design and delivery. Now that we've come this far, I think it's time to push the boat out even further. Let's start borrowing from other domains of psychology where people have done a much better job of shaping culture. That would be quite a departure from the regimented and evidence-rooted standards of medical practice, but a few trendsetters in the field are seeing very promising early outcomes. Exploring the possibilities of tactics like guerilla marketing and nudging is scary but exciting at the same time, and probably where the future of this endeavour lies.

Point #5

Finally, I hope that it's become self-evident that we cannot separate sport injury psychology from sport injury sociology. Injuries don't happen to people in a vacuum – they occur within a specific context at a specific point in time. That context is shaped by the physical environment (e.g., geography, resources, weather) as well as the culture of the sport, and athletes bring to that mix their own background and non-sport roles. We've also established that injury risk and recovery are influenced by the interaction of personal and situational factors, yet many of the social elements therein are still understudied. A better appreciation for how things like cultural norms, group dynamics, and communication styles can be internalized or act as externally imposed constraints would undoubtedly help us understand athletes' cognitions and behaviours. This is difficult to sort out, though, if you're not a member of the sport community in the first place. Many of those details are accessible only to those inside the circle, and most researchers simply are not. So, there's a huge opportunity here to listen to the *athlete voice* and learn from practitioners who are actively working in that cultural space, and this is something we need to see more of if we hope to fully support athletes through their injury experiences.

The Elephant in the Room

The five key points that I've picked out have been drawn from the conceptual side of our discussion about sport injury psychology, but there's an overarching issue that we really need to start talking about more openly. Astute readers will have noticed that, throughout the book, we've spoken mostly about athletes in a generic sense. Although we'd like to think that much of the information could be applied to anyone, and at the end of the day it probably can be to some extent, we've made a repetitive argument that not everyone's injury experience is the same. But through the chapters, we've not explicitly mentioned some of the key factors that likely play a big part in this, which might stand out as a little strange. The truth is, research in this area has been largely homogenous, focused primarily on groups of high-performance athletes in early adulthood from the global North. That's a big problem. The experiences of these athletes are perfectly valid, of course, but we know they're not going to be universally generalizable. How can we possibly think we've understood the context of injury, then, if we haven't accounted for the fact that the current evidence base is exclusive to a narrow range of those people we're hoping to help?

How about an illustration. We might, for example, consider sex/gender as a factor that could affect an athlete's injury risk or recovery. Plenty of evidence suggests that might be the case, particularly around anterior cruciate ligament (ACL) injuries. Studies have found that girls/women seem to incur ACL injuries at a significantly higher rate, and they're far less likely to return to sport afterwards.[3,4] This disparity can't be accounted for by purely biological differences, so there must be other factors at play.[5] There actually has been some exploration of differences between girls/women and boys/men in the injury psychology literature (around ACL and other kinds of injuries), but this has typically been done on a dichotomous distribution that doesn't necessarily differentiate between sex and the full spectrum of gender identity. We know that sport is a gendered environment that isn't always equitable (e.g., fewer resources for women's leagues),[5] and girls/women are notoriously underrepresented in sport medicine research.[6] Therefore, as Parsons and colleagues[5] so eloquently argued, sex and gender can be seen as both intrinsic and extrinsic risk factors (or personal and situational variables in post-injury parlance). Because injury research hasn't been approached from this perspective, though, it's unclear how big an effect it might have on girls'/women's injury experiences. It's really not as simple as asking whether women and men respond to injury the same way, we need to ask that question in the context of a sport environment that treats them differently.

And that's just one example. Many of the models we use to describe injury risk and rehabilitation list off a number of factors that have the potential to influence the way athletes think, feel, and act. These include their level of competition, access to resources, injury history or years of experience, etc. But what about the environmental pressures they face based on their culture, geography, or socio-economic status? How do we factor in biases that affect members of LGBTQ2+, BIPOC, or other marginalized communities? What about the influence of ageism and ableism on the way people are treated in sport and medicine? Imagine the psychological impact of these environmental factors and how they shape the lived experience of sport injury, even in the most basic terms. If life stress is a strong risk factor, then those who face additional challenges within and outside of sport are at a significant disadvantage, yet this hasn't been properly addressed in research or in practice. Inequitable treatment and barriers in the rehabilitation setting can dis-criminate as well, and there's a risk of exacerbating these problems through the blanket application of intervention strategies. I mean, it's hardly appropriate to advise someone to seek professional psychological support if that would be in-accessible to them. The fact that much of this hasn't been dealt with in the research literature to date is an extreme limitation that can't be overlooked. It's well past time that we, as researchers, practitioners, and policymakers, stop being satisfied with speaking in generalizations derived from small studies of easily recruited samples. We must instead focus on representation in our work to promote complete and more effective athlete care.

I realize that this is a lot to think about at the end of a book, and I know I haven't done the issue justice at all. The discussion could fill an entire volume of its own and would be better articulated by those who have lived these experiences firsthand. But in as much as it forms an important and necessary step in this field moving forward, it needed to be brought up. Now our job is to turn words into actions and integrate the principles of equity and social responsibility into research and athlete care.

A Final Word

How can we sum all of this up, then? Well, why don't we try this analogy: if you've ever played with Lego, then you may have had a similar experience to mine. Any time I got a new set, the first thing I did was build whatever it was supposed to be, maybe a submarine or a pirate ship. It worked well that first time and I had a lot of fun doing it, but pretty soon I'd start to think about what else could be made with the bricks. As I played, I would discover infinite ways to reassemble them and add bits from other sets – maybe one day I'd build a space station or a skyscraper instead. Once I understood how the individual pieces worked, I could fit them together in multiple ways depending on my objective at the time. Well, in a way, sport injury psychology is a little bit like that. There are some foundation pieces (i.e., fundamental principles) that we need to master first. We can't go mixing and matching bits of theory, for example. But, once we've got a handle on that and understand how interventions can be applied, we can select and adapt these elements to solve problems in our own sport environments. No two solutions will look completely the same, since each athlete's context will be unique to them, but we can combine the pieces in a variety of ways to achieve a positive outcome.

Sport injury psychology is a rapidly evolving field. There are many questions yet to be answered around patterns in risk and how best to apply interventions for recovery and prevention. We still need to refine our theories and continue to test the hypotheses they generate, and we really have to sort out some more robust research approaches. Yet, for all of these limitations, there's a wealth of information available to guide practice, whether you're a psychologist, a coach, a parent, or even an athlete. Hopefully, this book has given you a little insight into the role of psychosocial variables in injury risk and rehabilitation, and has left you with a few tips and tricks along the way. At the very least, I hope it's been an interesting story. Thanks for reading it.

Note

i There's precedent for this, albeit at the edge of science fiction. Asimov's Laws, or the Three Laws of Robotics, were devised by author Isaac Asimov to govern the development and behaviour of robotic technology.[1] Although these are undoubtedly a product of imagination, they're actually not so farfetched. Ethical codes are being written around the world to govern the development of Artificial Intelligence, some of which may be rooted in Asimov's Laws and will likely shape technology and its use for generations to come.[2]

References

1 Asimov I. Runaround. In: I Asimov (ed.). *I, Robot.* New York: Doubleday 1950.
2 BBC news. Robotic age poses ethical dilemma. Available at: http://news.bbc.co.uk/1/hi/technology/6425927.stm Accessed May 31, 2021.
3 Agel J, Rockwood T, Klossner D. Collegiate ACL injury rates across 15 sports: National Collegiate Athletic Association injury surveillance system data update (2004-2005 through 2012-2013). *Clin J Sport Med* 2016;26:518–523; doi:10.1097/JSM.0000000000000290.
4 Ardern CL, Taylor NF, Feller JA, et al. Fifty-five per cent return to competitive sport following anterior cruciate ligament reconstruction surgery: an updated systematic review and meta-analysis including aspects of physical functioning and contextual factors. *Br J Sports Med* 2014;48:1543–1552; doi:10.1136/bjsports-2013-093398.
5 Parsons JL, Coen SE, Bekker S. Anterior cruciate ligament injury: towards a gendered environmental approach. *Br J Sports Med.* Published Online First: 10 March 2021; doi: 10.1136/bjsports-2020-103173.
6 Costello JT, Bieuzen F, Bleakley CM. Where are all the female participants in Sports and Exercise Medicine research? *Eur J Sport Sci* 2014;14(8):847–851; doi: 10.1080/17461391.2014.911354.

INDEX